HUMAN RESPIRATORY SYNCYTIAL VIRUS INFECTION

Edited by **Bernhard Resch**

Human Respiratory Syncytial Virus Infection
Edited by Bernhard Resch

Published by InTech
Janeza Trdine 9, 51000 Rijeka, Croatia

Publishing Process Manager Ivana Zec

Technical Editor Teodora Smiljanic

Cover Designer InTech Design Team

Additional hard copies can be obtained from orders@intechopen.com

Human Respiratory Syncytial Virus Infection, Edited by Bernhard Resch
p. cm.
ISBN 978-953-307-718-5

For EU product safety concerns:
IN TECH d.o.o., Prolaz Marije Krucifikse Kozulić 3, 51000 Rijeka, Croatia,
info@intechopen.com or visit our website at intechopen.com.

Meet the editor

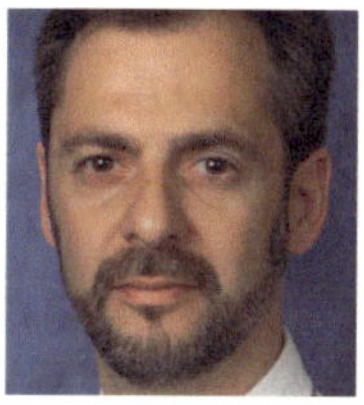

Born in Graz, Austria, Prof. Resch received his medical degree at the Karl-Franzens-University Graz in 1988. Following post-doc studies at the Division of Neonatology, and the Department of Pediatric Surgery of the University Hospital Graz, he became consultant of Pediatrics in 1997 and consultant of Neonatal and Pediatric Intensive Care Medicine in 2000. Since 2004, he is Professor of Pediatrics and since 2008, Head of the Research Unit of Neonatal Infectious Diseases and Epidemiology of the Medical University Graz. His main research fields include neonatal infectious diseases, RSV infection, and periventricular leukomalacia of the preterm infant. He is a member and board member of several scientific societies, presently head of the Austrian Society of Neonatology and Pediatric Intensive Care Medicine, and member of the editorial board of several international journals including "The Open Journal of Microbiology".

Contents

Preface XI

Part 1 **Pathophysiology of RSV Infection** 1

Chapter 1 **MHC Class I Ligands and Epitopes in HRSV Infection** 3
Daniel López

Chapter 2 **RSV Induced Changes in miRNA Expression in Lung** 19
Shirley R. Bruce and Joseph L. Alcorn

Chapter 3 **Animal Models of Respiratory Syncytial Virus Pathogenesis and Vaccine Development: Opportunities and Future Directions** 43
Amelia R. Woolums, Sujin Lee and Martin L. Moore

Chapter 4 **Structural and Functional Aspects of the Small Hydrophobic (SH) Protein in the Human Respiratory Syncytial Virus** 75
Siok Wan Gan and Jaume Torres

Chapter 5 **Cellular and Molecular Characteristics of RSV-Induced Disease in Humans** 97
Olivier Touzelet and Ultan F. Power

Chapter 6 **Detection of Bacteriophage in Droplets** 123
Phillipa Perrott and Megan Hargreaves

Part 2 **Epidemiologic and Diagnostic Aspects of RSV Infection** 145

Chapter 7 **Life-Threatening RSV Infections in Children** 147
Martin C.J. Kneyber

Chapter 8 **Epidemiology and Diagnosis of Human Respiratory Syncytial Virus Infections** 161
Javed Akhter and Sameera Al Johani

Part 3 Treatment and Prophylaxis of Human RSV Disease 177

Chapter 9 **Anti-Respiratory Syncytial Virus Agents from Phytomedicine 179**
Damian Chukwu Odimegwu, Thomas Grunwald and Charles Okechukwu Esimone

Chapter 10 **Treatment of Respiratory Syncytial Virus Infection: Past, Present and Future 197**
Dirk Roymans and Anil Koul

Preface

Respiratory syncytial virus (RSV) is the most significant cause of acute respiratory tract infections in infants and young children throughout the world. The World Health Organization estimates that one third of the 12.2 million annual deaths in children below 5 years are the result of acute infections of the respiratory tract, with RSV, Streptococcus pneumoniae, and Haemophilus influenzae as the predominant pathogens Severity of RSV outbreaks varies from year to year, perhaps in part because of a variation in circulating strains. Mortality associated with primary RSV infection in otherwise healthy children is estimated to be 0.005 to 0.02 percent, and is approximately 1 to 3 percent among hospitalized children. Repeated RSV infections are common in all age groups. RSV usually spreads by close contact with infected people or their infectious secretions, which tend to be profuse, especially in young children. RSV in nasal secretions of acutely infected infants remains infectious on countertops for more than 6 hours and on cloth and paper tissue for 30 minutes. Risk factors for acquisition of RSV bronchiolitis in infants and young children include birth between April and the end of September, day-care attendance, lack of breast-feeding, residence in crowded homes, multiple births, and presence of siblings. Risk factors associated with increased severity of RSV infection in healthy infants and children include male gender, low socioeconomic status, crowded living conditions, indoor smoke pollution, malnutrition, a family history of asthma or atopy, and lower cord serum RSV antibody titers. Children born with certain medical conditions including prematurity, bronchopulmonary dysplasia, congenital heart disease, neuromuscular impairment, cystic fibrosis, and immune deficiency syndromes have consistently been found to be at increased risk for severe RSV disease compared with children without these conditions and have been the primary risk groups considered for RSV prophylaxis with the humanized monoclonal antibody palivizumab. Another phenomenon following early RSV lower respiratory tract infection includes recurrent episodes of wheezing mimicking early childhood asthma during childhood. The prevalence of respiratory symptoms appears to diminish over the first years of life, but recent studies observed either reactive airway disease or lung function abnormality even until adolescence.

In this online access book on human RSV infections several distinguished authors contribute their experience on RSV. The book is divided in three sections representing a total of ten chapters. A major focus lies on the fascinating pathophysiology of RSV demonstrating recent and actual work on different mechanisms involved in the complex pathogenesis of the virus. A second section elucidates epidemiologic and diagnostic aspects of RSV infection covering a more clinical view of RSV disease. At last, treatment modalities including the search for a vaccine that is still not in sight are discussed and conclude this book, thus, drawing a bow that reaches from experimental models of RSV related lung disease over clinical aspects of disease to the latest news of therapeutic and prophylactic approaches to human RSV infection.

Bernhard Resch, MD
Professor of Pediatrics
Research Unit for Neonatal Infectious Diseases and Epidemiology
Division of Neonatology, Department of Pediatrics
Medical University of Graz
Austria

Part 1

Pathophysiology of RSV Infection

1

MHC Class I Ligands and Epitopes in HRSV Infection

Daniel López
Centro Nacional de Microbiología, Instituto de Salud "Carlos III"
Spain

1. Introduction

Human respiratory syncytial virus (HRSV) (Collins et al., 2007), a *Pneumovirus* of the *Paramyxoviridae* family is an enveloped virus containing a negative-sense, single-stranded RNA genome of 15.2 kilobases that is transcribed into 10mRNAs encoding 11 proteins because two overlapping open reading frames of M2 mRNA encode the M2-1 and M2-2 proteins. N is the nucleocapsid protein; L, the catalytic subunit of the RNA-dependent RNA polymerase, M2-1 transcription factor and the P phosphoprotein are components of the polymerase complex. M2-2 is a regulatory factor in RNA synthesis whereas M is the matrix protein. The non structural proteins NS1 and NS2 are antagonists of host type I interferons (IFN). Lastly F, G and SH are three transmembrane proteins.

HRSV is the single most important cause of serious lower respiratory tract illnesses such as bronchiolitis and pneumonia in infants and young children (Hall, 2001; Shay et al., 2001; Thompson et al., 2003). In these acute lower respiratory infections due to HRSV, the case fatality ratio in children younger than 1 year of industrialised or developing countries is the 0.7% and 2.1% respectively (Nair et al., 2010). Worldwide mortality from HRSV infection has been estimated in about 66,000 to 199,000 deaths annually in young children (Nair et al., 2010).

In addition, infections of this virus occur in people of all ages, but although usually mild infections are reported in healthy adults, HRSV poses a serious health risk in immunocompromised individuals (Ison & Hayden, 2002; Wendt & Hertz, 1995) and in the elderly (Falsey et al., 2005; Han et al., 1999). In the United States, HRSV is estimated to cause approximately 13,000 annual deaths among adults who are elderly or have underlying immunosuppressive and/or cardiopulmonary conditions (Falsey et al., 2005).

HRSV exists as a single serotype, but has two antigenic subgroups, A and B (Anderson et al., 1985; Mufson et al., 1985). The attachment G protein, a type II transmembrane glycoprotein with little homology to any other known viral protein is the major source of antigenic differences between the two HRSV subgroups. Between these subgroups A and B, the G protein varies by ~50% in amino acid sequence (Johnson et al., 1987). The nature of these differences indicates that the two subgroups represent two lines of divergent evolution, rather than variants that differ only at a few major antigenic sites.

Although the ciliated cells of the respiratory epithelium are the primary site of HRSV replication *in vivo* (reviewed in (Collins et al., 2007)), this virus can infect both human and murine immune system cells, mainly professional antigen-presenting cells (APCs). HRSV infection induces maturation in human and murine monocytes and macrophages (Becker et al., 1991a; Franke-Ullmann et al., 1995; Midulla et al., 1989; Panuska et al., 1990) and human plasmacytoid but not myeloid dendritic cells (Hornung et al., 2004). Upregulation of typical activation markers such as CD86 and MHC class II upon HRSV infection of mouse spleen B cells was also previously reported (Rico et al., 2009; Rico et al., 2010).

2. Innate and humoral immunity

The HRSV infection, as any other pathogenic illness, is controlled by the concerted activity of different layers from host immune system. Cells of innate immune response as neutrophils infiltrate deeply the airways of ventilated HRSV-infected infants as shown their high presence in broncho-alveolar lavage samples of these young patients (Everard et al., 1994). Also, abundant alveolar macrophages were found in the lower respiratory tract in HRSV infection (Becker et al., 1991b). In addition, the depletion of macrophages enhances virus titers in the HRSV-infected lung by significant inhibition of early inflammatory cytokines release (Pribul et al., 2008).

Although the humoral response plays no role in the course of a primary infection, the protection from subsequent HRSV infections is mediated through antibodies (Abs). In mice model, the depletion of B lymphocytes does not alter the clearance of virus in the primary infection but the rate of viral clearance after secondary infection was significantly decreased (Graham et al., 1991a). Decreased protection from secondary infection correlated with low titers of HRSV-specific Abs in the serum of exposed individuals (Mills et al., 1971). Also, newborn infants with high titers of maternal acquired Abs are less likely to severe bronchiolitis (Holberg et al., 1991). In high-risk infants the passive immunization with HRSV-specific Abs reduces hospitalization from HRSV infection (The IMpact-RSV Study Group, 1998).

Vaccination studies using individual HRSV proteins have shown presence of serum Abs induced by F, G, M2 and P proteins, but the protection was associated only to the two major surface glycoproteins (F and G proteins) (Connors et al., 1991). Two different structures of the HRSV F protein: an immature folded form, and other mature cleaved form found in virions have been described (Lawless-Delmedico et al., 2000; López et al., 1998). Although some neutralizing epitopes of the mature form are not found in the immature F protein, both forms induce Ab responses of comparable magnitude (Sakurai et al., 1999). Among different virus isolates, the G protein is the less conserved protein: only a 50% identity for G protein but a 90% for the F protein between the two antigenic subgroups of HRSV (Collins et al., 2007). Therefore, the majority of F-specific but few G-specific monoclonal Abs are cross-reactive (Collins et al., 2007) and thus, very few individual G-protein-specific monoclonal Abs efficiently neutralize HRSV infectivity.

Both immunoglobulin A and G play an important role in protection from HRSV infection. IgA is largely associated with mucosal immunity. As HRSV initially replicates in apical respiratory epithelial cells from the lung airways thus, IgA must be an important factor in protection from initial infection. Fast and specific IgA Ab secretion in the upper airways of primary HRSV-infected mice could be detected (Singleton et al., 2003). Increased infection in human adults correlated with decreased HRSV-specific IgA titers in nasal wash (Walsh &

Falsey, 2004). Also, the intranasal administration of HRSV-specific IgA prior to HRSV infection enhances the antiviral protection compared with untreated mice (Weltzin et al., 1994), although it is not as efficient as administration of HRSV-specific IgG to decrease overall pulmonary viral titers in animals (Fisher et al., 1999). In addition, decreased incidence of severe disease associated with lower-airway infection was found in both elderly and young individuals with high HRSV-neutralizing IgG Ab titers (Falsey & Walsh, 1998; Walsh & Falsey, 2004).

3. Cellular immunity

Both experimental models and studies in infected infants indicate the key role of cellular immunity in the control of infection and the virus-induced complex inflammatory processes and airway damage by HRSV. This includes both release of cytokines and chemokines and $CD4^+$ or $CD8^+$ responses.

3.1 Cytokines and chemokines

In the primary HRSV infection, the airway epithelial cells and lung-resident leukocytes secrete cytokines and chemokines quickly. These cell-signaling molecules recruit circulating leukocytes to the infected lung that release new cytokines mediating proinflammatory functions. Some of these chemokines and cytokines activate and recruit immune cells. In contrast, others cytokines and chemokines suppress or regulate the proinflammatory state associated to HRSV infection. In summary, this complex cocktail of cytokines, chemokines, and different immune system cells are all implicated in HRSV disease in humans. Even, differences in immunologic responses at birth may be determinant factor of the risk of RSV disease. Comparing cytokines secretion from cord blood samples after stimulation with lipopolysaccharide both healthy control children and hospitalized infants with HRSV, low IL-1β, IL-2, IL-4, IL-5, and IL-10 but high IL-6 and IL-8 responses were found in HRSV-infected young subjects (Juntti et al., 2009). In other studies, also reduced phytohemagglutinin-induced IL-13 response (Gern et al., 2006) and increased IL-4 secretion (Macaubas et al., 2003) were detected in umbilical cord blood cells of infants with risk of severe HRSV infection and asthma. High production of several Th2 cytokines such as IL-4, IL-5, and IL-13 has been associated with severe HRSV airway-disease in infants (Gern et al., 2006). Increased IL-4 was also observed in nasopharyngeal secretions of HRSV-infected children compared to control children (Murai et al., 2007). These results indicate that a Th2 polarization can enhance HRSV-associated illness. In addition, in other study an increased concentration of IL-17 associated to Th17 cells was detected in moderately ill patients as compared with severe HRSV cases but the mechanism was not elucidated (Larranaga et al., 2009). In this line recently, a role of HRSV NS1 protein in the suppression of Th17 response with subsequent decreased protective adaptive immunity had been proposed (Munir et al., 2011).

IFNs are proteins secreted by host cells in response to the presence of viruses among other intracellular pathogens. Different viruses generate IFN-suppressive proteins. HRSV nonstructural proteins NS1 and NS2 cooperatively interfere with the host antiviral cytokine response antagonizing the α/β IFN-induced response in infected epithelial cells as well as suppressing plasmacytoid dendritic cell maturation (Schlender et al., 2000).

3.2 T-cell mediated response

Although the immune mechanism involved in HRSV disease and protection is not well understood, humoral and cellular responses appear to play different roles in the antiviral protection, and resolution of HRSV infection as well as disease pathogenesis. The HRSV-specific antibodies are sufficient to prevent or limit the severity of infection but are not required for clearing primary infection (Graham et al., 1991a). However, T cell-mediated responses are necessary to abolish viral replication once HRSV infection is established, and for the clearance of virus-infected cells in primary infection (Anderson & Heilman, 1995).

Studies in mice have shown that F and G envelope proteins prime different subsets of $CD4^+$ T cells. In this system, G protein primes only $CD4^+$ T cells towards a Th2-type cytokine response (Johnson et al., 1998) while F protein primes both $CD4^+$ and $CD8^+$ T cells toward a Th1-type biased cytokine response (Alwan & Openshaw, 1993). In contrast, G protein primes a mixed Th1/Th2 $CD4^+$ T cell response in humans (De Graaff et al., 2004).

Using a murine HRSV-infected model in which the $CD4^+$ and $CD8^+$ T-lymphocyte subpopulations were depleted individually or together by injections of specific Abs, the role of both effector T cells was evaluated. This study showed that both $CD4^+$ and $CD8^+$ lymphocyte subsets are important in clearing a primary infection (Graham et al., 1991b). In addition, $CD4^+$ T cell responses play key roles in pulmonary pathology during infection. IFN-γ secreting $CD4^+$ T cells (Th1-type cytokine response) clear HRSV in low lung pathology, while viral clearance by IL-4 secreting $CD4^+$ cells (Th2-type cytokine response) is strongly associated with significant pulmonary damages, including eosinophilic infiltration (Alwan et al., 1992; Tang & Graham, 1997).

HRSV-specific cytolytic T lymphocytes have been detected in peripheral blood mononuclear cells from infants with bronchiolitis (Chiba et al., 1989; Isaacs et al., 1987). $CD8^+$ T cells with an activated effector cell phenotype could be isolated from bronchoalveolar lavage samples and blood of infants with a severe primary respiratory HRSV infection (Heidema et al., 2007). Although also, the HRSV infection suppresses lung $CD8^+$ T-lymphocyte effector activity by blocking IFN-γ secretion by the HRSV-specific T cells (Chang & Braciale, 2002). In this study, alteration the development of pulmonary CD8+ T-cell memory by interfering with TCR-mediated signaling was described (Chang & Braciale, 2002). Outstandingly, this fault in effector function was only identified in $CD8^+$ T cells from infected lung. In contrast, the effector $CD8^+$ T cells that had migrated from the draining lymph nodes to other secondary lymphoid organs had no insufficiency in their function. Moreover, the viral load after primary HRSV infection was significantly increased in the lungs of IFN-γ knockout mice compared with wild type mice (Lee et al., 2008). Thus, during primary HRSV infection the IFN-γ production is decisive to the development of protection against HRSV-associated disease. The poor induction of IFN-γ release by HRSV may contribute possibly to its weak immunogenicity and the frequent reinfection observed in the human host. In addition, the analysis of responses in congenic mice with different major histocompatibility complex (MHC) haplotypes indicated that susceptibility to sequelae after neonatal HRSV infection was predominantly inherited (Tregoning et al., 2010). Thus, MHC haplotype and its effect on $CD8^+$ T cell immune response play a central role in neonatal HRSV infection. In summary, all these results indicate clearly a key role of $CD8^+$ immune response in virus clearance.

Human cytotoxic T cells from normal not sick adults recognize almost six proteins: F, N, M, M2-1, NS2, and SH but little or no recognition of G, NS1 or P proteins of HRSV was found (Cherrie et al., 1992). As only the recognition of F and M2 proteins were associated with a recent infection, these data indicate the existence of a long term $CD8^+$ response against HRSV (Cherrie et al., 1992). In addition, F, N, and M2 proteins of this virus also induce cytolytic T responses in the mouse model (Kulkarni et al., 1993b),(Olson et al., 2008; Openshaw et al., 1990; Pemberton et al., 1987).

4. MHC class I epitopes

In cellular immunity, the recognition and killing of infected cells by $CD8^+$ cytolytic T lymphocytes (CTLs) first requires proteolytic degradation of newly synthesized viral proteins in the cytosol by the combined action of proteasomes and degradative peptidases (Shastri et al., 2002). This antigen processing generates short peptides of 8 to 12 residues that are translocated to the endoplasmic reticulum lumen by transporter associated with antigen processing (TAP), and subsequent N-terminal trimming by the metallo-aminoproteases ERAP1 and 2 is frequently required (Rock et al., 2004; Saveanu et al., 2005). Peptide binding to newly synthesized β2-microglobulin and MHC class I heavy chain generates stable peptide/MHC complexes. Usually, this interaction is made possible by two major anchor residues at position 2 and the C-terminus of the antigenic peptide (Parker et al., 1994; Rammensee et al., 1999) that are deeply accommodated into specific pockets of the antigen recognition site of the MHC class I molecule (Bjorkman et al., 1987a; Bjorkman et al., 1987b). Finally, the stable trimolecular peptide-MHC-β_2-microglobulin complexes are transported to the cell membrane and presented for CTL recognition (York et al., 1999).

Several HRSV epitopes restricted by different MHC class I molecules of the mouse (H-2) or human (HLA) have been identified using CTL from seropositive individuals or murine models respectively.

4.1 H-2 class I epitopes

A study from the early 1990s shown that the cytotoxic activity of lung $CD8^+$ lymphocytes correlated with a protective cellular immune response in BALB/c mice vaccinated with a recombinant virus expressing the M2 protein of HRSV (Kulkarni et al., 1993a). This protein was the only HRSV protein that induced resistance to virus infection in H-2^d mice (BALB/c) but not in H-2^b or H-2^k mice (Kulkarni et al., 1993a). The conserved peptide between subgroup A and B HRSV strains SYIGSINNI, which spans residues 82-90 of the HRSV M2 protein, was identified as the immunodominant K^d-restricted CTL epitope in H-2^d mice, and other two M2 peptides were also identified (the different H-2 class I epitopes of HRSV identified are summarized in Table 1)(Kulkarni et al., 1993b). Afterward, a new H-2K^d-restricted subdominant epitope with the amino acid sequence VYNTVISYI, spanning residues 127-135 of the same M2 protein, was also identified (Lee et al., 2007). In addition, the frequency of specific T cells responding to two H-2K^d-presented epitopes in the same protein following HRSV infection for both lymphoid and nonlymphoid tissues was evaluated. In the cellular response to HRSV infection the ratios of specific T lymphocytes for $M2_{82-90}$ (dominant) and $M2_{127-135}$ (subdominant) epitopes were either 3:1 in the spleen or 10:1 in the lung both in primary response, secondary infection, and memory (Lee et al., 2007).

Strain	H-2	Sequence [a]	Protein	Position	Reference
BALB/c	K^d	SYIGSINNI	Matrix 2	82-90	(Kulkarni et al., 1993b)
BALB/c	K^d	EYALGVVGV	Matrix 2	71-79	(Kulkarni et al., 1993b)
BALB/c	K^d	NYFEWPPHA	Matrix 2	26-34	(Kulkarni et al., 1993b)
BALB/c	K^d	VYNTVISYI	Matrix 2	127-135	(Lee et al., 2007)
BALB/c	K^d	KYKNAVTEL	Fusion	85-93	(Chang et al., 2001)
BALB/c	K^d	ELQLLMQSTPPTNNR	Fusion	92-106	(Jiang et al., 2002)
BALB/c	K^d	TYMLTNSEL	Fusion	249-257	(Johnstone et al., 2004)
BALB/c	K^d	TYMLTNSELL	Fusion	249-258	(Johnstone et al., 2004)
C57Bl/6	D^b	NAITNAKII	Matrix	187-195	(Rutigliano et al., 2005)

[a] The H-2K^d or D^b anchor motifs are underlined.

Table 1. Summary of H-2 class I epitopes of HRSV

To identify the epitope(s) responsible to the protective CTL response against HRSV F protein detected in BALB/c mice (Pemberton et al., 1987) a panel of overlapping synthetic peptides corresponding to the complete HRSV F protein sequence of A2 strain was used (Chang et al., 2001). The peptide spanning residues 85-93 of this protein was identified as the immunodominant H-2K^d-restricted epitope recognized by F-specific CD8$^+$ T cells from BALB/c mice. No HRSV F-specific CTL response was associated to H-2D^d or H-2L^d class I molecules (Chang et al., 2001).This F-specific CD8$^+$ T cell response was 10-fold lower than the dominant M2-specific response during primary HRSV infection. With the same strategy of screening a panel of overlapping synthetic peptides a second H-2K^d-restricted epitope for HRSV F-specific CD8$^+$ CTL was described (Jiang et al., 2002). This is a long 15-mer peptide from the F protein (92–106 residues), which in contrast to other murine HRSV epitopes not contain the known allele-specific motif for H-2K^d binding: Tyr at position 2 (P2) and aliphatic C-terminal residues (Table 1 and SYFPEITHI database: http://www.syfpeithi.de (Rammensee et al., 1999)). All 15 amino acids of this unusual epitope appear to be required for effective presentation to CTL. The interaction of 15-mer epitope with the presenting H-

$2K^d$ class I molecule was not studied. Thus, future studies are needed to clarify this intriguing protein structure.

The use of predictive methods for $H\text{-}2^d$ binding by means of web software tools enabled the identification of a new epitope in the F glycoprotein of the Long strain, F249–258, which is presented by K^d as a 9-mer (TYMLTNSEL) or a 10-mer (TYMLTNSELL) peptide (Johnstone et al., 2004). No hierarchy in $CD8^+$ T-lymphocyte responses to F85–93 and F249–258 epitopes was found *in vivo* during a primary response. In contrast, F85–93 was found dominant with respect to F249–258 in *in vivo* memory and secondary responses (Johnstone et al., 2004).

The majority of studies on the HRSV pathogenesis in mice have been performed in the BALB/c mice because are among the most permissive mice but several strains of mice are also susceptible to HRSV infection (Prince et al., 1979). Overlapping synthetic peptide strategy, spanning the F, G, and M proteins of HRSV were used to identify HRSV epitopes in $H\text{-}2^b$ mice (Rutigliano et al., 2005). An $H\text{-}2D^b$-restricted CTL epitope from the RSV M protein, corresponding to aa 187–195 (NAITNAKII) was identified (Rutigliano et al., 2005). In C57Bl/6 mice, M187–195-specific CTLs were activated with similar kinetics to the immunodominant epitope M2 82–90 in BALB/c mice.

4.2 HLA class I epitopes

The peptide ^{308}NPKASLLSL^{316} was the first human HRSV-specific CTL epitope identified from healthy adult volunteers using a panel of overlapping peptides spanning the HRSV nucleoprotein (Goulder et al., 2000). Later with a similar experimental strategy, other four viral nucleoprotein epitopes were found associated to HLA-A2 (Terrosi et al., 2007) or –B8 (Venter et al., 2003) positive donors (Table 2).

Overlapping peptide approach with the HRSV fusion protein shown the existence of two HLA-B57 and –Cw12-restricted CTL epitopes from infants who had just recovered from severe HRSV infection (Brandenburg et al., 2000). In the same way, HLA-A1-restricted CTL specific for the peptide RELPRFMNYT, spanning residues 109-118 of fusion protein, was detected in peripheral blood mononuclear cells from three healthy volunteers (Rock & Crowe, 2003).

Finally, five epitopes derived from the matrix, NS2 and matrix 2 proteins of HRSV were identified by selection of peptides with appropriate binding motifs, for four different HLA class I alleles (HLA-A1, -A3, -B44 and -B51) using the SYFPEITHI prediction software (Rammensee et al., 1999) from healthy donors (Table 2). All epitopes were detected in 4-5 different individuals suggesting that the dominant epitope was specifically presented by the respective HLA class I allele (Heidema et al., 2004).

Thirteen different HRSV CTL epitopes have been identified either healthy adult donors or sick infants (Table 2). They were presented by three HLA-A, five –B, and one –C class I molecules indicating broad cellular immune control against this virus. All $CD8^+$ epitopes were peptides with the canonical anchor motifs for the respective presenting molecule. The exception was the absence of HLA-A1 anchor motif (Asp or Glu at position 3 and aromatic C-terminal residue) in the ligand ^{109}RELPRFMNYT^{118} of the fusion protein (Rock & Crowe, 2003), indicating the complexity and plasticity of interactions in HLA-peptide complexes.

In summary, different CTL epitopes have been identified in five of six HRSV proteins previously described as recognized by human CD8+ T lymphocytes by Cherrie et al. (Cherrie et al., 1992). Only the identification of CTL epitopes from SH protein remains open and future studies are needed.

HLA	Sequence [a]	Protein	Position	Reference
A2	QLLSSSKYT	Nucleoprotein	16-24	(Terrosi et al., 2007)
A2	KMLKEMGEV	Nucleoprotein	137-145	(Terrosi et al., 2007)
B8	VMLRWGVLA	Nucleoprotein	258-266	(Venter et al., 2003)
A2	ILNNPKASL	Nucleoprotein	303-311	(Terrosi et al., 2007)
B7	NPKASLLSL	Nucleoprotein	308-316	(Goulder et al., 2000)
A1	RELPRFMNYT	Fusion	109-118	(Rock & Crowe, 2003)
B57	RARRELPRF	Fusion	118-126	(Brandenburg et al., 2000)
Cw12 [b]	IAVGLLLYC	Fusion	551-559	(Brandenburg et al., 2000)
B51	IPYSGLLLV	Matrix	195-203	(Heidema et al., 2004)
A1	YLEKESIYY	Matrix	229-237	(Heidema et al., 2004)
B44	AELDRTEEY	Matrix 2	64-72	(Heidema et al., 2004)
A3	RLPADVLKK	Matrix 2	151-159	(Heidema et al., 2004)
B51	LAKAVIHTI	NS2	41-49	(Heidema et al., 2004)

[a] The HLA anchor motifs are underlined.
[b] No data of HLA-Cw12 anchor motif.

Table 2. Summary of HLA class I epitopes of HRSV

5. HLA class I ligands

In most cases, the natural MHC class I ligand is assumed to be the one that has the canonical anchor sites, the minimal length, and the optimal antigenicity when tested as a synthetic peptide although some studies indicates that the extrapolation of either antigenicity or MHC binding strength is not sufficient to identify natural viral MHC class I ligands (Samino et al., 2004; Samino et al., 2006). All previous studies identifying several HRSV epitopes in mice and human were performed with synthetic peptides and no formal identification of natural epitopes was performed. Thus, the high-performance liquid chromatography (HPLC) coupled to high sensitivity mass spectrometry could be a useful technology to identify the endogenously processed HLA ligands derived from HRSV in infected cells.

The basic strategy of this experimental approach beginning with the isolation of HLA-bound peptide repertoires from cells either infected or not infected with HRSV. Next, both peptide pools are fractionated by HPLC in consecutive runs and under identical conditions to reduce alterations in the peptide elution patterns. Later, every HPLC fraction from each peptide pool is analyzed by MALDI-TOF mass spectrometry. Each spectrum of a single HPLC fraction of HRSV-infected cells is compared with the equivalent fraction of the uninfected cells. This technique allows the selection of peptides found only in the HRSV-infected cells. Next, the corresponding MS/MS spectrum of each differential peptide is obtained by ion-trap mass spectrometry and its amino acid sequence is assigned with bioinformatics tools. These sequences could be validated by comparison with the MS/MS spectrum of the corresponding synthetic peptide. With this experimental approach, the viral amino acid sequence AITNAKII, spanning residues 188-195 of the HRSV matrix protein was identified as endogenously processed and presented in infected human cells (Infantes et al., 2011). This natural ligand is a non canonical HLA-Cw4 ligand that uses alternative interactions to the anchor motifs previously described for its presenting HLA-Cw4 class I molecule (Table 3).

Interestingly, the M187-195 NAITNAKII nonamer has been described as an H-2D^b-restricted CTL epitope (Rutigliano et al., 2005) in the mouse model (Table 1). It has the canonical anchor motifs for D^b molecules: Asn at position 5 and aliphatic C-terminal residue (Falk et al., 1991). Therefore, two viral peptide species of different lengths that share the same antigenic core and differ only in the additional N-terminal residue were bound to either HLA-Cw4 or H-2D^b presenting molecules in the respective infected cells. Surprisingly, both the human octamer and the mouse nonamer bound efficiently to HLA-Cw4 molecules, in spite of the lack of canonical anchors for interaction with the presenting molecule.

In other study that involved culturing virus-infected cells with stable isotope-labeled amino acids expected to be anchor residues for the HLA allele of interest and then performing immunoprecipitation of HLA molecules and two-dimensional HPLC-mass spectrometry analysis, one HRSV ligand for each HLA-A2 or -B7 class I molecule was identified (Meiring et al., 2006) (Table 3). The ligand KLIHLTNAL (residues 33-41 of the NS1 protein) was presented by HLA-A2 whereas the peptide KARSTPVTL of the fusion protein was endogenously bound to HLA-B7 in human infected cells (Table 3).

Therefore, in the previous studies only one HRSV ligand restricted by a single HLA molecule was presented on the cell membrane surface. Thus, this is the rule? Or conversely, could a particular HLA molecule bind several ligands of this small virus simultaneously? To answer this question, HLA-B27 ligands isolated from large amounts of human healthy or HRSV-infected cells were compared using mass spectrometry technologies. This analysis demonstrated the existence of nine naturally processed HLA-B27 ligands from six different HRSV proteins in the same infected cells (Infantes et al., 2010) (Table 3). Thus, the nine detected ligands represent 2% of the proteome of this small virus, which is monitored by the same HLA class I allele. If these data are typical for all HLA class I molecules, the cellular immune response would monitor ~ 12% of the proteome of this viral pathogens in heterozygous HLA-A, -B and -C infected individuals. These data suggest that the cellular immune pressure could be high in some small viruses as HRSV.

HLA	Sequence [a]	Protein	Position	Reference
Cw4	AITNAKII	Matrix	188-195	(Infantes et al., 2011)
A2	KLIHLTNAL	NS1	33-41	(Meiring et al., 2006)
B7	KARSTPVTL	Fusion	551-559	(Meiring et al., 2006)
B27	HRQDINGKEM	Nucleoprotein	100-109	(Infantes et al., 2010)
B27	RRANNVLKNEM	Nucleoprotein	184-194	(Infantes et al., 2010)
B27	KRYKGLLPKDI	Nucleoprotein	195-205	(Infantes et al., 2010)
B27	SRSALLAQM	Matrix	76-84	(Infantes et al., 2010)
B27	VRNKDLNTL	Matrix	169-177	(Infantes et al., 2010)
B27	KRLPADVLKK	Matrix 2	150-159	(Infantes et al., 2010)
B27	GRNEVFSNK	Polymerase	2089-2097	(Infantes et al., 2010)
B27	LRNEESEKMAK	Phosphoprotein	198-208	(Infantes et al., 2010)
B27	HRFIYLINH	NS2	37-45	(Infantes et al., 2010)

[a] The HLA anchor motifs are underlined.

Table 3. Summary of natural HLA class I ligands of HRSV identified by mass spectrometry.

6. Perspectives of HLA-ligand-based vaccine development against HRSV

HRSV lacks effective approved vaccine or antiviral therapy. Worldwide, this virus remains one of the pathogens deemed most important for vaccine development (Hall, 1994). Over the last decades, several efforts have been made towards HRSV vaccine development using different experimental approaches (reviewed in (Murata, 2009)), including inactivated or live attenuated virus strains, vector-based, and viral protein subunit/DNA-based candidates. Also, against pathogens under cellular immune control as HRSV, the polyepitope vaccine approach could be valuable. This vaccine comprises a recombinant DNA construct inserted into a viral genome (generally vaccinia or adenovirus) encoding a chimerical protein where distinct HLA class I-restricted epitopes from one or more pathogens are expressed. Currently, polyepitope vaccine to coinduce multiple CTL responses directed towards a number of different protein target antigens are being used against diseases produced by different pathogens including arenavirus, Epstein Barr virus, HIV, malaria and even several cancers (reviewed in (Suhrbier, 2002)) but not with HRSV. These multiepitope vaccines are thermostable, safe, easy to manufacture, and cost effective. In this context, the identification of pathogen-derived peptides bound to HLA molecules by high resolution mass spectrometry is an emerging focus of HLA-ligand-based vaccine development (Ovsyannikova et al., 2007). In addition, as mutations that enable escape from host cellular immunity against HRSV do not appear to accumulate with time (Collins et al., 2007), thus this virus could be a candidate particularly adequate to the multiepitope vaccine therapeutic approach.

7. Conclusion

HRSV is the single most important cause of serious lower respiratory tract illnesses such as bronchiolitis and pneumonia in infants and young children. Mild infections of this virus occur in healthy adults but HRSV poses a serious health risk in immunocompromised individuals and in the elderly. Although the immune mechanisms involved in HRSV disease and protection are not fully understood the $CD8^+$ T lymphocytes are required to clear virus-infected cells. In last decades, several HRSV epitopes restricted by different MHC class I molecules of the mouse (H-2) or human (HLA) have been identified using murine models or CTL of seropositive individuals respectively. In recent years, using mass spectrometry analysis of complex HLA-bound peptide pools, physiologically processed HLA ligands from HRSV have been identified. This knowledge could be used in the peptide-based vaccine development.

8. Acknowledgment

This work was supported by grants provided by the FIPSE Foundation.

9. References

Alwan, W.H. & Openshaw, P.J. (1993). Distinct patterns of T- and B-cell immunity to respiratory syncytial virus induced by individual viral proteins. Vaccine *11*, 431-437.

Alwan, W.H.; Record, F.M. & Openshaw, P.J. (1992). CD4+ T cells clear virus but augment disease in mice infected with respiratory syncytial virus. Comparison with the effects of CD8+ T cells. Clin Exp. Immunol. *88*, 527-536.

Anderson, L.J. & Heilman, C.A. (1995). Protective and disease-enhancing immune responses to respiratory syncytial virus. J Infect. Dis. *171*, 1-7.

Anderson, L.J. et al. (1985). Antigenic characterization of respiratory syncytial virus strains with monoclonal antibodies. J Infect. Dis *151*, 626-633.

Becker, S.; Quay, J. & Soukup, J. (1991a). Cytokine (tumor necrosis factor, IL-6, and IL-8) production by respiratory syncytial virus-infected human alveolar macrophages. J Immunol. *147*, 4307-4312.

Becker, S.; Quay, J. & Soukup, J. (1991b). Cytokine (tumor necrosis factor, IL-6, and IL-8) production by respiratory syncytial virus-infected human alveolar macrophages. J Immunol. *147*, 4307-4312.

Bjorkman, P.J. et al. (1987a). Structure of the human class I histocompatibility antigen, HLA-A2. Nature *329*, 506-512.

Bjorkman, P.J. et al. (1987b). The foreign antigen binding site and T cell recognition regions of class I histocompatibility antigens. Nature *329*, 512-518.

Brandenburg, A.H. et al. (2000). HLA class I-restricted cytotoxic T-cell epitopes of the respiratory syncytial virus fusion protein. J Virol *74*, 10240-10244.

Chang, J. & Braciale, T.J. (2002). Respiratory syncytial virus infection suppresses lung $CD8^+$ T-cell effector activity and peripheral $CD8^+$ T-cell memory in the respiratory tract. Nat. Med. *8*, 54-60.

Chang, J.; Srikiatkhachorn, A. & Braciale, T.J. (2001). Visualization and characterization of respiratory syncytial virus F-specific $CD8^+$ T cells during experimental virus infection. J. Immunol. *167*, 4254-4260.

Cherrie, A.H. et al. (1992). Human cytotoxic T cells stimulated by antigen on dendritic cells recognize the N, SH, F, M, 22K, and 1b proteins of respiratory syncytial virus. J Virol. *66*, 2102-2110.

Chiba, Y. et al. (1989). Development of cell-mediated cytotoxic immunity to respiratory syncytial virus in human infants following naturally acquired infection. J Med Virol. *28*, 133-139.

Collins, P.L., Chanock, R.M., and Murphy, B.R. (2007). Respiratory Syncytial Virus. In Fields Virology, Lippincott Williams & Wilkins, ed., pp. 1443-1486.

Connors, M. et al. (1991). Respiratory syncytial virus (RSV) F, G, M2 (22K), and N proteins each induce resistance to RSV challenge, but resistance induced by M2 and N proteins is relatively short-lived. J Virol. *65*, 1634-1637.

De Graaff, P.M. et al. (2004). HLA-DP4 presents an immunodominant peptide from the RSV G protein to CD4 T cells. Virology *326*, 220-230.

Everard, M.L. et al. (1994). Analysis of cells obtained by bronchial lavage of infants with respiratory syncytial virus infection. Arch. Dis Child *71*, 428-432.

Falk, K. et al. (1991). Allele-specific motifs revealed by sequencing of self-peptides eluted from MHC molecules. Nature *351*, 290-296.

Falsey, A.R. et al. (2005). Respiratory syncytial virus infection in elderly and high-risk adults. N. Engl. J. Med. *352*, 1749-1759.

Falsey, A.R. & Walsh, E.E. (1998). Relationship of serum antibody to risk of respiratory syncytial virus infection in elderly adults. J Infect. Dis *177*, 463-466.

Fisher, R.G. et al. (1999). Passive IgA monoclonal antibody is no more effective than IgG at protecting mice from mucosal challenge with respiratory syncytial virus. J Infect. Dis *180*, 1324-1327.

Franke-Ullmann, G. et al. (1995). Alteration of pulmonary macrophage function by respiratory syncytial virus infection in vitro. J Immunol. *154*, 268-280.

Gern, J.E. et al. (2006). Bidirectional interactions between viral respiratory illnesses and cytokine responses in the first year of life. J Allergy Clin Immunol. *117*, 72-78.

Goulder, P.J. et al. (2000). Characterization of a novel respiratory syncytial virus-specific human cytotoxic T-lymphocyte epitope. J Virol *74*, 7694-7697.

Graham, B.S. et al. (1991a). Respiratory syncytial virus infection in anti-mu-treated mice. J Virol *65*, 4936-4942.

Graham, B.S. et al. (1991b). Role of T lymphocyte subsets in the pathogenesis of primary infection and rechallenge with respiratory syncytial virus in mice. J. Clin. Invest. *88*, 1026-1033.

Hall, C.B. (1994). Prospects for a respiratory syncytial virus vaccine. Science *265*, 1393-1394.

Hall, C.B. (2001). Respiratory syncytial virus and parainfluenza virus. N. Engl. J. Med. *344*, 1917-1928.

Han, L.L.; Alexander, J.P. & Anderson, L.J. (1999). Respiratory syncytial virus pneumonia among the elderly: an assessment of disease burden. J Infect. Dis *179*, 25-30.

Heidema, J. et al. (2004). Human CD8(+) T cell responses against five newly identified respiratory syncytial virus-derived epitopes. J. Gen. Virol. *85*, 2365-2374.

Heidema, J. et al. (2007). CD8+ T cell responses in bronchoalveolar lavage fluid and peripheral blood mononuclear cells of infants with severe primary respiratory syncytial virus infections. J Immunol. *179*, 8410-8417.

Holberg, C.J. et al. (1991). Risk factors for respiratory syncytial virus-associated lower respiratory illnesses in the first year of life. Am J Epidemiol *133*, 1135-1151.

Hornung, V. et al. (2004). Replication-dependent potent IFN-alpha induction in human plasmacytoid dendritic cells by a single-stranded RNA virus. J. Immunol. *173*, 5935-5943.

Infantes, S. et al. (2010). Multiple, non-conserved, internal viral ligands naturally presented by HLA-B27 in human respiratory syncytial virus-infected cells. Mol. Cell. Proteomics *9*, 1533-1539.

Infantes, S. et al. (2011). Unusual viral ligand with alternative interactions is presented by HLA-Cw4 in human respiratory syncytial virus-infected cells. Immunol. Cell Biol. *89*, 558-565.

Isaacs, D.; Bangham, C.R. & McMichael, A.J. (1987). Cell-mediated cytotoxic response to respiratory syncytial virus in infants with bronchiolitis. Lancet *2*, 769-771.

Ison, M.G. & Hayden, F.G. (2002). Viral infections in immunocompromised patients: what's new with respiratory viruses? Curr. Opin. Infect. Dis. *15*, 355-367.

Jiang, S. et al. (2002). Virus-specific CTL responses induced by an $H\text{-}2K^d$-restricted, motif-negative 15-mer peptide from the fusion protein of respiratory syncytial virus. J. Gen. Virol. *83*, 429-438.

Johnson, P.R. et al. (1987). The G glycoprotein of human respiratory syncytial viruses of subgroups A and B: extensive sequence divergence between antigenically related proteins. Proc. Natl Acad. Sci U. S. A *84*, 5625-5629.

Johnson, T.R. et al. (1998). Priming with secreted glycoprotein G of respiratory syncytial virus (RSV) augments interleukin-5 production and tissue eosinophilia after RSV challenge. Journal of Virology *72*, 2871-2880.

Johnstone, C. et al. (2004). Shifting immunodominance pattern of two cytotoxic T-lymphocyte epitopes in the F glycoprotein of the Long strain of respiratory syncytial virus. J. Gen. Virol. *85*, 3229-3238.

Juntti, H. et al. (2009). Cytokine responses in cord blood predict the severity of later respiratory syncytial virus infection. J Allergy Clin Immunol. *124*, 52-58.

Kulkarni, A.B. et al. (1993a). The cytolytic activity of pulmonary CD8+ lymphocytes, induced by infection with a vaccinia virus recombinant expressing the M2 protein of respiratory syncytial virus (RSV), correlates with resistance to RSV infection in mice. J. Virol. *67*, 1044-1049.

Kulkarni, A.B. et al. (1993b). Immunization of mice with vaccinia virus-M2 recombinant induces epitope-specific and cross-reactive K^d-restricted $CD8^+$ cytotoxic T cells. J. Virol. *67*, 4086-4092.

Larranaga, C.L. et al. (2009). Impaired immune response in severe human lower tract respiratory infection by respiratory syncytial virus. Pediatr Infect. Dis J *28*, 867-873.

Lawless-Delmedico, M.K. et al. (2000). Heptad-repeat regions of respiratory syncytial virus F1 protein form a six-membered coiled-coil complex. Biochemistry *39*, 11684-11695.

Lee, S. et al. (2007). Tissue-specific regulation of CD8+ T-lymphocyte immunodominance in respiratory syncytial virus infection. J. Virol. *81*, 2349-2358.

Lee, Y.M. et al. (2008). IFN-gamma production during initial infection determines the outcome of reinfection with respiratory syncytial virus. Am J Respir. Crit Care Med *177*, 208-218.

López, J.A. et al. (1998). Antigenic structure of human respiratory syncytial virus fusion glycoprotein. J. Virol. *72*, 6922-6928.

Macaubas, C. et al. (2003). Association between antenatal cytokine production and the development of atopy and asthma at age 6 years. Lancet *362*, 1192-1197.

Meiring, H.D. et al. (2006). Stable isotope tagging of epitopes: a highly selective strategy for the identification of major histocompatibility complex class I-associated peptides induced upon viral infection. Mol. Cell Proteomics. *5*, 902-913.

Midulla, F. et al. (1989). Respiratory syncytial virus infection of human cord and adult blood monocytes and alveolar macrophages. Am Rev Respir. Dis *140*, 771-777.

Mills, J. et al. (1971). Experimental respiratory syncytial virus infection of adults. Possible mechanisms of resistance to infection and illness. J Immunol. *107*, 123-130.

Mufson, M.A. et al. (1985). Two distinct subtypes of human respiratory syncytial virus. J Gen Virol *66 (Pt 10)*, 2111-2124.

Munir, S. et al. (2011). Respiratory syncytial virus interferon antagonist NS1 protein suppresses and skews the human T lymphocyte response. PLoS. Pathog. *7*, e1001336.

Murai, H. et al. (2007). IL-10 and RANTES are elevated in nasopharyngeal secretions of children with respiratory syncytial virus infection. Allergol. Int *56*, 157-163.

Murata, Y. (2009). Respiratory syncytial virus vaccine development. Clin Lab Med *29*, 725-739.

Nair, H. et al. (2010). Global burden of acute lower respiratory infections due to respiratory syncytial virus in young children: a systematic review and meta-analysis. Lancet *375*, 1545-1555.

Olson, M.R.; Hartwig, S.M. & Varga, S.M. (2008). The number of respiratory syncytial virus (RSV)-specific memory CD8 T cells in the lung is critical for their ability to inhibit RSV vaccine-enhanced pulmonary eosinophilia. J Immunol. *181*, 7958-7968.

Openshaw, P.J. et al. (1990). The 22, 000-kilodalton protein of respiratory syncytial virus is a major target for Kd-restricted cytotoxic T lymphocytes from mice primed by infection. J Virol. *64*, 1683-1689.

Ovsyannikova, I.G. et al. (2007). Mass spectrometry and peptide-based vaccine development. Clin Pharmacol. Ther. *82*, 644-652.

Panuska, J.R. et al. (1990). Productive infection of isolated human alveolar macrophages by respiratory syncytial virus. J Clin Invest *86*, 113-119.

Parker, K.C.; Bednarek, M.A. & Coligan, J.E. (1994). Scheme for ranking potential HLA-A2 binding peptides based on independent binding of individual peptide side-chains. J. Immunol. *152*, 163-175.

Pemberton, R.M. et al. (1987). Cytotoxic T cell specificity for respiratory syncytial virus proteins: fusion protein is an important target antigen. J. Gen. Virol. *68*, 2177-2182.

Pribul, P.K. et al. (2008). Alveolar macrophages are a major determinant of early responses to viral lung infection but do not influence subsequent disease development. J Virol *82*, 4441-4448.

Prince, G.A. et al. (1979). Respiratory syncytial virus infection in inbred mice. Infect. Immun. *26*, 764-766.

Rammensee, H.G. et al. (1999). SYFPEITHI: database for MHC ligands and peptide motifs. Immunogenetics *50*, 213-219.

Rico, M.A. et al. (2010). TLR4-independent upregulation of activation markers in mouse B lymphocytes infected by HRSV. Mol. Immunol. *47*, 1802-1807.

Rico, M.A. et al. (2009). Human respiratory syncytial virus infects and induces activation markers in mouse B lymphocytes. Immunol. Cell Biol. *87*, 344-350.

Rock, K.L.; York, I.A. & Goldberg, A.L. (2004). Post-proteasomal antigen processing for major histocompatibility complex class I presentation. Nat. Immunol. *5*, 670-677.

Rock, M.T. & Crowe, J.E. (2003). Identification of a novel human leucocyte antigen-A*01-restricted cytotoxic T-lymphocyte epitope in the respiratory syncytial virus fusion protein. Immunology *108*, 474-480.

Rutigliano, J.A. et al. (2005). Identification of an H-2D(b)-restricted CD8+ cytotoxic T lymphocyte epitope in the matrix protein of respiratory syncytial virus. Virology *337*, 335-343.

Sakurai, H. et al. (1999). Human antibody responses to mature and immature forms of viral envelope in respiratory syncytial virus infection: significance for subunit vaccines. J Virol *73*, 2956-2962.

Samino, Y. et al. (2004). An endogenous HIV envelope-derived peptide without the terminal NH_3+ group is physiologically presented by major histocompatibility class I molecules. J. Biol. Chem. *279*, 1151-1160.

Samino, Y. et al. (2006). A long N-terminal-extended nested set of abundant and antigenic major histocompatibility complex class I natural ligands from HIV envelope protein. J. Biol. Chem. *281*, 6358-6365.

Saveanu, L. et al. (2005). Concerted peptide trimming by human ERAP1 and ERAP2 aminopeptidase complexes in the endoplasmic reticulum. Nat. Immunol. *6*, 689-697.

Schlender, J. et al. (2000). Bovine respiratory syncytial virus nonstructural proteins NS1 and NS2 cooperatively antagonize alpha/beta interferon-induced antiviral response. J. Virol. *74*, 8234-8242.

Shastri, N.; Schwab, S. & Serwold, T. (2002). Producing nature's gene-chips: the generation of peptides for display by MHC class I molecules. Annu. Rev. Immunol. *20*, 463-493.

Shay, D.K. et al. (2001). Bronchiolitis-associated mortality and estimates of respiratory syncytial virus-associated deaths among US children, 1979-1997. J. Infect. Dis. *183*, 16-22.

Singleton, R. et al. (2003). Inability to evoke a long-lasting protective immune response to respiratory syncytial virus infection in mice correlates with ineffective nasal antibody responses. J Virol *77*, 11303-11311.

Suhrbier, A. (2002). Polytope vaccines for the codelivery of multiple CD8 T-cell epitopes. Expert. Rev Vaccines. *1*, 207-213.

Tang, Y.W. & Graham, B.S. (1997). T cell source of type 1 cytokines determines illness patterns in respiratory syncytial virus-infected mice. J Clin Invest *99*, 2183-2191.

Terrosi, C. et al. (2007). Immunological characterization of respiratory syncytial virus N protein epitopes recognized by human cytotoxic T lymphocytes. Viral Immunol. *20*, 399-406.

The IMpact-RSV Study Group (1998). Palivizumab, a humanized respiratory syncytial virus monoclonal antibody, reduces hospitalization from respiratory syncytial virus infection in high-risk infants. Pediatrics *102*, 531-537.

Thompson, W.W. et al. (2003). Mortality associated with influenza and respiratory syncytial virus in the United States. JAMA *289*, 179-186.

Tregoning, J.S. et al. (2010). Genetic susceptibility to the delayed sequelae of neonatal respiratory syncytial virus infection is MHC dependent. J Immunol. *185*, 5384-5391.

Venter, M. et al. (2003). Respiratory syncytial virus nucleoprotein-specific cytotoxic T-cell epitopes in a South African population of diverse HLA types are conserved in circulating field strains. J. Virol. *77*, 7319-7329.

Walsh, E.E. & Falsey, A.R. (2004). Humoral and mucosal immunity in protection from natural respiratory syncytial virus infection in adults. J Infect. Dis *190*, 373-378.

Weltzin, R. et al. (1994). Intranasal monoclonal immunoglobulin A against respiratory syncytial virus protects against upper and lower respiratory tract infections in mice. Antimicrob. Agents Chemother. *38*, 2785-2791.

Wendt, C.H. & Hertz, M.I. (1995). Respiratory syncytial virus and parainfluenza virus infections in the immunocompromised host. Semin. Respir. Infect. *10*, 224-231.

York, I.A. et al. (1999). Proteolysis and class I major histocompatibility complex antigen presentation. Immunol. Rev. *172*, 49-66.

2

RSV Induced Changes in miRNA Expression in Lung

Shirley R. Bruce and Joseph L. Alcorn
Department of Pediatrics, University of Texas Health Science Center at Houston, Houston, TX
USA

1. Introduction

The ability of Respiratory Syncytial Virus (RSV) to exist within the host cells of the lung depends on its ability to evade host antiviral defenses. Indeed, suppression of host cell immune defenses is not restricted to RSV but is a common mechanism of survival employed by most viruses. Viruses utilize a number of mechanisms to evade detection by the immune response including translational repression of host cell mRNA. One mechanism to alter translation of a specific mRNA is through binding of microRNAs (miRNAs) within the 3'-untranslated region (3'-UTR) of the target gene. Here, we will discuss mechanisms of translational repression by miRNAs during viral infection and will provide data on changes in miRNA expression during RSV infection of the lung.

1.1 Functions of the lung

The lung is a complex multicellular organ that has two main responsibilities; air exchange and pulmonary defense. The first responsibility is for exchange of oxygen with CO_2 between epithelial cells and capillaries in the lung alveolus. As oxygen enters the nasal passages, it passes through the trachea into the bronchi of each lung. From the bronchi, oxygen passes through much narrower bronchioles until it reaches the terminal alveoli, where actual exchange takes place. The alveolar surface is composed primarily of type I and type II alveolar epithelial cells which assist in gas exchange and in preventing alveolar collapse upon exhalation (West, 1990). Type I alveolar epithelial cells are large, thin cells that possess long cytoplasmic extensions. The cytoplasmic extensions allow type I cells to stretch along the large alveolar surface area, forming the air/blood barrier necessary for gas exchange. While type I cells cover 90% of the surface area within the alveoli, they only represent 8% of the total cells in an adult lung (Crapo et al., 1982). Type II epithelial cells are cuboidal in shape and much smaller than type I epithelial cells. They are typically found at the alveolar-septal junction and represent 15% of the cells lining the alveoli (Crapo et al., 1982). To prevent alveolar collapse upon exhalation, type II cells synthesize and secrete surfactant, which is composed of approximately 90% lipid and 10% protein (Haagsman & Diemel, 2001). The protein portion of surfactant is composed of four different surfactant proteins, A (SP-A), B (SP-B), C (SP-C) and D (SP-D), and these proteins are critical for the lungs primary functions of mediating gas exchange and the removal of infectious agents. The hydrophobic proteins SP-B and SP-C, along with the lipid portion of surfactant, function to reduce surface tension at the air liquid interface of the lung thereby maintaining alveolar stability and allowing gas exchange to occur (Haagsman & Diemel, 2001). The importance of SP-B in normal lung function is demonstrated by prematurely-born infants and by humans carrying genetic mutations of the SP-B gene that result in the lack of appropriate levels of the SP-B protein (Beers et al., 2000; Nogee et al., 1994). SP-B protein is produced late in the third trimester and infants born prior to 31 weeks of gestation are subject to respiratory dysfunction and respiratory distress syndrome (RDS) leading to increased morbidity and mortality of the neonate (Pryhuber et al., 1991). Full term infants born with a genetic defect in SP-B, which results in decreased expression of the SP-B protein, experience respiratory failure and lethal RDS succumbing by 6 months of age (Beers et al., 2000; Nogee et al., 1994).

The second responsibility of the lung is the removal or neutralization of infectious agents via the pulmonary innate and adaptive defenses (Wilmott et al., 1998). As a natural consequence of gas exchange, the lung is exposed to numerous environmental stimuli. Suspended within the inhaled air is an array of particulate matter and infectious agents that result in many respiratory illnesses. These infectious agents include bacterial and viral agents, as well as inert irritants found in the environment. The hydrophilic surfactant proteins SP-A and SP-D, produced by type II epithelial cells, aid in removal of infectious agents (see below) (Crouch & Wright, 2001). In addition, goblet cells within the lung produce a thin layer of mucous which helps trap foreign particles found in the air we breathe. Once foreign particles are trapped within the mucous, ciliated epithelium in the bronchi and bronchioles function to move mucus out of the lung and towards the pharynx (Murray, 2010). Also within the lung are a variety of secreted factors which target microbial agents for lysis and destruction as part of the innate immune response (Ganz, 2002).

1.2 Respiratory syncytial virus pathogenesis

One pathogenic agent encountered during breathing is RSV. RSV is a negative sense, single stranded, enveloped RNA virus of the family *Paramyxoviridea* (Domachowske & Rosenberg, 1999; Hacking & Hull, 2002). RSV infects epithelial cells of the lung, resulting in lower respiratory tract disease that can be particularly problematic for children, elderly adults and individuals with compromised immune systems (Englund et al., 1988; Griffin et al., 2002). A highly ubiquitous and contagious virus, RSV is the major respiratory pathogen in young children <1 year of age and virtually every individual has been infected with RSV at least once by the age of 3 (Black, 2003; Centers for Disease Control [CDC] 2004; Denny & Clyde 1986; Foy et al., 1973; Mufson et al., 1973; Parrott et al., 1973). In the United States up to 2.5% of children require hospitalization for RSV infections and epidemiological studies in children suggest an association between lower respiratory infection and persistent or recurrent respiratory obstruction (Mufson et al., 1973; Parrott et al., 1973). Prematurely-born infants have immature lungs and inadequate host defense mechanisms, resulting in increased susceptibility to pneumonia and bronchiolitis as a result of RSV infection.

When RSV infects airway epithelial cells in culture, no virus is produced in the initial 12 hours. An exponential growth phase follows this latent period, reaching a slight plateau at 34 hr, and then further exponential growth occurs until 48 h. Ultimately, lysis of the cell occurs with complete cellular destruction by 96 hr. During this relatively slow life cycle, most of the infectious virus remains cell-associated, with extracellular viral release upon death and lysis of the cell (Richman & Tauraso, 1971). In the lung, RSV infections generally last 8-15 days. Despite the prevalence of RSV infections, there are currently no adequate treatments. Palivizumab a monoclonal antibody directed against RSV surface fusion (F) protein (Subramanian et al., 1998), pharmacologic options (Frogel, 2008), and the antiviral drug Ribavirin show limited effectiveness (Ventre & Randolph, 2007).

The RSV genome is composed of 11 primary RNAs which encode major viral proteins (Domachowske & Rosenberg, 1999). Two of these proteins, the G protein and the F (fusion) protein, transmembrane proteins found within the envelope of the RSV viron, are important for viral infection. The G protein is the major attachment protein and the F protein is important for fusion between the viral envelope and the host membrane (Domachowske & Rosenberg, 1999; Hacking & Hull, 2002). The F protein is also involved in syncytial formation between adjacent cells, giving rise to the multinucleated cell-like structures that are characteristic of RSV infection (Domachowske & Rosenberg, 1999; Hacking & Hull, 2002). In addition to the G and F proteins, a small hydrophobic (SH) protein of unknown function is also located within the viral envelope. The matrix (M) protein is located in the inner layer of the viral envelope and although the function of the M protein is not know, it is presumed to play a role in virus assembly and budding similar to the M protein of other members of the *Paramyxoviridea* family (L. Rodriguez et al., 2004). The nucleocapsid (N), nucleocapsid phosphoprotein (P), and the polymerase (L) proteins form a single complex and this complex is important for RSV replication and transcription (Cowton et al., 2006). The RSV genome also contains several proteins that can inhibit or ameliorate the host response to infection. Two nonstructural proteins (NS1,NS2) are the most abundantly expressed proteins of the RSV genome, and these proteins have been shown to inhibit the response of host cells to interferon by inhibiting the activation of interferon regulatory factor 3, a transcription factor involved in IFN-β promoter activity (Bossert & Conzelmann 2002; Bossert et al., 2003). In addition, the G protein can be expressed in a truncated, secreted form that acts as a chemokine mimic. Secreted G protein competes with the chemokine fractalkine (Fkn) for binding to the CX3CR1 receptor (Tripp et al., 2001). Binding of Fkn to the CX3CR1 receptor induces migration of leukocytes to the site of infection and this migration can be subverted by the RSV G protein. While some RSV proteins can mitigate detection by the host cell immune response, components of the lung innate immunity, such as SP-A, can directly bind to the RSV F protein and mediate uptake of the virus by resident macrophages (Barr et al., 2000; Ghildyal et al., 1999).

1.3 Innate immune environment of the lung

As the first line of defense against invading pathogens, the innate immune system acts in an immediate non-specific manner to a variety of organisms. A physical barrier to pathogens is established by the airway epithelium and the cell-cell junctions between neighboring cells. Overlaying the airway epithelium is a layer of mucous which entraps foreign particles inhaled during breathing (Knowles & Boucher, 2002). The mucous forms a semi-permeable barrier that is not permeable to many pathogens however, still allows for exchange of gas and other nutrients. Mucins are the major component of respiratory mucous and have antiviral and anti-inflammatory properties (Thornton et al., 2008). Located within the mucous are polypeptide components including lysozyme, lactoferrin, protease inhibitors, defensins, and members of the collectin family of surfactant proteins SP-A and SP-B, all of which function to neutralizing foreign particles (Ganz, 2002; McCormack & Whitsett, 2002). Monocytes, macrophages, neutrophiles and epithelial cells secrete the enzyme lysozyme which lysis the bacterial cell wall of gram positive bacteria (Laible & Germaine, 1985). Lactoferrin is also secreted by neurophiles and binds iron in the environment thus depriving bacteria of essential nutrients

(Arnold et al., 1977). Defensins are a group of proteins produced by neutrophiles and epithelial cells of the respiratory system. They can bind to bacterial cells and some enveloped viruses forming pores in the microbial membrane. Formation of these pores compromises the integrity of the cell membrane allowing for the efflux of essential nutrients (Ganz, 2003). Finally, the hydrophilic proteins SP-A and SP-D, produced by type II epithelial cells, are also part of the lung's innate defense mechanism and serve to neutralize foreign particles and stimulate the immune response (Tino & Wright 1996; Wright & Youmans 1993).

The SP-A and SP-D proteins belong to a family of C-type lectins called collectin that function in the innate host defense of the lung (Crouch & Wright, 2001; Holmskov et al., 2003). Members of the collectin family of proteins are important in the innate response within the lung where they opsonize pathogens by non-specific binding to glycoconjugates and lipids present on the cell surface, facilitating phagocytosis by resident macrophages within the lung (Tino & Wright, 1996; Wright & Youmans, 1993). In addition, SP-A and SP-D can bind to receptors on the surface of macrophages to enhance phagocytosis of nonopsonized particles (Crouch & Wright, 2001). The importance of SP-A in the innate immune response to foreign pathogens is illustrated by transgenic mice that are deficient in SP-A. These mice were unable to efficiently clear bacterial infections, such as group *B streptococcus* and *Pseudomonas aeruginosa* (LeVine et al., 1997; LeVine et al., 1998). Furthermore, SP-A deficient mice infected with RSV exhibited increased RSV plaque forming units when compared with control mice (LeVine et al., 1999). These data suggest that SP-A is important in the lung's defense against RSV infections. Previous studies from our laboratory using alveolar type II cells in primary culture and the lung adenocarcinoma cell line NCI-H441 have shown that RSV infection alters SP-A protein production (Alcorn et al., 2005; Bruce et al., 2009). In the presence of RSV, SP-A mRNA increases approximately 3-fold however, the level of cellular and secreted SP-A protein decreases. The decrease in SP-A protein expression in lung epithelial cells during RSV infection results from translational inhibition of SP-A mRNA leading to reduced *de novo* SP-A protein synthesis (Bruce et al., 2009).

1.4 Host/virus interactions

Viruses are obligate, intracellular parasites with the sole purpose to replicate itself, usually at the expense of the host cell, and viruses are not considered to be of any great benefit to humans in general. The viral genomes of RNA viruses reside in the cytoplasm of host cells while the host genomes reside within the nucleus. The nuclear membrane physically separates the cellular location of these two genomes. However, the protein and RNA products produced from each genome can interact with one another, having consequences for the replication and survival of the virus and the host cell. Viruses have developed a number of mechanisms to circumvent detection by the innate and adaptive immune system of the host, in order to assure survival of virus progeny. Alternatively, the innate immune system of the host contains a number of mechanisms designed for early detection of viral infections. The constant evolutionary pressure upon the virus and the host for survival leads to different, novel and more effective strategies to win the race for continued existence. Viruses can mutate quickly in order to survive within the environment (Holmes, 2011). Their small genome and small number of proteins would allow the viruses to adapt quickly. Humans have a much larger genome and their ability to adapt to the environment would presumably occur at a much slower rate. Since viruses generally replicate at the expense of the host cell, the host cell must spend energy and resources to combat the virus. The host cell innate immune response is an early detection method used for this purpose.

The innate immune system of the host cell contains a number of mechanisms designed for early detection of viral infections. Through pattern recognition receptors (PRR) located within host cells, viral components such as DNA, RNA and proteins are recognized and the innate immune response activated (Akira et al., 2006). PRRs recognize pathogen associated molecular patterns (PAMPs) which distinguish host molecules from pathogen associated molecules (Kawai & Akira, 2009). Binding of PAMPs to toll-like receptors (TLR) are one mechanism by which pathogenic microorganisms are recognized. TLRs are transmembrane proteins that recognize ssRNA, dsRNA, DNA and viral envelope proteins. Activation of TLRs initiates production of type I Interferons (IFNs) which lowers the susceptibility of the cell to infection by altering metabolism and upregulating the expression of MHC class I and MHC class II molecules (Bonjardim et al., 2009). Retinoic acid-inducible gene I (Rig-I)-like receptors (RLRs) are a family of cytoplasmic proteins that recognize viral RNA (Kang et al., 2002; Yoneyama et al., 2004, 2005). As with TLR receptor signaling, RLR proteins also initiate production of type I IFNs. Finally, the cytoplasmic nucleotide oligomerization domain (NOD)-like receptors (NLRs), also recognize viral DNA and regulate interleukin-1β maturation (Muruve et al., 2008).

Viruses utilize a number of mechanisms to evade the host immune response. For example, some viruses are able to inhibit the action of interferons. Interferon expression inhibits protein synthesis and destroys RNA in infected cells, up-regulates MHC class I and MHC class II expression and stimulates the innate immune response by activating macrophages and natural killer cells (Fensterl & Sen, 2009). Human cytomegalovirus (HCMV), Varicella-Zoster virus (VZV), Kaposi's sarcoma-associated herpesvirus (KSHV) and Epstein-Barr virus (EBV) contain proteins expressed during the lytic cycle, which disrupt interferon signaling (Abendroth et al., 2000; Grundhoff & Sullivan, 2011; Sedmak et al., 1994). Secondly, viruses can alter MHC class I expression. For example, HCMV produces two proteins US2 and US11 which "dislocate" newly synthesized MHC class I molecules from the endoplasmic reticulum to the cytoplasm, where the MHC molecules are targeted for degradation by the proteosomal pathway (Wiertz et al., 1996a, 1996b). Here the virus interferes with the process of antigen presentation and downregulates the adaptive immune response. Some viruses produce their own cytokine mimics which can alter the immune response. Interleukin-10 (IL-10) is an anti-inflammatory cytokine which inhibits pro-inflammatory cytokines, including interferon, and suppresses antigen-presentation (Moore et al., 1993). EBV and HCMV produce homologous of IL-10 which can bind to IL-10 receptors and dampen the immune response during viral infection (Hsu et al., 1990; Raftery et al., 2004). In addition, both HIV-1 and RSV infection were shown to induce expression of IL-10 in the host cell, thus suppressing release of early immunoregulatory cytokines (Panuska et al., 1995; Schols & De Clercq, 1996). Decoy receptors for the human cytokines are produced by some viruses which effectively dilute the amount of cytokines available for the immune response. The molluscum contagiosum virus (MCV), a human pox virus, produces two proteins that bind the human cytokine IL-18. IL-18 is a pro-inflammatory cytokine which induces the innate immune system. Binding of IL-18 by these decoy receptors prevents IL-18 from binding to its normal receptor on the cell surface and prevents activation of the interferon pathway (Xiang & Moss, 1999). Some viruses are able to inhibit activation of the pattern recognition receptors on host cells. Influenza virus for example, has adapted to circumvent the activation of the RLR pathway of innate immune system activation. The influenza genome contains a nonstructural protein (NS1) which specifically inhibits TRIM25 ubiquitination of RIG-I, a member of the RLR pathway. In the absence of ubiquitination, RIG-I fails to activate type I interferon production which increases virulence of the virus (Gack et al., 2009). HCMV has incorporated a mimic of a MHC class I molecule. The HCMV UL18 protein looks like a MHC class I molecule and is displayed on the surface of cells infected with HCMV (Beck & Barrell, 1988). Once on the cell surface UL18 binds the LILRB1 inhibitory receptor on Natural Killer cells (NK) with higher affinity than the host cell MHC class I molecule (Chapman et al., 1999). During viral infection, many viruses have developed a mechanism to suppress the appearance of MHC class I molecules on the host cell surface. NK cells seek out cells which lack high levels of MHC class I molecules, which are presumably virally infected, and targets these cells for destruction. Since the UL18 protein interactions with the NK LILRB1 receptor, the cell is not targeted for destruction and the HCMV virus can complete its lifecycle. Finally, some viruses contain microRNAs within their genome which can target host cell genes involved in the immune response (discussed below).

1.5 miRNA processing and function

MicroRNAs (miRNAs) play an increasingly important role in gene expression and act at the level of mRNA stability and mRNA translation. Located within the genome, microRNAs are small, single stranded, noncoding RNAs of ~21-22 nt that regulate gene expression by altering mRNA stability and mRNA translation (R.C. Lee et al., 1993). In mammalian cells, the genes for miRNAs are found in intergenic chromosomal regions between known genes or in the intronic regions of mRNAs (Lagos-Quintana et al., 2001; A. Rodriguez et al., 2004) and are transcribed by RNA polymerase II and in some cases RNA polymerase III (Borchert et al., 2006). Furthermore, many miRNAs have been organized in clusters (Ambros, 2004). In some cases a single promoter can drive expression of several miRNAs, resulting in a polycistronic transcript which would presumably allow for their coordinated regulation (Aravin et al., 2003; Y. Lee et al., 2002). miRNAs are initially transcribed as a long primary transcript (pri-miRNA) that can fold into a hairpin secondary structure; the transcript is cleaved within the nucleus to a 70-100 nt pre-miRNA by the RNAse III Drosha (Y. Lee et al., 2003). Subsequently, the pre-miRNA is transported to the cytoplasm via the exportin 5 pathway where the pre-miRNA is further processed into an approximately 22 nt dsRNA by the RNAse III Dicer (Hutvagner et al., 2001; Yi et al., 2003). One strand of the dsRNA is incorporated into the multi-protein RNA induced silencing complex (RISC), where the miRNA exerts its effect on gene expression (Hutvagner & Zamore 2002; Mourelatos et al., 2002). The purpose of miRNAs is to inhibit protein expression of a gene by either targeting the mRNA for degradation or by preventing translation of the target mRNA (Ulvila et al., 2010). Degradation of the mRNA occurs when the miRNA forms a perfect RNA/RNA hybrid with its target mRNA. In mammalian cells however, miRNAs generally form an imperfect RNA/RNA hybrid within the 3′-UTR of its target mRNA. This imperfect binding within the 3′-UTR interfers with and inhibits translation of the mRNA presumably by sequestering the mRNA away from the translational machinery in translationally silent regions of the cytoplasm known as p-bodies (Pillai et al., 2005). While miRNAs are generally thought to inhibit protein expression, recent evidence shows that in some cases, miRNAs can also increase protein production (Vasudevan et al., 2007). During cell cycle arrest miR-369-3 and let-7 were shown to stimulate translation of their target mRNAs while the same miRNAs inhibited translation of their target mRNAs during cellular proliferation. This suggests that the function of at least some miRNAs can be altered during the cell cycle, oscillating between a repressive and a stimulatory function. While miRNAs act as fine tuning regulators of important biological processes such as apoptosis, proliferation, and differentiation miRNAs can also regulate interactions between host and virus. miRNAs involved in regulating host-virus interactions can be derived from the virus, in the case of nuclear DNA viruses, or derived from the host cell (Ulvila et al., 2010).

2. miRNA expression during viral infection

The use of small non-coding RNAs to interfere with gene expression is observed in diverse organisms, from mammals to drosophila to plants (Stram & Kuzntzova, 2006). In plants, these small RNAs are vital to the plant's immune response to viruses and bacteria, and some plant viruses have evolved mechanisms to downregulate the inductive effect of these small RNAs on antiviral innate immunity (Lucy et al., 2000; Voinnet, 2001). The role of small RNAs in the innate immune response of mammals is still poorly understood although, great progress has been achieved over the past few years. Our understanding of how miRNAs aid in the innate immune response is enhanced by the use of microarray miRNA analysis.

2.1 Changes in host miRNAs

The first report of these small non-coding RNAs in animals was in the nematode *Caenorhabditis elegans (C. elegans)* where these non-coding RNAs were shown to be important for proper development (R.C. Lee et al., 1993). In *C. elegans* proteins produced from the *lin-14* and *lin-28* mRNAs must be decreased in order for proper development and specification of cell fates during the early larval stages. The *lin-4* miRNA directed against the 3′-UTRs of these two mRNAs can repress protein production and was shown to do so after translation initiation. *C. elegans* that contain *lin-4* miRNA mutations are unable to downregulate protein expression from *lin-14* and *lin-28* mRNAs resulting in reiteration of early larval developmental stages (R.C. Lee et al., 1993; Wightman et al., 1993).

Not only do miRNAs regulate gene expression of endogenous mRNAs, but endogenous human miRNAs can interact with some viral genomes to alter viral gene expression. In one report examining the liver specific human miR-122, it was shown that miR-122 binds to the 5′ region of the hepatitis C genome (HCV), that mutations within the HCV miR-122 binding sites reduced translation of the HCV mRNA, and that binding of miR-122 within the HCV genome increased the yield of infectious HCV virus (Jangra et al., 2010). Since viral genomes are by necessity small, this would suggest that at least some viral genomes can utilize endogenous miRNAs to their advantage, decreasing the need to incorporate the sequences for some translational control elements within the viral genome. Alternatively, in a human hepatoma cell line, treatment with Interferon β (IFNβ) identified eight IFNβ-induced miRNAs with complementarity to the HCV genome (Pedersen et al., 2007). Five miRNA mimics corresponding to the IFNβ induced miRNAs were able to inhibit HCV replication and thus infection by HCV. Additionally, miR-122 which was previously shown to increase translation of HCV, was downregulated by IFNβ treatment (Pedersen et al., 2007). These results indicate that an increase in IFNβ production induced by the cells immune response to pathogens can abrogate HCV infection.

One of the most studied viruses, protein expression from the human immunodeficiency virus type 1(HIV-1) is regulated by host cellular miRNAs during their latency period. Resting CD4+ T cells exhibit increased levels of human miR-28, miR-125b, miR-150, miR-223 and miR-328 when compared to activated CD4+ T cells. These cellular miRNAs are predicted to target the 3′ ends of HIV-1 mRNAs. Huang, et.al showed that that inhibition of these miRNAs resulted in increased HIV-1 protein translation in resting CD4+ T cells transfected with HIV-1 (Huang et al., 2007). Their data suggests that cellular host miRNAs contribute to the latency of HIV-1 in resting CD4+ T cells. Type III latency of EBV, but not type I latency, showed increased expression of host cell miR-155 in B cells (Jiang et al., 2006; Kluiver et al., 2006). Furthermore, miR-155 was shown to target a number of transcriptional regulatory factors (Yin et al., 2008). In addition to miR-155, EBV was shown to increase expression of cellular miR-146, miR-200, miR-429, miR-29b, and miR-10b (Anastasiadou et al., 2010; Cameron et al., 2008; Ellis-Connell et al., 2010; G. Li et al., 2010). Kaposi's sarcoma-associated herpesvirus (KSHV), herpes simplex virus-1 and HCMV induce expression of miR-132 in their host cells and increased expression of miR-132 decreases expression of interferon-stimulated genes (Lagos et al., 2010), indicating that the viruses are attempting to suppress the initial innate immune response. Alternatively, increased host cell miRNA levels have been shown to decrease viral replication; the replication of primate foamy virus was repressed by human miR-32 (Lecellier et al., 2005). In addition, depletion of Dicer function, a protein involved in miRNA processing, in mice increased their susceptibility to infection with Vesicular stomatitis virus, likely from improper processing of miR-24 and miR-93 (Otsuka et al., 2007). Host cellular miRNAs can modulate expression of protein components of the innate immune response and in some cases, viruses have adapted ways to either exploit these miRNAs for their own survival or to counteract the effects of these miRNAs.

2.2 Virally encoded miRNAs

Not only are miRNAs found within the genome of the host cell, but DNA viruses which replicate in the nucleus, such as members of the herpes virus and polyomavirus families, have been found to encoded viral miRNAs (vmiRNAs) within the viral genome. RNA viruses, which replicate in the cytoplasm, have not been found to contain vmiRNAs within their genomes. The most likely explanation for the presence of vmiRNAs within the genome of DNA viruses, but not RNA viruses, is the need to initially process the pre-miRNAs by the nuclear enzyme Drosha. These vmiRNAs target components of the innate immune system, apoptotic factors and regulators of the host cell cycle (Boss & Renne, 2010). Inhibition of these pathways promotes viability and proliferation of the host cell, allowing for continued viral replication and synthesis. Moreover, production of vmiRNAs directed against host cell components illustrates the complex relationship between viruses and their host cells as each tries to ameliorate the damage caused by the other.

miRNAs derived from the viral genome are processed by the same pathway and in the same manner in which host cell miRNAs are processed. The first viral vmiRNAs were discovered in the genome of EBV (Pfeffer et al., 2004). Latent infection of a Burkitt's lymphoma cell line with EBV revealed the presence of five EBV encoded small RNAs with the characteristic stem-loop structure observed with mammalian miRNAs. Also, these vmiRNAs have been show to target the human mRNAs encoding the pro-apoptotic protein Bim and the p53 up-regulated modulator of apoptosis (PUMA) (Choy et al., 2008; Marquitz et al., 2011). Currently, at least 44 mature vmiRNAs have been identified in the EBV genome (Grundhoff & Sullivan, 2011). The human adenovirus genome, which produces a mild respiratory infection, contains several small vmiRNAs, one of which neutralizes the anti-viral action of interferon (Kitajewski et al., 1986; Reich et al., 1966). In addition, HCMV is reported to contain at least 11 vmiRNAs precursors which putatively target genes involved in T-cell activation and other inflammatory reactions (Grey et al., 2005; Stern-Ginossar et al., 2007) and the Kaposi Sarcoma Virus encodes at least 12 pre-miRNAs which target genes involved in the immune response and in cellular proliferation (Cai et al., 2005; Samols et al., 2007). In these examples, the viral genome contains vmiRNAs which allow the virus to escape detection by the host immune response. Thus, virally encoded or cellular miRNAs, altered after infection, may modulate viral replication.

3. miRNA expression profile in the lung during RSV infection

Our laboratory is interested in the expression of SP-A during RSV infection. SP-A is important in the innate immune response against invading pathogens and recognizes glycoconjugates and lipids present on the cell surface of these organisms. Through opsinization, SP-A targets these organisms for destruction by resident macrophages. Once these pathogens are phagocytosed by macrophages and dendritic cells within the lung epithelium, the pathogens can be processed and their peptides presented to components of the adaptive immune response (Tino & Wright, 1996; Wright & Youmans, 1993). The inability of SP-A to target these organisms early in the infection could lead to increased pathogenicity, prolonged infection and increased morbidity. We found that RSV infection of type II pulmonary epithelial cells results in a 3-fold increase in SP-A mRNA, an attempt by the host cell to upregulate the innate immune response to this pathogen. However, the amount of SP-A protein produced during RSV infection decreases up to 60% when compared to uninfected cells. This decrease in SP-A protein resulted from translational inhibition of the mRNA which was specific to the SP-A mRNA and not a global translational repression of all cellular mRNAs (Bruce et al., 2009). The disparity between increase SP-A mRNA and decreased SP-A protein is puzzling and suggests that during viral infection, RSV is blocking enhanced expression of this component of the innate immune response. How this translational block is occurring is currently unknown. RSV is an RNA virus and not likely to contain conanical miRNAs that could target host mRNAs that encode components of the innate immune response. For example, virally encoded proteins could potentially act as transcriptional factors that change cellular miRNA levels, which could alter the course of infection by RSV. Since miRNAs play pivotal roles in development and in the innate immune response and miRNAs exert their function through translational inhibition, we investigated whether RSV infection would alter the miRNA profile of primary type II epithelial cells derived from human fetal lung explants. Using miRNA microarray analysis performed by LC Sciences, Houston, TX, we compared the miRNA profile of primary type II epithelial cells from fetal lung extracts treated in the absence and presence of RSV infection.

3.1 miRNAs normally expressed in lung type II cells

Previously, the miRNA profiles of the mouse lung and of the human A549 cell line, a human lung carcinoma cell line, have been reported (Jiang et al., 2005). However, the miRNA expression profile of primary human fetal lung type II epithelial cells has not been reported. Baseline expression of the miRNA profile of type II epithelial cells from fetal lung explants were performed using Affymetrix chips that contained probes for 856 mature human miRNAs from the miRBase version 12 database. The florescent expression results of miRNAs from type II epithelial cells from three fetal lung samples (gestational age 19-21 weeks) were averaged. To rule out any dye labeling bias, two of the samples were Cy3 labeled and one of the samples was Cy5 labeled. These studies revealed the presence of 184 miRNAs with an average florescent signal strength ranging from a high of 48,314 to a low of 50, from all three samples. The top 25 highest expressed miRNAs, are shown in Figure 1.

No.	miRNA	Average Signal Strength
1	miR-21	48314
2	let-7a	27336
3	let-7f	26117
4	miR-26a	26102
5	let-7d	21538
6	let-7c	20250
7	miR-200c	19115
8	let-7e	17697
9	miR-23b	17694
10	miR-23a	16717
11	let-7g	15064
12	miR-92a	14256
13	miR-200b	14217
14	let-7b	13890
15	miR-26b	13226
16	miR-125a-5p	12878
17	miR-1246	12147
18	miR-125b	10021
19	let-7i	9929
20	miR-27b	9067
21	miR-1826	9045
22	miR-30d	8613
23	miR-15b	8417
24	miR-30b	8010
25	miR-92b	7820

Fig. 1. Average signal strength of the highest expressed miRNAs in human alveolar type II epithelial cells.

Several miRNAs from the let-7 family (let-7a, let-7f, let-7d, let-7c, let-7e, let-7g, let-7b and let-7i), known to be involved in development, differentiation and cell proliferation were highly expressed from the fetal lung explants (Peter, 2009). The let-7 family members are expressed late in embryonic development and regulate a number of genes involved in early embryonic development (Schulman et al., 2005). Previous miRNA results using the A549 cell line did not reveal high level expression of the let-7 miRNAs consistent with higher expression in developing tissue as compared with cancer cell lines which are often times dedifferentiated (Jiang et al., 2005). In addition to the let-7 family, several members of the miR-200 family, miR-200b and miR-200c, were also highly expressed. Members of the miR-200 family play a key role in the epithelial-to-mesenchymal transition (S.M. Park et al., 2008). This suggests that the human type II epithelial cells grown in primary culture more faithfully represent the miRNA expression profile seen during fetal lung development, as opposed to cell lines, and serves as the basis for examining changes in miRNA expression of human type II cells during different treatments.

3.2 miRNAs whose level increase during RSV infection

To determine the differential miRNA expression profile of fetal human type II epithelial cells to RSV infection, cells were treated in the absence or presence of RSV (M.O.I.=1) for two hours and RNA harvested 24 hrs later. RSV infection resulted in a significant increase (p-value <0.01) in 37 miRNAs with 11 showing a two-fold or greater increase (Figure 2).

No.	miRNA	Human Pulmonary Type II Signal Strength	RSV Treated Pulmonary Type II Signal Strength	Fold Change Increase
1	miR-654-5p	19.62	427.98	21.8
2	miR-663	508.08	4,709.58	9.3
3	miR-149*	141.47	811.71	5.7
4	miR-29c	27.63	144.46	5.2
5	miR-638	1,482.68	4,636.37	3.1
6	miR-1469	232.43	587.35	2.5
7	miR-19b	165.53	413.60	2.5
8	miR-15a	271.71	646.77	2.4
9	miR-181d	165.22	377.95	2.3
10	miR-30e	203.56	411.82	2.0
11	miR-1915	369.23	723.68	2.0

Fig. 2. Human alveolar type II epithelial cell miRNAs that increase 2-fold or greater during RSV infection.

miR-654-5p showed the greatest change at an approximate 22-fold increase followed by miR-663 with an approximately 9-fold increase in the presence of RSV. Using the miRBase databank, we determined the chromosomal location of the miRNAs that showed a 2-fold or greater change in the presence of RSV (Figure 3) (Griffiths-Jones et al., 2008). Seven of the miRNAs were located in intergenic regions or within the intron of processed transcripts.

UPREGULATED miRNAs

miRNA	Chrom	Region	Gene	
miR-654-5p	14	Intergenic	None	Cluster
miR-663	20	Intronic	Processed Transcript	
miR-149*	2	Intronic	Glypican-1	
miR-29c	1	Intergenic	None	Cluster
miR-638	19	Intronic	Dynamin 2	
miR-1469	15	Intronic	Nuclear Receptor subfamily 2	
miR-19b	13	Intronic	Processed Transcript	Cluster
miR-19b	X	Intergenic	None	Cluster
miR-15a	13	Intronic	Processed Transcript	Cluster
miR-181d	19	Intergenic	None	Cluster
miR-30e	1	Intronic	Putative Protein Coding	Cluster
miR-1915	10	Intronic	Uncharacterized Protein	

DOWNREGULATED miRNAs

miRNA	Chrom	Region	Gene	
miR-122	18	Intergenic	None	Cluster
miR-421	X	Intergenic	None	Cluster
miR-183	7	Intergenic	None	Cluster
miR-1268	15	Intergenic	None	
miR-182	7	Intergenic	None	Cluster
miR-331-3p	12	Intergenic	None	Cluster

Fig. 3. Genomic location of human miRNAs that change during RSV infection.

Those miRNAs found in intergenic regions are miR-654-5p, miR-29c, miR-19b and miR-181d. Located on chromosome 14, miR-654-5p is found in an intergenic region comprising a cluster of 16 different miRNAs. All of the miRNAs located in this cluster are expressed at low or undetectable levels in human lung epithelial type II cells and miR-654-5p is the only miRNA in this cluster upregulated during RSV infection, suggesting that this miRNA has its own promoter and is not transcribed as part of a polycystronic mRNA. Several of the miRNAs identified in our differential microarray analysis reside in intron containing, processed transcripts that do not contain open reading frames and are thus not translated. The three miRNAs located in the introns of processed transcripts are miR-663, miR-19b and miR-15a. Previously, the presence of processed yet untranslated mRNA transcripts has presented a conundrum as to their physiological importance however, the identification of miRNAs within the introns of these transcripts could suggest that these types of transcripts may be "hot spots" for other unidentified miRNAs. Two copies of miR-19b are found in the human genome, one on chromosome 13 and this copy is found in an intron of a processed transcript and the second copy is located on the X chromosome in an intergenic region. Three of the miRNAs, miR-149*, miR-638 and miR-1469 are located in intronic regions of known genes and one miRNA, miR-1915 is located in the intron of an uncharacterized protein. miR-149* is located on chromosome 2 in the intron of the glypican 1 (GPC-1) gene which encodes a cell surface proteoglycan. GPC-1 is important for TGF-beta1 induced cell growth inhibition (J. Li et al., 2004). Located within an intron of the dynamin 2 (DPN2) gene is miR-638. DPN2 is present in many different cell types, is a GTPase and is involved in endocytosis (Durieux et al., 2010). Finally, miR-1469 is located on chromosome 15 in an intron of the nuclear receptor subfamily 2, group F, member 2 (NR2F2) gene. NR2F2 is a ligand inducible transcription factor of the steroid thyroid hormone superfamily and plays an important role in lung development. In the mouse, NR2F2 is detected in both the proximal and distal lung (Kimura et al., 2002). Whether the upregulation of the three miRNAs, located in the introns of known genes, is a consequence of increased transcription of these genes during RSV infection is unknown. It would be interesting to determine whether the mRNAs of the GPC-1, DPN2 and NR2F2 genes also increase during RSV infection.

3.3 Viral targets of miRNAs increased during RSV infection

The increase in miRNA expression during RSV infection could serve to regulate viral and/or host cell mRNA expression. For example the PB1 mRNA of the H1N1 influenza A virus was recently shown to be a target of miR-654. The influenza PB1 protein is part of a complex involved in transcription initiation and elongation of viral genes (Ulmanen et al., 1981). Binding of miR-654 to the PB1 mRNA was through imperfect base pairing between the miRNA and the mRNA which typically results in translational repression in mammalian cells. However, binding of miR-654 to the PB1 mRNA resulted in mRNA degradation rather than translational repression (Song et al., 2010). In this example, miRNAs are acting as anti-viral agents by inhibiting viral expression. Similarly, increased expression of miR-149* and miR-638 was observed during HCV infection of a hepatoma cell line and inhibition of miR-149* and miR-638 increased HCV entry into the cell line as measured by luciferase assay. In addition, inhibition of miR-638 resulted in increased HCV mRNA but inhibition of miR-149* decreased HCV abundance (Liu et al., 2010). Finally, in concordance with the RSV results, a keratinocyte cell line infected with human papillomavirus type 11 (HPV-11) also showed upregulation of miR-149*, miR-638, and miR-663 (Dreher et al., 2010).

3.4 Cellular targets of miRNAs that increase during RSV infection

Several algorithms are available for predicting cellular targets of miRNAs however, relatively few confirmed mRNA targets have been identified. RAC-alpha serine/threonine-protein kinase (Akt1) and E2F1 (a transcription factor) both play a role in apoptosis (Liu et al., 2001; Polager & Ginsberg, 2008). Overexpression of miR-149* was shown to directly regulate the 3′-UTR of these two mRNAs resulting in decreased mRNA and protein levels and increased apoptosis in cell lines (Lin et al., 2010). Apoptosis is an important host cell mechanism to regulate viral infection and the increase in miR-149* is one avenue to increase apoptosis of infected cells. Activator protein 1 (AP-1) a transcription factor which regulates genes in response to various stimuli including cytokines, bacterial infections and viral infections is a direct target of miR-663 (Hess et al., 2004; Tili et al., 2010a) and miR-663 also targets the 3′-UTR of transforming growth factor beta 1 (TGFbeta1) (Tili et al., 2010b) a cytokine involved in cell growth, differentiation and proliferation. Cyclin E expression, which is necessary for cell cycle progession from G1 to S phase, is regulated by miR-29C (Ding et al., 2011). In addition, miR-29C directly suppresses p85 alpha (regulatory subunit of PI3 kinase) and CDC42 (Rho family GTPase), two proteins that negatively regulate p53 another cell cycle regulatory protein (S.Y. Park et al., 2009). B-cell lymphoma 2 (BCL-2) a protein involved in regulating apoptosis, breast cancer type 1 susceptibility (BRCA1) a protein involved in the repair of DNA double strand breaks and BMI1 a protein involved in transcriptional repression are directly regulated by miR-15a (Bhattacharya et al., 2009; Cimmino et al., 2005; Zhu et al., 2009). Finally, ubiquitin-conjugating enzyme E2I (UBE2I or UBC9) an enzyme responsible for targeting proteins for degradation is targeted by miR-30e (Wu et al., 2009).

3.5 miRNAs whose level decrease during RSV infection

Thirty four miRNAs were shown to significantly decrease (p-value <0.01) in the presence of RSV infection with six showing a decrease of 2-fold or more (Figure 4).

Unlike what we observed with miRNAs that increased in the presence of RSV, none of the miRNAs which decreased by 2-fold or more were located within introns of known genes. Indeed, all of the miRNAs were located in intergenic regions (Figure 3). The largest decrease was with miR-122 which showed a 7-fold decrease followed by miR-421 with a 4-fold decrease. The decrease in miR-122 is interesting as decreased expression of miR-122 was also observed during HCV infection of a hepatoma cell line (Liu et al., 2010) and during Borna disease virus (BDV) infection of human oligodendralglial cells (Qian et al., 2010). miR-122 is abundantly expressed in the liver and plays a role in HCV replication by binding to sites within the HCV 5′-UTR and stimulating HCV accumulation in vivo. When miR-122 was sequestered in liver cells, replication of HCV RNAs was inhibited (Jopling et al., 2005). Conversely, overexpression of miR-122 blocked replication, transcription and protein synthesis of BDV in oligodendralglial cells (Qian et al., 2010) and inhibited Hepatitis B virus expression in hepatoma cells (Qiu et al., 2010). These data suggest that miR-122 can have contrasting effects on expression of different viruses. Several members of the let-7 family of miRNAs were decreased in the presence of RSV (data not shown). Whether this represents an attempt to inhibit cellular differentiation is unknown however, the amount of decrease in the presence of RSV, while statistically significant, was less than 2-fold.

No.	miRNA	Human Pulmonary Type II Signal Strength	RSV Treated Pulmonary Type II Signal Strength	Fold Change Decrease
1	miR-122	529.32	76.89	-6.9
2	miR-421	123.75	28.95	-4.3
3	miR-183	2,481.76	1,046.96	-2.4
4	miR-1268	177.12	76.53	-2.3
5	miR-182	4,513.70	2,127.39	-2.1
6	miR-331-3p	275.98	135.27	-2.0

Fig. 4. Human alveolar type II epithelial cell miRNAs that decrease 2-fold or greater during RSV infection.

3.6 Cellular targets of miRNAs that decrease during RSV infection

Two of the miRNAs that decrease 2-fold or more during RSV infection have known mRNA targets. First, miR-122 was shown to bind the 3'-UTR of cationic amino acid transporter (CAT-1) resulting in decreased protein abundance of CAT-1 protein (Jopling et al., 2006). In addition, miR-122 has been shown to directly target interleukin-1 alpha (IL-1A) (Gao et al., 2009). IL-1A activates the immune response shortly after infection stimulating proliferation of fibroblasts and lymphocytes as well as chemotaxis of neutrophils (Boraschi et al., 1990; Ozaki et al., 1987). Also, the CUTL1 mRNA which encodes a transcriptional repressor that regulates genes specifying terminal differentiation, is also directly regulated by miR-122 (Xu et al., 2010). Second, miR-421 was shown to regulate the androgen receptor (AR), a transcription factor important for male sexual characteristics (Ostling et al., 2011) and Ataxia-Telangiectasia mutated (ATM) a serine/threonine protein kinase involved in cell cycle arrest, DNA repair and/or apoptosis (Hu et al., 2010).

4. Conclusion

The innate immune response is our first line of defense against invading pathogens and is important for activating the immune response early during infection. Viruses, which are obligate intracellular parasites, must subvert the innate immune response in order to replicate and survive. The constant battle between the host and the virus for survival necessitates the continued evolution of new and better avenues of gene regulation. One fairly recent identified avenue of gene regulation is that of miRNAs which can regulate gene expression at the level of mRNA stability and/or translational efficiency (R.C. Lee et al., 1993). miRNAs can be encoded by the host genome or in some cases, within the viral genome (Boss & Renne 2010). In order to fully understand the intricate interaction of the host and the viral genomes during infection, the impact of miRNAs on changes in gene regulation is an important consideration. In the present study, we determined the miRNA expression pattern from primary fetal lung type II epithelial cells and identified changes in miRNA expression that occurs during RSV infection. RSV infection significantly increased 37 miRNAs and significantly decreased 34 miRNAs. Suggesting that changes in miRNA levels could alter cellular protein levels and affect the course of pathogen associated infections.

One component of the innate immune system within the lung is SP-A. Because SP-A can bind to glycocongugates and lipids on the surface of pathogens, it plays an important role in eliminating these pathogens early during infection (Tino & Wright, 1996; Wright & Youmans, 1993). The divergent results between the increase in SP-A mRNA and the decrease in SP-A protein during RSV infection prompted us to investigates whether changes in miRNA levels occur during RSV infection (Bruce et al., 2009). Using the MicroInspector bioinformatics tool, we checked the 3'-UTR of the SP-A mRNA against the miRNAs that increased at least 2-fold, during RSV infection (Rusinov et al., 2005). Several putative miR-638 and miR-149* binding sites were identified. Whether these miRNAs directly regulate the SP-A mRNA is currently unknown and future directions within the laboratory, will seek to address this question.

The change in cellular miRNA expression profile resulting from several viral infections has recently been investigated. Here we add to this knowledge by investigating the change in cellular miRNA expression of type II lung epithelial cells in the presence of RSV infection. Comparing our results with the results of other viral infections has identified common miRNAs whose expression change in regard to these different viral infections. In the presence of infection with a DNA virus (HPV-11) or an RNA virus (RSV, HCV) miR-149* and miR-638 both increase in concentration within the cell (Dreher et al., 2010; Liu et al., 2010). When cells were infected with the RSV or HCV virus, the level of miR-663 increased within the cell (Liu et al., 2010). The increase in these miRNAs does not appear to be random, but rather a specific attempt by the cell to inhibit replication, transcription, protein synthesis or entry of the virus into the host cell. Commonalities in the changing expression of specific miRNAs during viral infection, suggests that these miRNAs may have antiviral effects. Augmenting expression of these antiviral miRNAs could be an avenue to treat viral infections and could have a global affect on viral infection, resulting in a broad-spectrum avenue to defend against viral invasion. Evaluation of changes in miRNA expression, resulting from additional viral infections, may clarify the miRNAs which exhibit anti-viral effects, and will further our understanding of the host/viral interactions that occur during infection.

5. Acknowledgment

This research was funded in part by NIH-NHLBI (R01-068116) to J. Alcorn.

6. References

Abendroth, A., B. Slobedman, et al. (2000). "Modulation of major histocompatibility class II protein expression by varicella-zoster virus." J Virol 74(4): 1900-7.

Akira, S., S. Uematsu, et al. (2006). "Pathogen recognition and innate immunity." Cell 124(4): 783-801.

Alcorn, J. L., J. M. Stark, et al. (2005). "Effects of RSV infection on pulmonary surfactant protein SP-A in cultured human type II cells: contrasting consequences on SP-A mRNA and protein." Am J Physiol Lung Cell Mol Physiol 289(6): L1113-22.

Ambros, V. (2004). "The functions of animal microRNAs." Nature 431(7006): 350-5.

Anastasiadou, E., F. Boccellato, et al. (2010). "Epstein-Barr virus encoded LMP1 downregulates TCL1 oncogene through miR-29b." Oncogene 29(9): 1316-28.

Aravin, A. A., M. Lagos-Quintana, et al. (2003). "The small RNA profile during Drosophila melanogaster development." Dev Cell 5(2): 337-50.

Arnold, R. R., M. F. Cole, et al. (1977). "A bactericidal effect for human lactoferrin." Science 197(4300): 263-5.

Barr, F. E., H. Pedigo, et al. (2000). "Surfactant protein-A enhances uptake of respiratory syncytial virus by monocytes and U937 macrophages." Am J Respir Cell Mol Biol 23(5): 586-92.

Beck, S. and B. G. Barrell (1988). "Human cytomegalovirus encodes a glycoprotein homologous to MHC class-I antigens." Nature 331(6153): 269-72.

Beers, M. F., A. Hamvas, et al. (2000). "Pulmonary surfactant metabolism in infants lacking surfactant protein B." Am J Respir Cell Mol Biol 22(3): 380-91.

Bhattacharya, R., M. Nicoloso, et al. (2009). "MiR-15a and MiR-16 control Bmi-1 expression in ovarian cancer." Cancer Res 69(23): 9090-5.

Black, C. P. (2003). "Systematic review of the biology and medical management of respiratory syncytial virus infection." Respir Care 48(3): 209-31; discussion 231-3.

Bonjardim, C. A., P. C. Ferreira, et al. (2009). "Interferons: signaling, antiviral and viral evasion." Immunol Lett 122(1): 1-11.

Boraschi, D., L. Villa, et al. (1990). "Differential activity of interleukin 1 alpha and interleukin 1 beta in the stimulation of the immune response in vivo." Eur J Immunol 20(2): 317-21.

Borchert, G. M., W. Lanier, et al. (2006). "RNA polymerase III transcribes human microRNAs." Nat Struct Mol Biol 13(12): 1097-101.

Boss, I. W. and R. Renne (2010). "Viral miRNAs: tools for immune evasion." Curr Opin Microbiol 13(4): 540-5.

Bossert, B. and K. K. Conzelmann (2002). "Respiratory syncytial virus (RSV) nonstructural (NS) proteins as host range determinants: a chimeric bovine RSV with NS genes from human RSV is attenuated in interferon-competent bovine cells." J Virol 76(9): 4287-93.

Bossert, B., S. Marozin, et al. (2003). "Nonstructural proteins NS1 and NS2 of bovine respiratory syncytial virus block activation of interferon regulatory factor 3." J Virol 77(16): 8661-8.

Bruce, S. R., C. L. Atkins, et al. (2009). "Respiratory syncytial virus infection alters surfactant protein A expression in human pulmonary epithelial cells by reducing translation efficiency." Am J Physiol Lung Cell Mol Physiol 297(4): L559-67.

Cai, X., S. Lu, et al. (2005). "Kaposi's sarcoma-associated herpesvirus expresses an array of viral microRNAs in latently infected cells." Proc Natl Acad Sci U S A 102(15): 5570-5.

Cameron, J. E., Q. Yin, et al. (2008). "Epstein-Barr virus latent membrane protein 1 induces cellular MicroRNA miR-146a, a modulator of lymphocyte signaling pathways." J Virol 82(4): 1946-58.

CDC (2004). Respiratory Syncytial Virus Fact Sheet, National Center for Infectious Diseases Respiratory and Enteric Viruses Branch.

Chapman, T. L., A. P. Heikeman, et al. (1999). "The inhibitory receptor LIR-1 uses a common binding interaction to recognize class I MHC molecules and the viral homolog UL18." Immunity 11(5): 603-13.

Choy, E. Y., K. L. Siu, et al. (2008). "An Epstein-Barr virus-encoded microRNA targets PUMA to promote host cell survival." J Exp Med 205(11): 2551-60.

Cimmino, A., G. A. Calin, et al. (2005). "miR-15 and miR-16 induce apoptosis by targeting BCL2." Proc Natl Acad Sci U S A 102(39): 13944-9.

Cowton, V. M., D. R. McGivern, et al. (2006). "Unravelling the complexities of respiratory syncytial virus RNA synthesis." J Gen Virol 87(Pt 7): 1805-21.

Crapo, J. D., B. E. Barry, et al. (1982). "Cell number and cell characteristics of the normal human lung." Am Rev Respir Dis 126(2): 332-7.

Crouch, E. and J. R. Wright (2001). "Surfactant proteins a and d and pulmonary host defense." Annu Rev Physiol 63: 521-54.

Denny, F. W. and W. A. Clyde, Jr. (1986). "Acute lower respiratory tract infections in nonhospitalized children." J Pediatr 108(5 Pt 1): 635-46.

Ding, D. P., Z. L. Chen, et al. (2011). "miR-29c Induces Cell Cycle Arrest in Esophageal Squamous Cell Carcinoma by Modulating Cyclin E expression." Carcinogenesis.

Domachowske, J. B. and H. F. Rosenberg (1999). "Respiratory syncytial virus infection: immune response, immunopathogenesis, and treatment." Clin Microbiol Rev 12(2): 298-309.

Dreher, A., M. Rossing, et al. (2010). "Differential expression of cellular microRNAs in HPV-11 transfected cells. An analysis by three different array platforms and qRT-PCR." Biochem Biophys Res Commun 403(3-4): 357-62.

Durieux, A. C., B. Prudhon, et al. (2010). "Dynamin 2 and human diseases." J Mol Med 88(4): 339-50.

Ellis-Connell, A. L., T. Iempridee, et al. (2010). "Cellular microRNAs 200b and 429 regulate the Epstein-Barr virus switch between latency and lytic replication." J Virol 84(19): 10329-43.

Englund, J. A., C. J. Sullivan, et al. (1988). "Respiratory syncytial virus infection in immunocompromised adults." Ann Intern Med 109(3): 203-8.

Fensterl, V. and G. C. Sen (2009). "Interferons and viral infections." Biofactors 35(1): 14-20.

Foy, H. M., M. K. Cooney, et al. (1973). "Incidence and etiology of pneumonia, croup and bronchiolitis in preschool children belonging to a prepaid medical care group over a four-year period." Am J Epidemiol 97(2): 80-92.

Frogel, M. P. (2008). "In the trenches: a pediatrician's perspective on prevention and treatment strategies for RSV disease." Manag Care 17(11 Suppl 12): 7-12, discussion 18-9.

Gack, M. U., R. A. Albrecht, et al. (2009). "Influenza A virus NS1 targets the ubiquitin ligase TRIM25 to evade recognition by the host viral RNA sensor RIG-I." Cell Host Microbe 5(5): 439-49.

Ganz, T. (2002). "Antimicrobial polypeptides in host defense of the respiratory tract." J Clin Invest 109(6): 693-7.

Ganz, T. (2003). "Defensins: antimicrobial peptides of innate immunity." Nat Rev Immunol 3(9): 710-20.

Gao, Y., Y. He, et al. (2009). "An insertion/deletion polymorphism at miRNA-122-binding site in the interleukin-1alpha 3' untranslated region confers risk for hepatocellular carcinoma." Carcinogenesis 30(12): 2064-9.

Ghildyal, R., C. Hartley, et al. (1999). "Surfactant protein A binds to the fusion glycoprotein of respiratory syncytial virus and neutralizes virion infectivity." J Infect Dis 180(6): 2009-13.

Grey, F., A. Antoniewicz, et al. (2005). "Identification and characterization of human cytomegalovirus-encoded microRNAs." J Virol 79(18): 12095-9.

Griffin, M. R., C. S. Coffey, et al. (2002). "Winter viruses: influenza- and respiratory syncytial virus-related morbidity in chronic lung disease." Arch Intern Med 162(11): 1229-36.

Griffiths-Jones, S., H. K. Saini, et al. (2008). "miRBase: tools for microRNA genomics." Nucleic Acids Res 36(Database issue): D154-8.

Grundhoff, A. and C. S. Sullivan (2011). "Virus-encoded microRNAs." Virology 411(2): 325-43.

Haagsman, H. P. and R. V. Diemel (2001). "Surfactant-associated proteins: functions and structural variation." Comp Biochem Physiol A Mol Integr Physiol 129(1): 91-108.

Hacking, D. and J. Hull (2002). "Respiratory syncytial virus--viral biology and the host response." J Infect 45(1): 18-24.

Hess, J., P. Angel, et al. (2004). "AP-1 subunits: quarrel and harmony among siblings." J Cell Sci 117(Pt 25): 5965-73.

Holmes, E. C. (2011). "What does virus evolution tell us about virus origins?" J Virol 85(11): 5247-51.

Holmskov, U., S. Thiel, et al. (2003). "Collections and ficolins: humoral lectins of the innate immune defense." Annu Rev Immunol 21: 547-78.

Hsu, D. H., R. de Waal Malefyt, et al. (1990). "Expression of interleukin-10 activity by Epstein-Barr virus protein BCRF1." Science 250(4982): 830-2.

Hu, H., L. Du, et al. (2010). "ATM is down-regulated by N-Myc-regulated microRNA-421." Proc Natl Acad Sci U S A 107(4): 1506-11.

Huang, J., F. Wang, et al. (2007). "Cellular microRNAs contribute to HIV-1 latency in resting primary CD4+ T lymphocytes." Nat Med 13(10): 1241-7.

Hutvagner, G., J. McLachlan, et al. (2001). "A cellular function for the RNA-interference enzyme Dicer in the maturation of the let-7 small temporal RNA." Science 293(5531): 834-8.

Hutvagner, G. and P. D. Zamore (2002). "A microRNA in a multiple-turnover RNAi enzyme complex." Science 297(5589): 2056-60.

Jangra, R. K., M. Yi, et al. (2010). "Regulation of hepatitis C virus translation and infectious virus production by the microRNA miR-122." J Virol 84(13): 6615-25.

Jiang, J., E. J. Lee, et al. (2005). "Real-time expression profiling of microRNA precursors in human cancer cell lines." Nucleic Acids Res 33(17): 5394-403.

Jiang, J., E. J. Lee, et al. (2006). "Increased expression of microRNA-155 in Epstein-Barr virus transformed lymphoblastoid cell lines." Genes Chromosomes Cancer 45(1): 103-6.

Jopling, C. L., K. L. Norman, et al. (2006). "Positive and negative modulation of viral and cellular mRNAs by liver-specific microRNA miR-122." Cold Spring Harb Symp Quant Biol 71: 369-76.

Jopling, C. L., M. Yi, et al. (2005). "Modulation of hepatitis C virus RNA abundance by a liver-specific MicroRNA." Science 309(5740): 1577-81.

Kang, D. C., R. V. Gopalkrishnan, et al. (2002). "mda-5: An interferon-inducible putative RNA helicase with double-stranded RNA-dependent ATPase activity and melanoma growth-suppressive properties." Proc Natl Acad Sci U S A 99(2): 637-42.
Kawai, T. and S. Akira (2009). "The roles of TLRs, RLRs and NLRs in pathogen recognition." Int Immunol 21(4): 317-37.
Kimura, Y., T. Suzuki, et al. (2002). "Retinoid receptors in the developing human lung." Clin Sci (Lond) 103(6): 613-21.
Kitajewski, J., R. J. Schneider, et al. (1986). "Adenovirus VAI RNA antagonizes the antiviral action of interferon by preventing activation of the interferon-induced eIF-2 alpha kinase." Cell 45(2): 195-200.
Kluiver, J., E. Haralambieva, et al. (2006). "Lack of BIC and microRNA miR-155 expression in primary cases of Burkitt lymphoma." Genes Chromosomes Cancer 45(2): 147-53.
Knowles, M. R. and R. C. Boucher (2002). "Mucus clearance as a primary innate defense mechanism for mammalian airways." J Clin Invest 109(5): 571-7.
Lagos-Quintana, M., R. Rauhut, et al. (2001). "Identification of novel genes coding for small expressed RNAs." Science 294(5543): 853-8.
Lagos, D., G. Pollara, et al. (2010). "miR-132 regulates antiviral innate immunity through suppression of the p300 transcriptional co-activator." Nat Cell Biol 12(5): 513-9.
Laible, N. J. and G. R. Germaine (1985). "Bactericidal activity of human lysozyme, muramidase-inactive lysozyme, and cationic polypeptides against Streptococcus sanguis and Streptococcus faecalis: inhibition by chitin oligosaccharides." Infect Immun 48(3): 720-8.
Lecellier, C. H., P. Dunoyer, et al. (2005). "A cellular microRNA mediates antiviral defense in human cells." Science 308(5721): 557-60.
Lee, R. C., R. L. Feinbaum, et al. (1993). "The C. elegans heterochronic gene lin-4 encodes small RNAs with antisense complementarity to lin-14." Cell 75(5): 843-54.
Lee, Y., C. Ahn, et al. (2003). "The nuclear RNase III Drosha initiates microRNA processing." Nature 425(6956): 415-9.
Lee, Y., K. Jeon, et al. (2002). "MicroRNA maturation: stepwise processing and subcellular localization." EMBO J 21(17): 4663-70.
LeVine, A. M., M. D. Bruno, et al. (1997). "Surfactant protein A-deficient mice are susceptible to group B streptococcal infection." J Immunol 158(9): 4336-40.
LeVine, A. M., J. Gwozdz, et al. (1999). "Surfactant protein-A enhances respiratory syncytial virus clearance in vivo." J Clin Invest 103(7): 1015-21.
LeVine, A. M., K. E. Kurak, et al. (1998). "Surfactant protein-A-deficient mice are susceptible to Pseudomonas aeruginosa infection." Am J Respir Cell Mol Biol 19(4): 700-8.
Li, G., Z. Wu, et al. (2010). "MicroRNA-10b induced by Epstein-Barr virus-encoded latent membrane protein-1 promotes the metastasis of human nasopharyngeal carcinoma cells." Cancer Lett 299(1): 29-36.
Li, J., J. Kleeff, et al. (2004). "Glypican-1 antisense transfection modulates TGF-beta-dependent signaling in Colo-357 pancreatic cancer cells." Biochem Biophys Res Commun 320(4): 1148-55.
Lin, R. J., Y. C. Lin, et al. (2010). "miR-149* induces apoptosis by inhibiting Akt1 and E2F1 in human cancer cells." Mol Carcinog 49(8): 719-27.
Liu, X., Y. Shi, et al. (2001). "Downregulation of Akt1 inhibits anchorage-independent cell growth and induces apoptosis in cancer cells." Neoplasia 3(4): 278-86.

Liu, X., T. Wang, et al. (2010). "Systematic identification of microRNA and messenger RNA profiles in hepatitis C virus-infected human hepatoma cells." Virology 398(1): 57-67.

Lucy, A. P., H. S. Guo, et al. (2000). "Suppression of post-transcriptional gene silencing by a plant viral protein localized in the nucleus." EMBO J 19(7): 1672-80.

Marquitz, A. R., A. Mathur, et al. (2011). "The Epstein-Barr Virus BART microRNAs target the pro-apoptotic protein Bim." Virology 412(2): 392-400.

McCormack, F. X. and J. A. Whitsett (2002). "The pulmonary collectins, SP-A and SP-D, orchestrate innate immunity in the lung." J Clin Invest 109(6): 707-12.

Moore, K. W., A. O'Garra, et al. (1993). "Interleukin-10." Annu Rev Immunol 11: 165-90.

Mourelatos, Z., J. Dostie, et al. (2002). "miRNPs: a novel class of ribonucleoproteins containing numerous microRNAs." Genes Dev 16(6): 720-8.

Mufson, M. A., H. D. Levine, et al. (1973). "Epidemiology of respiratory syncytial virus infection among infants and children in Chicago." Am J Epidemiol 98(2): 88-95.

Murray, J. F. (2010). "The structure and function of the lung." Int J Tuberc Lung Dis 14(4): 391-6.

Muruve, D. A., V. Petrilli, et al. (2008). "The inflammasome recognizes cytosolic microbial and host DNA and triggers an innate immune response." Nature 452(7183): 103-7.

Nogee, L. M., G. Garnier, et al. (1994). "A mutation in the surfactant protein B gene responsible for fatal neonatal respiratory disease in multiple kindreds." J Clin Invest 93(4): 1860-3.

Ostling, P., S. K. Leivonen, et al. (2011). "Systematic analysis of microRNAs targeting the androgen receptor in prostate cancer cells." Cancer Res 71(5): 1956-67.

Otsuka, M., Q. Jing, et al. (2007). "Hypersusceptibility to vesicular stomatitis virus infection in Dicer1-deficient mice is due to impaired miR24 and miR93 expression." Immunity 27(1): 123-34.

Ozaki, Y., T. Ohashi, et al. (1987). "Potentiation of neutrophil function by recombinant DNA-produced interleukin 1a." J Leukoc Biol 42(6): 621-7.

Panuska, J. R., R. Merolla, et al. (1995). "Respiratory syncytial virus induces interleukin-10 by human alveolar macrophages. Suppression of early cytokine production and implications for incomplete immunity." J Clin Invest 96(5): 2445-53.

Park, S. M., A. B. Gaur, et al. (2008). "The miR-200 family determines the epithelial phenotype of cancer cells by targeting the E-cadherin repressors ZEB1 and ZEB2." Genes Dev 22(7): 894-907.

Park, S. Y., J. H. Lee, et al. (2009). "miR-29 miRNAs activate p53 by targeting p85 alpha and CDC42." Nat Struct Mol Biol 16(1): 23-9.

Parrott, R. H., H. W. Kim, et al. (1973). "Epidemiology of respiratory syncytial virus infection in Washington, D.C. II. Infection and disease with respect to age, immunologic status, race and sex." Am J Epidemiol 98(4): 289-300.

Pedersen, I. M., G. Cheng, et al. (2007). "Interferon modulation of cellular microRNAs as an antiviral mechanism." Nature 449(7164): 919-22.

Peter, M. E. (2009). "Let-7 and miR-200 microRNAs: guardians against pluripotency and cancer progression." Cell Cycle 8(6): 843-52.

Pfeffer, S., M. Zavolan, et al. (2004). "Identification of virus-encoded microRNAs." Science 304(5671): 734-6.

Pillai, R. S., S. N. Bhattacharyya, et al. (2005). "Inhibition of translational initiation by Let-7 MicroRNA in human cells." Science 309(5740): 1573-6.

Polager, S. and D. Ginsberg (2008). "E2F - at the crossroads of life and death." Trends Cell Biol 18(11): 528-35.

Pryhuber, G. S., W. M. Hull, et al. (1991). "Ontogeny of surfactant proteins A and B in human amniotic fluid as indices of fetal lung maturity." Pediatr Res 30(6): 597-605.

Qian, J., A. Zhai, et al. (2010). "Modulation of miR-122 on persistently Borna disease virus infected human oligodendroglial cells." Antiviral Res 87(2): 249-56.

Qiu, L., H. Fan, et al. (2010). "miR-122-induced down-regulation of HO-1 negatively affects miR-122-mediated suppression of HBV." Biochem Biophys Res Commun 398(4): 771-7.

Raftery, M. J., D. Wieland, et al. (2004). "Shaping phenotype, function, and survival of dendritic cells by cytomegalovirus-encoded IL-10." J Immunol 173(5): 3383-91.

Reich, P. R., B. G. Forget, et al. (1966). "RNA of low molecular weight in KB cells infected with adenovirus type 2." J Mol Biol 17(2): 428-39.

Richman, A. V. and N. M. Tauraso (1971). "Growth of respiratory syncytial virus in suspension cell culture." Appl Microbiol 22(6): 1123-5.

Rodriguez, A., S. Griffiths-Jones, et al. (2004). "Identification of mammalian microRNA host genes and transcription units." Genome Res 14(10A): 1902-10.

Rodriguez, L., I. Cuesta, et al. (2004). "Human respiratory syncytial virus matrix protein is an RNA-binding protein: binding properties, location and identity of the RNA contact residues." J Gen Virol 85(Pt 3): 709-19.

Rusinov, V., V. Baev, et al. (2005). "MicroInspector: a web tool for detection of miRNA binding sites in an RNA sequence." Nucleic Acids Res 33(Web Server issue): W696-700.

Samols, M. A., R. L. Skalsky, et al. (2007). "Identification of cellular genes targeted by KSHV-encoded microRNAs." PLoS Pathog 3(5): e65.

Schols, D. and E. De Clercq (1996). "Human immunodeficiency virus type 1 gp120 induces anergy in human peripheral blood lymphocytes by inducing interleukin-10 production." J Virol 70(8): 4953-60.

Schulman, B. R., A. Esquela-Kerscher, et al. (2005). "Reciprocal expression of lin-41 and the microRNAs let-7 and mir-125 during mouse embryogenesis." Dev Dyn 234(4): 1046-54.

Sedmak, D. D., A. M. Guglielmo, et al. (1994). "Cytomegalovirus inhibits major histocompatibility class II expression on infected endothelial cells." Am J Pathol 144(4): 683-92.

Song, L., H. Liu, et al. (2010). "Cellular microRNAs inhibit replication of the H1N1 influenza A virus in infected cells." J Virol 84(17): 8849-60.

Stern-Ginossar, N., N. Elefant, et al. (2007). "Host immune system gene targeting by a viral miRNA." Science 317(5836): 376-81.

Stram, Y. and L. Kuzntzova (2006). "Inhibition of viruses by RNA interference." Virus Genes 32(3): 299-306.

Subramanian, K. N., L. E. Weisman, et al. (1998). "Safety, tolerance and pharmacokinetics of a humanized monoclonal antibody to respiratory syncytial virus in premature infants and infants with bronchopulmonary dysplasia. MEDI-493 Study Group." Pediatr Infect Dis J 17(2): 110-5.

Thornton, D. J., K. Rousseau, et al. (2008). "Structure and function of the polymeric mucins in airways mucus." Annu Rev Physiol 70: 459-86.

Tili, E., J. J. Michaille, et al. (2010). "Resveratrol decreases the levels of miR-155 by upregulating miR-663, a microRNA targeting JunB and JunD." Carcinogenesis 31(9): 1561-6.

Tili, E., J. J. Michaille, et al. (2010). "Resveratrol modulates the levels of microRNAs targeting genes encoding tumor-suppressors and effectors of TGFbeta signaling pathway in SW480 cells." Biochem Pharmacol 80(12): 2057-65.

Tino, M. J. and J. R. Wright (1996). "Surfactant protein A stimulates phagocytosis of specific pulmonary pathogens by alveolar macrophages." Am J Physiol 270(4 Pt 1): L677-88.

Tripp, R. A., L. P. Jones, et al. (2001). "CX3C chemokine mimicry by respiratory syncytial virus G glycoprotein." Nat Immunol 2(8): 732-8.

Ulmanen, I., B. A. Broni, et al. (1981). "Role of two of the influenza virus core P proteins in recognizing cap 1 structures (m7GpppNm) on RNAs and in initiating viral RNA transcription." Proc Natl Acad Sci U S A 78(12): 7355-9.

Ulvila, J., D. Hultmark, et al. (2010). "RNA silencing in the antiviral innate immune defence--role of DEAD-box RNA helicases." Scand J Immunol 71(3): 146-58.

Vasudevan, S., Y. Tong, et al. (2007). "Switching from repression to activation: microRNAs can up-regulate translation." Science 318(5858): 1931-4.

Ventre, K. and A. G. Randolph (2007). "Ribavirin for respiratory syncytial virus infection of the lower respiratory tract in infants and young children." Cochrane Database Syst Rev(1): CD000181.

Voinnet, O. (2001). "RNA silencing as a plant immune system against viruses." Trends Genet 17(8): 449-59.

West, J. (1990). Respiratory Physiology - The Essentials. Baltimore, Williams and Wilkins.

Wiertz, E. J., T. R. Jones, et al. (1996). "The human cytomegalovirus US11 gene product dislocates MHC class I heavy chains from the endoplasmic reticulum to the cytosol." Cell 84(5): 769-79.

Wiertz, E. J., D. Tortorella, et al. (1996). "Sec61-mediated transfer of a membrane protein from the endoplasmic reticulum to the proteasome for destruction." Nature 384(6608): 432-8.

Wightman, B., I. Ha, et al. (1993). "Posttranscriptional regulation of the heterochronic gene lin-14 by lin-4 mediates temporal pattern formation in C. elegans." Cell 75(5): 855-62.

Wilmott, R., M. Fiedler, et al. (1998). Host Defense Mechanisms. Disorders of the Respiratory Tract in Children. Philadelphia, W.B. Saunders Company: 238-264.

Wright, J. R. and D. C. Youmans (1993). "Pulmonary surfactant protein A stimulates chemotaxis of alveolar macrophage." Am J Physiol 264(4 Pt 1): L338-44.

Wu, F., S. Zhu, et al. (2009). "MicroRNA-mediated regulation of Ubc9 expression in cancer cells." Clin Cancer Res 15(5): 1550-7.

Xiang, Y. and B. Moss (1999). "IL-18 binding and inhibition of interferon gamma induction by human poxvirus-encoded proteins." Proc Natl Acad Sci U S A 96(20): 11537-42.

Xu, H., J. H. He, et al. (2010). "Liver-enriched transcription factors regulate microRNA-122 that targets CUTL1 during liver development." Hepatology 52(4): 1431-42.

Yi, R., Y. Qin, et al. (2003). "Exportin-5 mediates the nuclear export of pre-microRNAs and short hairpin RNAs." Genes Dev 17(24): 3011-6.

Yin, Q., J. McBride, et al. (2008). "MicroRNA-155 is an Epstein-Barr virus-induced gene that modulates Epstein-Barr virus-regulated gene expression pathways." J Virol 82(11): 5295-306.

Yoneyama, M., M. Kikuchi, et al. (2005). "Shared and unique functions of the DExD/H-box helicases RIG-I, MDA5, and LGP2 in antiviral innate immunity." J Immunol 175(5): 2851-8.
Yoneyama, M., M. Kikuchi, et al. (2004). "The RNA helicase RIG-I has an essential function in double-stranded RNA-induced innate antiviral responses." Nat Immunol 5(7): 730-7.
Zhu, J. Y., T. Pfuhl, et al. (2009). "Identification of novel Epstein-Barr virus microRNA genes from nasopharyngeal carcinomas." J Virol 83(7): 3333-41.

3

Animal Models of Respiratory Syncytial Virus Pathogenesis and Vaccine Development: Opportunities and Future Directions

Amelia R. Woolums[1], Sujin Lee[2,3] and Martin L. Moore[2,3]
[1]*Department of Large Animal Medicine*
University of Georgia College of Veterinary Medicine, Athens, GA
[2]*Department of Pediatrics, Emory University School of Medicine, Atlanta, GA*
[3]*Children's Healthcare of Atlanta, Atlanta, GA*
USA

1. Introduction

Human respiratory syncytial virus (HRSV) is the leading cause of respiratory failure and viral death in infants (Thompson et al., 2003). In HRSV bronchiolitis, plugs of mucus, epithelial cell debris, and innate inflammatory cells obstruct the airways leading to pulmonary obstruction (Aherne et al., 1970; Lugo and Nahata, 1993). In autopsy lung tissues from fatal HRSV disease cases, epithelial damage and mechanical airway obstruction are implicated as key features of HRSV pathogenesis (Johnson et al., 2007; Welliver et al., 2007). Although laboratory animal models of HRSV pathogenesis have been widely used to determine pathogenic mechanisms of HRSV infection, the commonly used lab strains of HRSV do not cause airway epithelial cell desquamation, airway mucus production, or lung dysfunction in mice (Moore et al., 2009a; Peebles et al., 2001). However, some strains of HRSV (e.g. line 19 and clinical isolate A2001/2-20) were shown to cause airway mucus expression and lung dysfunction in mice, and clinical isolates can cause airway epithelial cell desquamation in mice (Moore et al., 2009a; Stokes et al., 2011). The fusion (F) glycoprotein of HRSV strain line 19 was implicated in the mechanism of line 19-induced airway mucus (Moore et al., 2009a). Variation in HRSV glycoprotein sequence may contribute to disease variation observed clinically. The pathogenesis of HRSV is likely due to a combination of host and viral genetic determinants. HRSV strain-specific virulence in mice facilitates mechanistic studies of HRSV pathogenesis and may provide more robust challenge models to test whether vaccines have potential to prevent HRSV disease.

Currently, there are no vaccines for prevention of HRSV disease. There are several obstacles to developing successful vaccines for HRSV, including immunological immaturity of infants, interference of immunogenicity by maternal Abs, and relatively poor immune responses to HRSV. In the 1960s, a formalin-inactivated HRSV (FI-HRSV) vaccine tragically resulted in enhanced disease in infants upon natural HRSV infection (Kapikian et al., 1969; Kim et al., 1969). Reasons for this may be formation of carbonyl groups on vaccine antigens due to formaldehyde treatment and/or poor Toll-like receptor stimulation by inactivated HRSV (Delgado et al., 2009; Moghaddam et al., 2006). Another significant obstacle in vaccine development is the lack of stringent challenge animal models. Mice and cotton rats are semi-permissive for HRSV infection, and species other than the chimpanzee are not particularly advantageous over mice and cotton rats (Belshe et al., 1977; Coates and Chanock, 1962; Prince et al., 1978; Prince and Porter, 1976). The lack of robust HRSV replication and disease in rodents has led to false hopes of vaccine efficacy.

Bovine RSV (BRSV) is closely related to HRSV and causes a similar disease in young calves. The pathogenesis and biology of BRSV are highly similar to HRSV. Successful BRSV vaccines are in use, and the vaccinology of BRSV has relevance for HRSV vaccine strategies. Another model of HRSV pathogenesis in the natural host is pneumonia virus of mice (PVM), a pneumovirus that is a natural pathogen of murids. PVM causes a dose-dependent lethal infection in mice with pathologic features resembling severe HRSV bronchiolitis. The caveat of using BRSV and PVM models for vaccine advancement is that the antigens are not specifically HRSV. Future studies testing HRSV vaccine efficacy would benefit greatly from HRSV-BRSV and HRSV-PVM chimeric viruses. Chimeric HRSV-BRSV viruses have been generated by RSV reverse genetics, and additional chimeras could be useful as robust challenge strains (Buchholz et al., 2000). Such a chimeric approach is taken in the HIV and influenza vaccine fields to overcome limits on host restriction.

2. Pathologic features of HRSV, BRSV, and PVM in their natural hosts

2.1 Pathologic features of natural HRSV infection in infants

Pathologic features of HRSV infection have not been extensively characterized because few reports have described autopsy findings in immunocompetent humans infected with HRSV. Furthermore, HRSV-infected patients who die often do so after days to weeks of intensive therapy which may include mechanical ventilation, oxygen therapy, and other interventions which can superimpose non-HRSV induced pathology (DeVincenzo, 2007). However, an informative report described lesions in an HRSV-infected child who died in an automobile accident, along with lesions from 3 archived cases from 1931-1949, prior to the initiation of modern intensive care practices (Johnson et al., 2007). Immunohistochemical (IHC) staining revealed viral antigen in bronchiolar epithelial cells, including ciliated cells. Intrabronchiolar syncytia were present in one patient. Viral antigen was also identified in type I and type II alveolar epithelial cells. Debris in airways consisted of fibrin and mucus along with sloughed epithelial cells and macrophages that stained positive for HRSV. Peribronchiolar and periarteriolar inflammation was characterized by mononuclear and lymphocytic infiltration. Organized lymphoid aggregates were often present, and bronchial arteries were congested. Neutrophils could be seen migrating into bronchioles and along the bronchiolar epithelium. Eosinophils were occasionally present in the peribronchiolar infiltrate. In the pulmonary parenchyma, interstitial inflammation was present, with marked vascular congestion. Three patients had intraalveolar leakage of fibrin with infiltration of macrophages and occasional neutrophils. One patient had severe pneumonitis with rare focal necrosis and hemorrhage. In these children with natural HRSV infection, bronchiolar-associated lymphoid tissue (BALT) was prominent and often hyperplastic (Johnson et al., 2007).

Immunohistochemical staining to characterize the phenotype of infiltrating cells was undertaken in one case. In this patient, the BALT consisted largely of $CD20^+$ B cells with some $CD3^+$ T cells and $CD68^+$ monocytes. In contrast, $CD3^+$ T cells were most prominent in the spaces between pulmonary arterioles and small distal airways; they were also found in the bronchiolar epithelium and in the alveolar interstitium. Despite the presence of T and B cells, the prominent pathologic changes of fatal HRSV infection were widespread viral antigen in airway and alveolar epithelia and mechanical obstruction of airways.

A second report describing histopathologic changes in infants with fatal HRSV-induced disease who were not subjected to prolonged mechanical ventilation or antiviral or anti-inflammatory therapy revealed similar findings to those in of Johnson et al. (Welliver et al., 2007). In tissues from nine patients who died due to severe lower respiratory tract infection and which were positive on IHC staining for HRSV, the terminal bronchioles were plugged with sloughed epithelial cells with abundant viral antigen identified by IHC. Bronchiolar walls were infiltrated with neutrophils and macrophages. As compared to tissues from children infected with influenza, HRSV-induced bronchiolar epithelial damage seemed much greater, and the amount of viral antigen present was increased. In contrast to the single case in which T cell subsets were evaluated by Johnson et al., $CD4^+$ or $CD8^+$ cells were infrequently identified by IHC staining of bronchioles and alveoli (Welliver et al., 2007). Staining for CD16 was used to identify neutrophils and macrophages and found to be extensive in HRSV-infected children. Staining for the apoptosis marker caspase 3 was strongly positive in bronchiolar epithelial cells. The conclusion of Welliver et al. was that children dying of severe acute HRSV infection suffered from bronchiolar obstruction due to widespread death and sloughing of epithelial cells. An excessive immune response mediated by T cells did not seem to be involved because of relatively few T cells found in these tissues. Although immune responses play important roles in HRSV pathogenesis, these two pathology studies taken together show that severe, unchecked HRSV disease in infants is a pulmonary disease associated with virus-induced epithelial damage leading to airway obstruction and *not* associated with immunopathology per se, e.g. excessive T cells or cytokine storm (DeVincenzo, 2007; Johnson et al., 2007; Welliver et al., 2007).

2.2 Pathologic features of BRSV infection in calves

Pathologic changes in the lungs of calves that die or are euthanized due to natural BRSV infection share many similarities with those described for children with fatal HRSV infection. Bronchitis and bronchiolitis with necrosis and sometimes hyperplasia of the bronchiolar epithelium is present, with lumina of bronchioles containing sloughed epithelial cells, neutrophils, mononuclear cells, and proteinaceous debris (Bryson et al., 1983; Elazhary et al., 1982; Pirie et al., 1981). Viral antigen is identified in bronchiolar and alveolar epithelial cells by IHC. Mononuclear cells are present in the bronchiolar lamina propria and surrounding bronchioles (Bryson et al., 1983; Pirie et al., 1981). Alveolar inflammation is also present, with neutrophils, monocytes, and macrophages in alveolar lumina and in the interstitium. Edema is present in alveolar lumina as well as interstitially, sometimes with hemorrhage and emphysema. Syncytia in bronchiolar and alveolar lumina are frequent (Bryson et al., 1983; Pirie et al., 1981). From these reports it appears that neutrophils play a larger role in the response to BRSV, although this may be in part due to frequent co-infection with mycoplasmas or other bacterial respiratory pathogens in calves in some reports (Bryson et al., 1983; Pirie et al., 1981). However, experimentally induced cases of BRSV infection where bacterial co-infection was not present were also characterized by bronchiolar epithelial necrosis and sloughing, with infiltration of neutrophils, lymphocytes, and mononuclear cells into bronchiolar and alveolar lumina (Bryson et al., 1983; McNulty et al., 1983). As noted for fatal HRSV, death of BRSV-infected bronchiolar and alveolar epithelial cells is associated with apoptosis (Viuff et al., 2002; Welliver et al., 2007).

As for HRSV, there is evidence that immune responses to BRSV infection can contribute to disease severity in at least some individuals. Although there are relatively few detailed studies of pathogenesis of naturally occurring disease due to BRSV infection, research by two different groups indicated a role for mast cell degranulation and mediator release in disease severity (Jolly et al., 2004; Kimman et al., 1989b). Unfortunately neither of these groups measured BRSV-specific IgE in affected calves so it is not clear if mast cell degranulation was triggered by virus-specific IgE or through other mechanisms. Other research has shown that BRSV-specific IgE concentration in blood or pulmonary efferent lymph can be strongly correlated with disease severity in BRSV infection, and that transcription of IL-4 mRNA is associated with IgE production (Gershwin et al., 2000).

2.3 Pathologic features of experimental PVM infection of mice

Like HRSV and BRSV, PVM is a member of the genus *Pneumovirus* within the family *Paramyxoviridae*. The PVM genome has 29-62% nucleotide identity to HRSV and BRSV, which are closely related to each other (Krempl et al., 2005). PVM is a natural respiratory pathogen of murids, and laboratory mouse strains are highly susceptible to experimental PVM infection (Rosenberg et al., 2005). PVM challenge of mice showed that changes in bronchial epithelial cells were evident as early as day 1 post-infection and were characterized by granular changes in the cytoplasm with lifting and stripping of the bronchial epithelium and shedding of cellular debris into bronchial lumina (Carthew and Sparrow, 1980). Plugs of cellular debris and neutrophils were evident by day 4 post-infection, as were severe alveolar congestion and edema, with infiltration of neutrophils and macrophages into alveolar spaces and the interstitium. In contrast to HRSV and BRSV, syncytial cells were not described in airways or alveoli. By day 7 post-infection alveolar spaces were filled with neutrophils, macrophages, and lymphocytes. IHC staining for PVM revealed virus in bronchial epithelial cells by day 2 post-infection, and virus in alveolar epithelial cells by day 4 post-infection. Virus was no longer evident by IHC staining after day 7 post-infection. As has been noted for BRSV (Gershwin et al., 1998) and HRSV (Stokes et al., 2011), pathologic changes in mice infected with PVM depend on the virulence of the challenge isolate; challenge of mice with the virulent strain J3666 induces more severe pathology than does challenge with strain 15 (Domachowske et al., 2002). Overall, the histopathology of severe HRSV, BRSV, and PVM infection in the natural host show striking similarities in 1) viral tropism for airway and alveolar epithelial cells, 2) airway epithelial desquamation, 3) obstruction of airways with mixtures of mucus, fibrin, and cells (epithelial debris and inflammatory cells), and 4) prominent neutrophil and macrophage inflammation in bronchiolar, alveolar, and interstitial spaces.

3. Animal models of HRSV pathogenesis

3.1 Mouse models of HRSV infection: Different HRSV strains

3.1.1 HRSV A2 strain mouse model

Mice are semi-permissive for HRSV replication, and BALB/c mice are one of the more susceptible strains (Prince et al., 1979). The A2 and Long strains are antigenic subgroup A reference strains. A2 was isolated in Australia in 1961, and Long was isolated in Baltimore in 1956. A hallmark of experimental pulmonary HRSV infection of mice is mononuclear cell lung infiltrates. The A2 strain has been used to elucidate roles T cells play in HRSV clearance, immunopathology, and immune modulation. Intranasal A2 strain infection of BALB/c mice induces IFN-γ and T cell-mediated clearance and immunopathology. Viral titers peak approximately 4 days post-infection and lymphocytic inflammation peaks one week post-infection. The peak lung T cell response of BALB/c mice to A2 infection is 6-12 days post-infection, and IFN-γ-expressing $CD8^+$ T cells peak before HRSV-specific $CD8^+$ T cells (Chang and Braciale, 2002; Chang et al., 2001; Hussell and Openshaw, 1998). $CD4^+$ and $CD8^+$ T cells exacerbate A2-induced illness and mediate virus clearance (Graham et al., 1991). $Foxp3^+$ CD4 T cells (Tregs) coordinate $CD8^+$ T cell recruitment, downregulate $CD8^+$ T cell TNF-α production, and limit disease severity (ruffled fur) in HRSV A2-infected BALB/c mice (Fulton et al., 2010). The A2 strain has been used to define $CD8^+$ T cell responses to specific HRSV epitopes (Lee et al., 2007; Ruckwardt et al., 2010). Although A2 infection of mice does not replicate human disease, the strain is important in the field as a reference strain, the basis of current reverse genetics systems, for HRSV protein structure studies, and for vaccine development (Collins et al., 1995; Jin et al., 1998; McLellan et al., 2011).

A2 HRSV inhibits T cell function in mice. During the CTL response to HRSV, approximately half of HRSV-specific $CD8^+$ T cells in the lungs of BALB/c mice produce IFN-γ, compared to influenza virus infection where nearly all influenza-specific $CD8^+$ T cells in the lung are IFN-γ^+ (Chang and Braciale, 2002). These data are in agreement with HRSV suppression of T cell proliferation *in vitro* (Preston et al., 1992, 1995; Roberts et al., 1986). HRSV inhibition of T cell responses may be an important reason why HRSV does not confer adequate immunity.

3.1.2 HRSV strain line 19 infection of mice

RSV strain line 19 is an antigenic subgroup A strain derived from a RSV clinical isolate obtained at the University of Michigan in 1967 (Herlocher et al., 1999). "Line 19" has been used as the name of a HRSV strain used by the Lukacs lab at the University of Michigan and other groups (Lukacs et al., 2006). The genome sequence of this line 19 was reported, and it is highly similar to the Long strain of HRSV (Moore et al., 2009a). The lack of nucleotide differences between line 19 and Long, particularly in the hypervariable regions of the G gene an in intergenic regions, raises the question of whether this line 19 is a passage variant of the Long strain. It may be that line 19 and Long derive from the same clinical isolate or nearly identical isolates circulating in Baltimore in 1956 (Long) and Ann Arbor in 1967 (line 19). However, it is interesting that the Long strain was adapted to mice by serial passage in the brains of suckling mice in the 1960s at the University of Michigan, and mouse passage number 19 in this study was noted as virulent (Cavallaro and Maassab, 1966). Whether currently used line 19 represents the 1967 Michigan clinical isolate (Herlocher et al., 1999) or mouse-adapted Long (Cavallaro and Maassab, 1966) is not as important as the fact that line 19 is a good tool to study HRSV-induced pulmonary pathophysiology in mouse models.

The pathogenesis of HRSV line 19 differs from the pathogenesis of HRSV A2 (Lukacs et al., 2006). Similar to A2, line 19 induces high levels of IFN-γ in the lung (Lukacs et al., 2006; Tekkanat et al., 2001). A2 replicates in HEp-2 cells and in the lungs of BALB/c mice to higher titers than line 19 (Lukacs et al., 2006). In contrast to A2, line 19 infection of BALB/c mice increases IL-13 levels in the lungs (Lukacs et al., 2006; Tekkanat et al., 2001). Line 19 infection causes mucus production and airway hyperresponsiveness (AHR) in BALB/c mice, whereas A2 does not (Lukacs et al., 2006; Tekkanat et al., 2001). Line 19 infection-induced mucus and AHR are IL-13-dependent and STAT6-dependent (Lukacs et al., 2006; Tekkanat et al., 2001). Line 19-induced AHR is ameliorated by neutralization of the chemokine CCL5 (RANTES), and CCL5 production in the lung was shown to be IL-13-dependent in line 19-infected mice (Tekkanat et al., 2002).

More recently, the Lukacs group has identified a role for the cytokine IL-17 in RSV pathogenesis. IL-17 is produced by $CD4^+$ TH_{17} cells and has been associated with bacterial infections, neutrophilic inflammation, and pro-allergic airway inflammation (Alcorn et al., 2010). Mice deficient in toll-like receptor 7 (TLR7), an innate immune system molecule recognizing single stranded RNA in endosomes (a common feature of virus infection), had greater lung IL-17 levels than wild-type mice after HRSV line 19 infection, and neutralization of IL-17 in line 19-infected TLR7-deficient mice reduced airway mucin expression (Lukacs et al., 2010). Bone marrow-derived dendritic cells (DCs) from TLR7-deficient mice expressed higher levels of IL-23 (an IL-17-promoting cytokine) in response to line 19 infection in vitro than wild-type DCs (Lukacs et al., 2010). These data suggest that the innate TLR response to HRSV restricts a pathogenic IL-17 response. IL-17 was found in tracheal aspirates of infants with severe RSV illness, and line 19-infected IL-17-deficient mice had less airway mucin expression than control mice (Mukherjee et al., 2011). These studies indicate that TH_{17}-type inflammation contributes to pulmonary mucus in the pathogenesis of HRSV. Previous reports implicated IL-4 and TH_2-type lung inflammation in severe HRSV disease, although this association has not been consistent (Brandenburg et al., 2000; Garofalo et al., 2001; Legg et al., 2003; Roman et al., 1997). The overall picture from the literature is that the balance of canonical TH_1 (IFN-γ) and TH_2 (IL-4) cytokines does not correlate with HRSV disease severity. The findings from the Lukacs group suggest that IL-17 (TH_{17}) should be considered in assessing the role of host immune responses in HRSV pathogenesis.

3.1.3 HRSV clinical isolate infection of mice

HRSV is an RNA virus with a mutation rate of 3.3×10^{-3} substitutions/site/year, equivalent to human influenza A virus (Jenkins et al., 2002). The A2 and Long reference HRSV strains have been passaged extensively in vitro and do not fully represent circulating HRSV. Viral disease depends exquisitely on viral strains. Small changes in viral gene sequences can have a large impact on pathogenesis. For example, elevated virulence of 1918 and avian influenza strains hinges on few amino acids differences (Hatta et al., 2001; Tumpey et al., 2005; Yu et al., 2008). Virulence in animal models of virus infection invariably depends on viral strains, across virus families (Ahmed and Oldstone, 1988; Borisevich et al., 2006). Relatively minor differences between viral strains also play important roles in complex human diseases. Examples include papillomavirus types (e.g. HPV-16) strongly associated with cervical cancer and hepatitis c virus genotypes associated with acute or persistent infection (Howley et al., 1989; Lehmann et al., 2004). Recently, a group of rhinoviruses (RV group C) was associated with half of all RV hospitalizations in young children, especially for asthma exacerbation (Miller et al., 2009).

HRSV clinical isolate strain 13018-8 was used to study the effects of HRSV on mouse DCs (Gonzalez et al., 2008). This HRSV caused maturation of mouse DCs, but the DCs were then unable to activate antigen-specific T cells in vitro, regardless of the antigen specificity (Gonzalez et al., 2008). The authors did not compare strain 13018-08 to a laboratory HRSV strain. The findings advance a mechanism (inhibition of DC-T cells immunological synapse formation) for HRSV suppression of T cell function (Gonzalez et al., 2008). HRSV clinical isolates exhibit varied pathogenesis phenotypes in BALB/c mice (Stokes et al., 2011). Out of six antigenic subgroup A isolates tested, three increased IL-13 levels in the lungs of BALB/c mice, and two (A2001/2-20 and A1997/12-35) induced greater IL-13 levels and weight loss than HRSV line 19 (Stokes et al., 2011). The clinical isolates had higher lung viral load than A2 and line 19 one day post-infection, viral antigen at this time point was localized to the bronchiolar epithelium, and there was corresponding histologic evidence of damage to the bronchiolar epithelium in mice infected with clinical isolates (Stokes et al., 2011). HRSV A2001/2-20 increased airway mucus expression and increased breathing effort in BALB/c mice whereas A2001/3-12 did not despite these two isolates exhibiting equivalent lung viral loads over a time course (Stokes et al., 2011). As with line 19, airway mucus induced in BALB/c mice by A2001/2-20 was IL-13-dependent (Stokes et al., 2011; Tekkanat et al., 2001).

3.2 HRSV infection of cotton rats

The cotton rat *Sigmodon hispidus* is one of the best small animal models of HRSV infection. Whereas infant but not adult ferrets are susceptible to HRSV, cotton rats are susceptible to HRSV infection throughout life (Prince et al., 1978; Prince and Porter, 1976). The virtues of cotton rats for HRSV research were recently reviewed and include approximately 100-fold more permissiveness to HRSV infection than mice (Boukhvalova et al., 2009). A disadvantage is that there are few reagents available for the cotton rats relative to mice. Cotton rats are susceptible to upper and lower respiratory tract infection with HRSV (Prince et al., 1978). HRSV replicated to relatively high titers in the nasal turbinates and lungs of naïve cotton rats (Prince et al., 1990; Prince et al., 1986; Prince et al., 1978). HRSV antigen was detected in nasal, bronchial, and bronchiolar epithelial cells (Prince et al., 1978). HRSV infection caused proliferative rhinitis, bronchiolitis, and the pulmonary infiltration of lymphocytes and neutrophils (Prince et al., 1986; Prince et al., 1978). The cotton rat model was used to study the Ab-mediated clearance of HRSV, and the data indicate that IgG-mediated HRSV clearance does not require antibody-dependent cellular cytotoxicity or complement (Prince et al., 1990). HRSV infection increased cotton rat lung mRNA steady state levels of RANTES, IP-10, MIP-1β, GRO, IFN-α, IFN-γ, IL-6, IL-10, and TNF-α (Blanco et al., 2002). GRO is a homolog of the human IL-8 chemokine and functions to recruit neutrophils. IP-10 is a chemokine that is known to attract T cells and NK cells. In cotton rat treated with a TLR3 agonist then infected with HRSV, it was shown that type I IFN responses can augment lung inflammation in this model (Boukhvalova et al., 2010).

An interesting recent study performed with HRSV Long strain showed that HRSV treatment of mouse peritoneal and alveolar macrophages induces these macrophages to become alternatively activated to express TH_2 cytokines IL-4 and IL-13, and infection of cotton rats with HRSV Long increased markers of alternatively activated macrophages (Shirey et al., 2010). Although the role of TH_2 cytokines in HRSV pathogenesis has been controversial, most studies have focused on a T cell source of these cytokines, e.g. by stimulation of patient peripheral blood mononuclear cells (PBMCs). Basophils can produce IL-4 in HRSV-infected mice, but these cells are rare (Moore et al., 2009b). The finding that macrophages can express TH_2 cytokines in response to HRSV (Shirey et al., 2010) is potentially very important because T_H2 cytokines (especially mucus-associated IL-13) are thought to contribute to HRSV disease and, as noted above, HRSV, BRSV, and PVM lung pathology in the natural host is characterized by prominent macrophage accumulation in bronchiolar and alveolar spaces.

3.3 Neonatal lamb model of HRSV infection

Neonatal (2-3 days of age) lambs were given a high dose of intrabronchial HRSV A2 infection (Olivier et al., 2009). Clinically, the lambs exhibited fever and, and some had a moderate cough (Olivier et al., 2009). Histopathology showed suppurative bronchiolitis with epithelial desquamation and cellular debris and neutrophils in airway lumina. HRSV antigen was detected by IHC, and it was fairly extensive in the bronchiolar epithelium and in alveolar regions where syncytia were evident (Olivier et al., 2009). In a second study from the Ackermann group, immune responses of newborn lambs infected with HRSV A2 were examined (Sow et al., 2011). A2 infection caused lung accumulation of neutrophils, macrophages, and $CD4^+$ and $CD8^+$ cells (Sow et al., 2011). Interestingly, IFN-α was not detected by RT-PCR, and lung IFN-β levels were actually lower in infected animals than in mock-infected animals, suggesting that HRSV suppressed type I IFN responses in this model (Sow et al., 2011). Cytokines and chemokines increased by HRSV A2 infection in the lungs of newborns lambs were TNF-α (day 3 post-infection), IL-10 (day 3 post-infection), IFN-γ (day 6 post-infection), IL-8 (day 6 post-infection), and MCP-1 (in macrophage-enriched laser capture microdissection regions day 6 post-infection). RT-PCR assays for IL-4, IL-13, and IL-17 mRNA levels gave results below the limit of detection (Sow et al., 2011). As in the pathology study of severe HRSV disease in infants noted above, there was evidence of widespread apoptosis in lungs of HRSV A2-infected newborn lambs (Sow et al., 2011; Welliver et al., 2007). New lambs appear to model HRSV disease closely, although PAS staining was not reported nor mucus evident in the airways in the histology micrographs.

3.4 Non-human primate models of HRSV infection

HRSV was originally isolated from chimpanzees, and this species is the only non-human primate model for HRSV that provides significantly greater permissivity than cotton rats. Young chimpanzees are productively infected with HRSV and exhibit upper respiratory tract illness, but adult squirrel monkeys, newborn rhesus monkeys, and infant cebus monkeys shed low virus levels and do not show clinical disease (Belshe et al., 1977). Bonnet monkeys can be infected with HRSV. However, a high HRSV dose resulted in viral titers similar to those seen in cotton rats, and the infected monkeys did not have clinical disease (Simoes et al., 1999). Chimpanzees can be valuable for HRSV vaccine evaluation (Teng et al., 2000). However high cost, regulatory issues, and genetic variability are major constraints.

3.5 Primary cell culture models of HRSV infection

Although cell and tissue culture systems lack an intact immune system, they can provide information about virus-host interactions, including immune pathways. Human airway epithelial (HAE) cells derived from surgery can be cultured at an air-liquid interface to produce a differentiated, polarized mucociliary epithelium. In this system, HRSV specifically infects ciliated epithelial cells via the apical membrane (Zhang et al., 2002). HRSV was shed from the apical surface, and there was no cytopathic effect (CPE) (Zhang *et al.*, 2002). However, it is possible that loosely adherent syncytia were washed off the apical surface in collection of supernatants for viral titration. Sendai virus (a paramyxovirus) readily causes syncytia in an elegant HAE system of well-differentiated pediatric bronchial epithelial cells (WD-PBEC) (Villenave et al., 2010). In non-polarized monolayers of primary pediatric bronchial epithelial cells, HRSV A2 replicated to higher titers and caused greater CPE than HRSV clinical isolates (Villenave et al., 2011). HRSV infection of primary epithelial cells results in the secretion of the chemokine IL-8 that is involved in neutrophil recruitment (Mellow et al., 2004; Villenave et al., 2011). In addition to epithelial cells, primary immune cells provide information about HRSV-host interactions. HRSV infects human monocyte-derived immature DCs inefficiently (Le Nouen et al., 2009). In a co-culture system of human DCs and T cells, it was shown that the HRSV NS1 protein (a type I IFN antagonist) suppressed CD8 T cell activation and proliferation, skews the CD4 T cell phenotype to T_H2-type responses, and suppresses markers of DC maturation (Munir et al., 2011). Also in this DC-T cell co-culture system, comparison of influenza A virus, human parainfluenzavirus type 3 (HPIV3), HRSV A2, and human metapneumovirus (HMPV) revealed that HRSV and HMPV uniquely fail to stimulate CCR7 expression by DC, resulted in impaired DC migration (Le Nouen et al., 2011). DCs are key for initiating adaptive immune responses in lymph nodes. Therefore, HRSV suppression of DC migration may underlie the relatively (compared to influenza viruses) poor immunity elicited by HRSV infection.

4. Challenges to HRSV vaccine development

4.1 Inhibition of pediatrics vaccines by maternal antibodies

Since hospitalization rates for HRSV infected children peak at 2 to 6 months of age, immunization for this age will be required for the prevention of severe HRSV disease (Boyce et al., 2000; Shay et al., 1999). However, there are several hurdles to develop HRSV vaccine in infants. One of the major obstacles is the inhibitory influence of maternal antibody (MatAb) on neonatal immunization (Crowe, 1998; Siegrist, 2003). Evidence of MatAb-mediated immune suppression in human studies has been well described in other infections such as measles, parainfluenza viruses (PIV) and influenza viruses (Albrecht et al., 1977; Crowe, 1998). Although underlying mechanisms by which MatAb suppresses infant responses to vaccination are not fully defined, possible hypothesized mechanisms are 1) Fc dependent phagocytosis, 2) neutralization of live viral vaccines, and 3) epitope masking by MatAb. First, inhibitory influence by MatAb could be mediated by Fc-dependent phagocytosis. The internalization of MatAb and antigen complex by antigen-presenting cells (APC) results in the inhibition of infant B cells in both human and mice. However, a study using FcγR knockout mice demonstrated that the existence of FcγR-independent inhibitory mechanisms (Karlsson et al., 1999). Next, the hypothesis that MatAb neutralizes the live viral vaccine has been widely believed (Albrecht et al., 1977). MatAb can inhibit viral replication of live attenuated HRSV in mice (Crowe, 2001a). Notably, MatAb does not affect the induction of T cell responses to HRSV or measles virus (Crowe et al., 2001; Gans et al., 1999). Lastly, as mentioned above, the hypothesis of B cell epitope specific masking has been postulated based on the possibility of the existence of an Fc-independent mechanism. Evidence of MatAb epitope masking is that MatAb to the V3 loop of HIV gp120 inhibited induction of Ab responses only to V3 but not to other epitopes (Jelonek et al., 1996). Similar results were observed in human infants (Kurikka et al., 1996; Nohynek et al., 1999). Several strategies should be considered to overcome the obstacles mediated by MatAb to effective vaccination of infants. First, novel immunization routes can be tested to determine whether vaccination route can modulate susceptibility to inhibition by MatAb. Second, infant T cell vaccines can be considered. According to previous observations, MatAb inhibits infant Ab responses but not infant T cell responses (Gans et al., 1999; Pabst et al., 1999).)

4.2 Non-durable immunity induced by natural HRSV infection

RSV elicits innate and adaptive immune responses that fail to establish long-lasting immunity because reinfection occurs throughout life (Collins et al., 2006). HRSV neutralizing Ab (nAb) can prevent RSV infection. Serum nAb titer is the best immune correlate of protection in humans, and a serum nAb titer of 1:300 is a benchmark for protection (Collins et al., 2006; Group, 1998; Prince et al., 1985). The RSV G and F proteins are virion surface glycoprotein spikes and the only known targets of RSV nAbs (Collins et al., 2006). Local secretory IgA also correlates with protection from RSV disease (Collins et al., 2006; Walsh, 1993). However, natural RSV infection is poorly immunogenic in children < 6 months old. Rates of detectable neutralizing Ab responses to natural infection in this age group are 50-75% (Brandenburg et al., 1997; Murphy et al., 1986a; Wagner et al., 1989; Welliver et al., 1980). In infants, immunological immaturity and suppression of immune responses by matAbs contribute to poor immunogenicity (Crowe, 2001c; Crowe and Williams, 2003). Seronegative infants and children can mount strong anti-G and anti-F Ab responses, although neonates produce poor Ab responses perhaps due to fewer somatic hypermutations in Ab genes (Shinoff et al., 2008; Weitkamp et al., 2005; Williams et al., 2009; Wright et al., 2000). Immunity to HRSV in adults is also non-durable. A striking example is a study in which HRSV nAbs were titrated in 457 cord blood samples in the Danish National Birth Cohort (DNBC) from 1998 to 2003 in order to study the temporal relationship between maternally-derived nAb and the seasonality of HRSV infant hospitalizations (Stensballe et al., 2009). The titer of nAb in cord blood oscillated. NAb titers were highest a few months after the annual HRSV winter epidemic and lowest just before the HRSV season, suggesting a cyclic model in which nAb titers in mothers (which are transferred to infants) wane after six months contributing to the next epidemic which boosts nAb titers for another six months. (Stensballe et al., 2009). In addition to low and non-durable Ab responses, the cellular immune response to HRSV infection is inhibited. As discussed above, HRSV inhibits T cell function in mice and in human DC-T cell co-cultures, and the HRSV NS1 protein (IFN antagonist) was implicated in suppression of T cell activation (Chang and Braciale, 2002; Le Nouen et al., 2011; Munir et al., 2011). Suboptimal immunity to HRSV infection is important for vaccine development because it implies that intranasal delivery of a live attenuated HRSV will not be effective. The degrees to which 1) matAb in infants, 2) immature immune system in infants, 3) immune modulation by HRSV, and 4) lack of optimal assays to measure HRSV immune responses and protection in patients contribute to the interpretation of poor immunogenicity in the vaccine target population needs to be elucidated.

4.3 Instability of live attenuated HRSV vaccines

Live HRSV vaccine candidates with attenuating mutations have been created by traditional methods of cold-adaptation (cold passage, *cp*) and chemical mutagenesis to yield temperature-sensitive (*ts*) HRSV mutants that replicate at temperatures similar to the upper respiratory tract but not at higher temperatures (Collins and Murphy, 2005). These mutations were defined by sequencing, and mutant HRSV strains that harbor *cpts* mutations have been generated by reverse genetics and tested as vaccine candidates. Leading live attenuated HRSV vaccine candidates and HRSV vaccine development have been reviewed (Collins and Murphy, 2005; Crowe, 2001b; Graham, 2011). Attenuating mutations are not necessarily additive, but addition of attenuating mutations into an already attenuated RSV vaccine candidate can decrease the rate of reversion to less attenuated genotypes, thereby increasing "genetic stability" (Collins and Murphy, 2005). A leading vaccine candidate (rA2cp248/404/1030ΔSH) was adequately attenuated in infants, but one third of isolates from nasal washes of vaccinees contained HRSV with loss of attenuation, evidence of reversion to wild-type, confirmed by sequence analysis (Karron et al., 2005). A strategy was explored to stabilize the "248" point mutation in the viral polymerase gene by mutagenizing the codon to encode an attenuating mutation with more than one nucleotide difference from the wild type (Luongo et al., 2009), as more nucleotide differences per degree of attenuation will be less likely to revert to wild-type. However, in the case of the 248 point mutation, this was not possible due to sequence constraints (Luongo et al., 2009). Instability of live vaccine strains has been an issue with poliovirus. Codon "de-optimization" of poliovirus by titration of CpG dinucleotides into the genome has produced viruses with tunable fitness, a strategy that may work for HRSV (Burns et al., 2009).

4.4 Formalin-inactivated HRSV vaccination

HRSV was discovered in 1956 (Chanock et al., 1957; Chanock, 1956). Once HRSV was recognized to be a common cause of upper and lower respiratory tract disease in infants and children, efforts were undertaken to develop a vaccine. In 1966, a formalin-inactivated whole virus RSV vaccine adsorbed to alum adjuvant (FI-HRSV) was administered to children (Kapikian et al., 1969; Kim et al., 1969). The following winter, compared to unvaccinated children, those who received FI-HRSV had a higher incidence of hospitalization and greater LRI severity due to HRSV (Kapikian et al., 1969; Kim et al., 1969). Two FI-HRSV-immunized infants died, and HRSV was recovered from lung sections (Kim et al., 1969). FI-HRSV enhanced respiratory disease (ERD) can be recapitulated using mice, cotton rats, calves, and non-human primates by FI-HRSV vaccination and HRSV challenge (Delgado et al., 2009; Gershwin et al., 1998; Graham et al., 1993; Johnson et al., 2004a; Moghaddam et al., 2006; Prince et al., 1986) Key features of FI-HRSV ERD are 1) failure to protect against HRSV replication, 2) an Ab response lacking in virus-neutralizing Abs, 3) a poor HRSV-specific $CD8^+$ T cell response, 4) an immunopathologic T_H2 immune response, and 5) immune complex deposition (Graham et al., 1993; Murphy and Walsh, 1988; Olson and Varga, 2007; Polack et al., 2002). HRSV G protein is implicated in ERD because priming with HRSV G-expressing vaccinia virus (vac-G) followed by HRSV challenge results in ERD whereas vac-F primes for protection (Srikiatkhachorn and Braciale, 1997). Vac-G-mediated ERD and FI-HRSV ERD act through different immune mechanisms, and G is not required for FI-RSV ERD (Johnson et al., 2004a; Johnson et al., 2004b). Nevertheless, vac-G studies revealed the potential for G to cause ERD. What causes FI-HRSV ERD? One hypothesis is that formalin disrupts antigenicity. Formalin causes formation of reactive carbonyl groups on HRSV proteins, and chemical reduction of these groups reduces FI-HRSV ERD (Moghaddam et al., 2006). Another mechanism invokes nonfunctional Ab responses in the absence of appropriate adjuvant, particularly TLR agonists. Co-formulation of ERD-causing inactivated HRSV vaccines with CpG ODN (a TLR9 agonist), MPL (a TLR4 agonist), and other adjuvants ameliorates ERD (Boukhvalova et al., 2006; Delgado et al., 2009; Mapletoft et al., 2008; Oumouna et al., 2005).

It appears that vaccination with FI-HRSV induced excessive activation of T_H2 cells, as measured by increased expression of cytokines including IL-4, IL-5, and IL-10, and relatively decreased expression of cytokines including IFN-γ and IL-2, by circulating or tissue lymphocytes following HRSV infection. The strong T_H2 response to FI-HRSV may suppress the anti-viral T_H1 response and development of cytotoxic T lymphocytes (CTL), mechanisms that limit viral replication in the normal response to HRSV infection. Immune pathways activated by T_H2 cells likely also contributed to the influx of eosinophils seen in the lungs of the two children who died as a result of FI-HRSV enhanced disease, which may have contributed to the excessive inflammatory response. However, utilization of eosinophil-deficient mice revealed that eosinophils are not required for ERD in mice induced by either vac-G and HRSV challenge or FI-PVM antigens and PVM challenge (Castilow et al., 2008; Percopo et al., 2009).

4.5 Extrapolation of vaccine efficacy from animal models

One of the challenges in determining how FI-HRSV caused ERD, and in determining how to safely and effectively vaccinate children with any type of HRSV vaccine, is limitations of animal models of HRSV infection. The strengths and weaknesses of the different models have been reviewed (Bem et al., 2011; Openshaw and Tregoning, 2005). Mouse models of HRSV infection and vaccination have been used widely, and they offer unparalleled opportunities to manipulate and dissect the immune response. However, because mice are not natural hosts of HRSV and are not very permissive to infection, relatively large amounts of virus must be administered to cause even mild disease. This may account for the fact that vaccination strategies that have appeared promising in mice have often not held up in subsequent research using non-human primate models or in human clinical trials. At this time it appears that no animal model will perfectly predict safety and efficacy of candidate HRSV vaccines. Thus candidate vaccines will always require careful and deliberate stepwise testing beginning with immunocompetent adults, then moving to seropositive children, then to seronegative children, to seropositive infants, and then to seronegative infants (Polack and Karron, 2004; Schickli et al., 2009). This pathway is time consuming, expensive, and fraught with the possibility of profound disappointment. Because of this, increased use of animal models of natural pneumovirus infection could provide a more efficient and fruitful testing ground for screening candidate vaccines and novel vaccination strategies before they are tested in non-human primates and in human clinical trials.

5. Vaccines for BRSV

Bovine HRSV and HRSV share many clinical and pathologic similarities in their respective hosts. Although no vaccine for human HRSV has yet been approved for use, vaccines for BRSV have been marketed since the 1980's. Because of the similarities between HRSV and BRSV, it should be possible to gain insight regarding factors that impact safety, efficacy, and duration of immunity in individuals vaccinated either in the presence or absence of circulating neutralizing antibodies using the BRSV model. Many published studies have shown that commercially available BRSV vaccines can induce protection against experimentally induced or naturally occurring BRSV disease (Durham and Hassard, 1990; Ellis et al., 2001; Van Donkersgoed et al., 1990b; Vangeel et al., 2007b; Verhoeff and van Nieuwstadt, 1984; West et al., 1999b; Xue et al., 2010).

Like HRSV vaccine ERD, BRSV vaccine ERD following natural BRSV infection has been identified; the problem has been associated with both live (Kimman et al., 1989a) and inactivated (Schreiber et al., 2000) BRSV vaccines. Kimman et al described a field outbreak of BRSV where disease appeared to be enhanced in calves that were vaccinated intramuscularly with commercially available modified-live BRSV vaccine while they were in an early stage of BRSV infection, as indicated by the retrospective identification of serum BRSV-specific IgM in calves at the time they were vaccinated. Disease was clinically evident at 1 to 2 weeks post vaccination and was more severe in vaccinated calves than in other calves on the farm that were not vaccinated. Schreiber et al described an episode of apparent vaccine ERD in calves given a commercially available vaccine inactivated with beta propiolactone and adjuvanted with alum and saponin and given by intramuscular injection. In an episode of natural BRSV infection that occurred 4 months after the last BRSV vaccination was given on this farm, older calves that had not been vaccinated and that had lower neutralizing Ab titers had less severe disease than younger calves that had been vaccinated and had higher neutralizing Ab titers. Notably, 11 of 35 vaccinated calves died during the outbreak, as compared to none of 24 unvaccinated calves. Histopathologic evaluation of lung tissue of vaccinated calves that died revealed changes consistent with BRSV infection but with infiltration of eosinophils, which are not frequently found in lung tissue of calves with severe BRSV disease that is not related to vaccination (Bryson et al., 1979; Pirie et al., 1981). The identification of eosinophils in lung tissue of calves evaluated in the study by Schreiber et al supported the concept that vaccination induced immune pathways supporting eosinophil recruitment, possibly related to production T_H2 cytokines such as IL-5 or release of chemokines such as eotaxin. The incident of vaccine-mediated ERD described by Schreiber et al was somewhat unusual in that some of the calves with vaccine ERD had higher serum neutralizing Ab titers than unvaccinated calves that had less severe disease. This is in contrast to the vaccine ERD induced in children given FI-HRSV in the 1960's (Murphy et al., 1986b), and indicates that it is possible for vaccine-induced immunopathologic mechanisms to be strong enough to overwhelm protective mechanisms. In most studies, inactivated BRSV vaccines induce low levels of neutralizing antibodies relative to total BRSV-specific antibody (Ellis et al., 1995; Gershwin et al., 1998).

The responses of calves vaccinated with FI-BRSV to BRSV challenge have been evaluated by at least 4 different groups (Antonis et al., 2003; Gershwin et al., 1998; Mohanty et al., 1981; West et al., 1999a). ERD followed challenge in some (Antonis et al., 2003; Gershwin et al., 1998) but not other (Mohanty et al., 1981; West et al., 1999a) studies. Gershwin's group showed that the amount of viral protein in the FI-BRSV vaccine was associated with induction of vaccine ERD, with vaccine containing relatively smaller amounts of viral protein being associated with ERD (Kalina et al., 2005). When FI-BRSV vaccine enhanced disease has been identified in cattle, it has been associated with production of high concentrations of non-neutralizing antibodies in serum (Gershwin et al., 1998), low levels of virus-specific IFN-γ production by PBMCs (Woolums et al., 1999), high concentrations of BRSV-specific serum IgE and low concentrations of BRSV-specific IgG1 in lung washes, and influx of eosinophils into lung tissue (Antonis et al., 2003; Kalina et al., 2004). These findings are consistent with what has been deduced regarding immunopathogensis of FI-HRSV vaccination from materials available from children vaccinated in the clinical trials in the 1960's, as well as from non-human primate and rodent models of FI-HRSV enhanced disease. All together, the extensive literature on BRSV vaccine ERD and similarities to HRSV vaccine ERD suggests that the BRSV model is relevant to HRSV vaccine safety. In the bovine model, BRSV vaccine ERD and efficacy can be studied in the context of natural infection.

Although BRSV vaccine ERD has been well-studied, extensive research and clinical experience indicate that BRSV vaccination can be safe and effective (Ellis et al., 1995; Ellis et al., 2005; Van Donkersgoed et al., 1990a; Vangeel et al., 2007a; Vangeel et al., 2009; Verhoeff and van Nieuwstadt, 1984; West et al., 1999b; Xue et al., 2010). In studies of resistance to experimental challenge, vaccination of calves with low or absent concentrations of serum neutralizing antibodies can protect them from virulent challenge. In a thorough evaluation of humoral and cellular immune responses following BRSV challenge of seronegative calves vaccinated with commercially available modified live vaccines given by intramuscular injection, serum BRSV-specific IgG concentration on days 4 - 7 post challenge and BRSV-specific IFN-γ production by PBMCs on the day of challenge best predicted protection against lung pathology (West et al., 1999b). Nasal fluid concentrations of BRSV-specific IgA at day 8 post-challenge were also significantly associated with protection against lung pathology, but inclusion of this outcome in the final statistical model did not improve prediction of protection. Vaccination with some inactivated vaccines has also provided good protection from virulent challenge without disease enhancement, proving that it is possible to use inactivated BRSV vaccines safely and effectively (Ellis et al., 1995; Ellis et al., 2005). Given the identification of both protection and enhanced disease in calves vaccinated with inactivated BRSV vaccines, it is likely that the formulation of the vaccine (as related to method of viral inactivation, concentration of viral protein, and nature of adjuvants and other components included) is critical to the outcome following BRSV infection of calves vaccinated with inactivated vaccines. Other factors such as host genetics and relative severity of viral challenge may also be involved.

Because disease due to BRSV is usually most severe in calves under 6 months of age, vaccines administered in the field need to be effective in calves with circulating antibodies of maternal origin. This is also true for HRSV vaccines. More research is needed to define how calves with maternal antibodies can be most effectively and safely vaccinated against BRSV. Work to date indicates that intramuscular (Harmeyer et al., 2006) or intranasal (Vangeel et al., 2007a) vaccination with modified live vaccines given to calves with moderate to high levels of serum maternal antibodies can be protective as measured by decreased severity of clinical signs and/or decreased duration of viral shedding post challenge. A small amount of information suggests that modified live but not inactivated vaccine given intranasally may be superior to intramuscular or subcutaneous vaccination in calves with maternal antibody (Kimman et al., 1989c). However, modified live intranasal vaccination of calves with circulating maternal antibodies did not protect them from disease associated with virulent BRSV challenge 4.5 months after vaccination in one study (Ellis et al., 2010). The efficacy of vaccination in individuals with maternal antibody likely depends on a combination of factors including the nature of vaccine administered, the route of administration, the timing and number of doses administered prior to challenge, the concentration of serum neutralizing antibodies circulating at the time of vaccination, and the severity of challenge, including the titer and virulence of the challenge isolate.

Clinical trials testing BRSV vaccination efficacy have been described since the 1980's. Many evaluated the impact of BRSV vaccination on all (undifferentiated) respiratory disease; fewer have evaluated protection against disease following BRSV infection specifically. In trials evaluating the impact of BRSV vaccination on undifferentiated respiratory disease, BRSV vaccine included in a panel of vaccines given to at-risk cattle decreased disease in some but not all groups of cattle (Van Donkersgoed et al., 1990a). Trials evaluating the impact of BRSV vaccination on disease after BRSV infection are more informative about the risks and benefits of BRSV vaccination. Most such trials have been carried out in Europe; in one excellent example involving 530 calves on 27 farms, calves on farms where all calves were vaccinated with a modified live BRSV vaccine by intramuscular route had significantly decreased rates of BRSV infection and disease, compared to farms where calves were not vaccinated. Farms where half the calves were vaccinated had significantly decreased rates of disease but not infection (Verhoeff and van Nieuwstadt, 1984).

6. Candidate HRSV vaccines

HRSV vaccine candidates and development have been reviewed thoroughly, so here we selectively point out novel strategies (Anderson et al., 2010; Collins and Murphy, 2005; Crowe, 2001b; Kneyber and Kimpen, 2004; Moore and Peebles, 2006). Live attenuated vaccines have not successfully found a balance of immunogenicity and safety. Adjuvants have potential to achieve immunogenicity. CpG oligodeoxynucleotides (CpG ODN, a TLR 9 agonist) and monophosphoryl lipid (MPL, a TLR 4 agonist) adjuvants enhance immune responses to experimental HRSV vaccines (Boukhvalova et al., 2006; Mapletoft et al., 2008; Neuzil et al., 1997; Oumouna et al., 2005). A novel oil-in-water nanoemulsion adjuvanted inactivated HRSV vaccine showed promise in mice (Lindell et al., 2011). Virus-like particles (VLPs) are supramolecular assemblages of antigenic proteins in a repetitive, particulate structure (Jennings and Bachmann, 2008). Licensures of two VLP vaccines (papilloma virus and hepatitis B virus) reflect the potential of VLP vaccines. Viral proteins presented as VLPs are highly immunogenic and induce protective humoral, cellular, and mucosal immune responses (Kang et al., 2009; Quan et al., 2007) Recent studies with Venezuelan equine encephalitis virus replicon particles (VRPs) expressing HRSV G or F as well as HRSV G-expressing Newcastle disease VLPs suggest that HRSV nonreplicating VLP-like vaccines, even without adjuvants, are immunogenic, effective, and do not cause ERD (Mok et al., 2007; Murawski et al., 2009). These G- and/or F-expressing VLPs lack immunomodulatory NS proteins, so they may less interfere with host immune responses than live attenuated vaccines that do express NS proteins. Unfortunately, live attenuated viruses lacking NS proteins were over-attenuated (Jin et al., 2003).

7. Molecular epidemiology of HRSV

A better understanding of HRSV molecular epidemiology will be informative for vaccine development. HRSV has one serotype, within which there are two antigenic subgroups, A and B, defined by reactivity to monoclonal Abs (Collins et al., 2006). Amino acid changes in variable regions of the HRSV attachment glycoprotein (G) occur in response to immune pressure (Botosso et al., 2009; Cane and Pringle, 1992, 1995; Gaunt et al., 2011; Zlateva et al., 2005). Within antigenic subgroups, HRSV strains can be further classified into clades, and clades can be divided into subtypes based on nt sequence of a hypervariable region of the G gene (Cane, 2001; Peret et al., 2000; Peret et al., 1998). The classification of HRSV strains is *antigenic subgroup > clade > subtype > isolate/strain*. Phylogenetic analysis of a hypervariable region of the G gene revealed that subgroup A strains can be divided into seven clades (GA1-GA7) and subgroup B strains can be divided into four clades (GB1-GB4) (Peret et al., 2000; Peret et al., 1998). These clades have held up as distinct clusters of circulating HRSV in communities around the world, and new clades are being described (Agenbach et al., 2005; Botosso et al., 2009; Cane, 2001; Matheson et al., 2006; Parveen et al., 2006; Peret et al., 2000; Peret et al., 1998; Scott et al., 2006). HRSV subtypes exhibit >96% nt similarity within hypervariable G and thus represent closely related isolates (Peret et al., 1998). Annual HRSV epidemics consist of one dominant subtype accounting for approximately 50% of isolates, and a variable number of less prevalent subtypes in a small number of clades (Cane, 2001; Peret et al., 2000; Peret et al., 1998; Sullender, 2000). The Dominant HRSV subtype in a given location is replaced in one or two HRSV seasons (Cane, 2001; Peret et al., 2000; Peret et al., 1998). Although immune selection appears to drive mutation in the HRSV G protein by positive selection, these mutations are not progressive antigenic drift as in influenza (Botosso et al., 2009; Cane and Pringle, 1995; Hay et al., 2001). Rather, it appears that positively selected sites flip-flop over time (Botosso et al., 2009), suggesting an antigenic toggling in G as immunity in the population rises and falls to circulating strains.

NAbs to HRSV bind either the viral G or F protein (Collins et al., 2006). Responses to HRSV F protein are generally cross-neutralizing to diverse HRSV strains whereas Abs to G are generally more subgroup- and clade-specific. HRSV induces Abs in humans and mice that bind epitopes conserved between all HRSV strains, and these Abs cross-neutralize strains. Palivizumab, a monoclonal nAb given prophylactically to humans, binds to the F protein and binds all HRSV strains (Meissner and Long, 2003). Despite nAbs that neutralize all HRSV strains tested, strain-specific Abs likely contribute to protection. It has been clearly demonstrated that the antigenic subgroup (A or B) is important for Ab responses. Ab responses to the G protein are largely subgroup-specific whereas Ab responses to the F protein are cross-reactive between subgroups A and B (Sullender, 2000; Sullender et al., 1998). Sera from HRSV antigenic subgroup A strain-infected individuals neutralizes subgroup A strains *in vitro* better than subgroup B strains (Cane, 2001; Sullender, 2000). For this reason, bivalent vaccines containing G and/or F proteins from representative subgroup A and B strains have been developed and tested in animals (Cheng et al., 2001; Whitehead et al., 1999). In addition to subgroup-specific Abs to the G protein, HRSV induces clade- or subtype-specific Abs (Beeler and van Wyke, 1989; Johnson et al., 1987; Scott et al., 2007). The neutralizing titer (reciprocal of dilution required to inhibit infectivity) of pooled adult human HRSV anti-serum varies between 320 and 2,560 for different subgroup A strains (Beeler and van Wyke, 1989). This suggests that (G-expressing e.g. live attenuated) vaccines based on one subgroup A strain will induce varied and suboptimal immunity to circulating subgroup A strains. Studies have shown that HRSV induces poor nAb titers in infants, and < 50% of young infants with culture-documented HRSV infection have detectable nAbs (Brandenburg et al., 1997; Wright et al., 2002; Wright et al., 2007). However, these studies used one subgroup A strain (A2) as the challenge strain for *in vitro* neutralization assays.

8. Conclusion and future directions

A major goal of studying RSV pathogenesis is to facilitate vaccines by elucidating virus-host interactions at the level of immunity and by providing challenge models to test candidate vaccines. The pathology of HRSV in infants resembles that of BRSV in calves and PVM in mice. The major features of this pathogenesis are 1) viral tropism for airway and alveolar epithelial cells, 2) airway epithelial desquamation, 3) obstruction of airways with mixtures of mucus, fibrin, and cells (epithelial debris and inflammatory cells), and 4) prominent neutrophil and macrophage inflammation in bronchiolar, alveolar, and interstitial spaces. Despite limitations, there are tractable non-chimpanzee animal models of HRSV pathogenesis that recapitulate key features of this pathogenesis. These include HRSV strain line 19 and HRSV clinical isolate infection of BALB/c mice, infection of cotton rats, and infection of newborn lambs. Each has advantages and caveats. Robust pathology and pulmonary dysfunction are endpoints that could prove useful for vaccine evaluation. Experimental BRSV and PVM infection in the natural host provide fully permissive comparative models of HRSV pathogenesis. In addition to comparative virology and pathogenesis, the BRSV field parallels HRSV with an extensive literature of vaccinology that includes inactivated virus ERD as well as numerous successful vaccines. Collaboration in these fields could facilitate insights into HRSV vaccines. Challenges such as MatAb, poor immunogenicity, immune modulation, and immature neonatal immunity exist in both infants and calves. One difference is that the molecular epidemiology of BRSV shows less virus variation than HRSV. Similarly, swine influenza exhibits low comparative variation, owing to the fact that these animals are culled, so the dynamics of immunity in the population differ from humans. One way to take advantage of the BRSV system would be to test HRSV vaccines in calves by challenging with chimeric BRSV viruses expressing the HRSV antigen(s).

9. Acknowledgment

This work was supported by the following funding sources: Children's Healthcare of Atlanta (Moore and Lee), NIH 1R01AI087798 (Moore), Georgia Research Alliance (Moore), Pifzer Animal Health (Woolums), Merck Animal Health (Woolums), Merial (Woolums), and Prince Agri-Products (Woolums).

10. References

Agenbach, E., Tiemessen, C.T., and Venter, M. (2005). Amino acid variation within the fusion protein of respiratory syncytial virus subtype A and B strains during annual epidemics in South Africa. *Virus Genes* Vol. 30, No. 2, pp. 267-278.

Aherne, W., Bird, T., Court, S.D., Gardner, P.S., and McQuillin, J. (1970). Pathological changes in virus infections of the lower respiratory tract in children. *J Clin Pathol* Vol. 23, No. 1, pp. 7-18.

Ahmed, R., and Oldstone, M.B. (1988). Organ-specific selection of viral variants during chronic infection. *J Exp Med* Vol. 167, No. 5, pp. 1719-1724.

Albrecht, P., Ennis, F.A., Saltzman, E.J., and Krugman, S. (1977). Persistence of maternal antibody in infants beyond 12 months: mechanism of measles vaccine failure. *J Pediatr* Vol. 91, No. 5, pp. 715-718.

Alcorn, J.F., Crowe, C.R., and Kolls, J.K. (2010). TH17 cells in asthma and COPD. *Annual Review of Physiology* Vol. 72, No. pp. 495-516.

Anderson, R., Huang, Y., and Langley, J.M. (2010). Prospects for defined epitope vaccines for respiratory syncytial virus. *Future Microbiol* Vol. 5, No. 4, pp. 585-602.

Antonis, A.F., Schrijver, R.S., Daus, F., Steverink, P.J., Stockhofe, N., Hensen, E.J., Langedijk, J.P., and van der Most, R.G. (2003). Vaccine-induced immunopathology during bovine respiratory syncytial virus infection: exploring the parameters of pathogenesis. *J Virol* Vol. 77, No. 22, pp. 12067-12073.

Beeler, J.A., and van Wyke, C.K. (1989). Neutralization epitopes of the F glycoprotein of respiratory syncytial virus: effect of mutation upon fusion function. *J Virol* Vol. 63, No. 7, pp. 2941-2950.

Belshe, R.B., Richardson, L.S., London, W.T., Sly, D.L., Lorfeld, J.H., Camargo, E., Prevar, D.A., and Chanock, R.M. (1977). Experimental respiratory syncytial virus infection of four species of primates. *J Med Virol* Vol. 1, No. 3, pp. 157-162.

Bem, R.A., Domachowske, J.B., and Rosenberg, H.F. (2011). Animal models of human respiratory syncytial virus disease. *Am J Physiol Lung Cell Mol Physiol* Vol. 301, No. 2, pp. L148-156.

Blanco, J.C., Richardson, J.Y., Darnell, M.E., Rowzee, A., Pletneva, L., Porter, D.D., and Prince, G.A. (2002). Cytokine and chemokine gene expression after primary and secondary respiratory syncytial virus infection in cotton rats. *J Inf Dis* Vol. 185, No. 12, pp. 1780-1785.

Borisevich, V., Seregin, A., Nistler, R., Mutabazi, D., and Yamshchikov, V. (2006). Biological properties of chimeric West Nile viruses. *Virology* Vol. 349, No. 2, pp. 371-381.

Botosso, V.F., Zanotto, P.M., Ueda, M., Arruda, E., Gilio, A.E., Vieira, S.E., Stewien, K.E., Peret, T.C., Jamal, L.F., Pardini, M.I., Pinho, J.R., Massad, E., Sant'anna, O.A., Holmes, E.C., and Durigon, E.L. (2009). Positive selection results in frequent reversible amino acid replacements in the G protein gene of human respiratory syncytial virus. *PLoS Pathog* Vol. 5, No. 1, pp. e1000254.

Boukhvalova, M.S., Prince, G.A., and Blanco, J.C. (2009). The cotton rat model of respiratory viral infections. *Biologicals* Vol. 37, No. 3, pp. 152-159.

Boukhvalova, M.S., Prince, G.A., Soroush, L., Harrigan, D.C., Vogel, S.N., and Blanco, J.C. (2006). The TLR4 agonist, monophosphoryl lipid A, attenuates the cytokine storm associated with respiratory syncytial virus vaccine-enhanced disease. *Vaccine* Vol. 24, No. 23, pp. 5027-5035.

Boukhvalova, M.S., Sotomayor, T.B., Point, R.C., Pletneva, L.M., Prince, G.A., and Blanco, J.C. (2010). Activation of interferon response through toll-like receptor 3 impacts viral pathogenesis and pulmonary toll-like receptor expression during respiratory syncytial virus and influenza infections in the cotton rat Sigmodon hispidus model. *J Interferon Cytokine Res* Vol. 30, No. 4, pp. 229-242.

Boyce, T.G., Mellen, B.G., Mitchel, E.F., Jr., Wright, P.F., and Griffin, M.R. (2000). Rates of hospitalization for respiratory syncytial virus infection among children in medicaid. *J Pediatr* Vol. 137, No. 6, pp. 865-870.

Brandenburg, A.H., Groen, J., Steensel-Moll, H.A., Claas, E.C., Rothbarth, P.H., Neijens, H.J., and Osterhaus, A.D. (1997). Respiratory syncytial virus specific serum antibodies in infants under six months of age: limited serological response upon infection. *J Med Virol* Vol. 52, No. 1, pp. 97-104.

Brandenburg, A.H., Kleinjan, A., van Het, L.B., Moll, H.A., Timmerman, H.H., de Swart, R.L., Neijens, H.J., Fokkens, W., and Osterhaus, A.D. (2000). Type 1-like immune response is found in children with respiratory syncytial virus infection regardless of clinical severity. *J Med Virol* Vol. 62, No. 2, pp. 267-277.

Bryson, D.G., McFerran, J.B., Ball, H.J., and Neill, S.D. (1979). Observations on outbreaks of respiratory disease in calves associated with parainfluenza type 3 virus and respiratory syncytial virus infection. *Vet Rec* Vol. 104, No. 3, pp. 45-49.

Bryson, D.G., McNulty, M.S., Logan, E.F., and Cush, P.F. (1983). Respiratory syncytial virus pneumonia in young calves: clinical and pathologic findings. *Am J Vet Res* Vol. 44, No. 9, pp. 1648-1655.

Buchholz, U.J., Granzow, H., Schuldt, K., Whitehead, S.S., Murphy, B.R., and Collins, P.L. (2000). Chimeric bovine respiratory syncytial virus with glycoprotein gene substitutions from human respiratory syncytial virus (HRSV): effects on host range and evaluation as a live-attenuated HRSV vaccine. *J Virol* Vol. 74, No. 3, pp. 1187-1199.

Burns, C.C., Campagnoli, R., Shaw, J., Vincent, A., Jorba, J., and Kew, O. (2009). Genetic inactivation of poliovirus infectivity by increasing the frequencies of CpG and UpA dinucleotides within and across synonymous capsid region codons. *J Virol* Vol. 83, No. 19, pp. 9957-9969.

Cane, P.A. (2001). Molecular epidemiology of respiratory syncytial virus. *Rev Med Virol* Vol. 11, No. 2, pp. 103-116.

Cane, P.A., and Pringle, C.R. (1992). Molecular epidemiology of respiratory syncytial virus: rapid identification of subgroup A lineages. *J Virol Methods* Vol. 40, No. 3, pp. 297-306.

Cane, P.A., and Pringle, C.R. (1995). Evolution of subgroup A respiratory syncytial virus: evidence for progressive accumulation of amino acid changes in the attachment protein. *J Virol* Vol. 69, No. 5, pp. 2918-2925.

Carthew, P., and Sparrow, S. (1980). A comparison in germ-free mice of the pathogenesis of Sendai virus and mouse pneumonia virus infections. *J Pathol* Vol. 130, No. 3, pp. 153-158.

Castilow, E.M., Legge, K.L., and Varga, S.M. (2008). Cutting edge: Eosinophils do not contribute to respiratory syncytial virus vaccine-enhanced disease. *J Immunol* Vol. 181, No. 10, pp. 6692-6696.

Cavallaro, J.J., and Maassab, H.F. (1966). Adaptation of respiratory syncytial (RS) virus to brain of suckling mice. *Proc Soc Exp Biol Med* Vol. 121, No. 1, pp. 37-41.

Chang, J., and Braciale, T.J. (2002). Respiratory syncytial virus infection suppresses lung CD8+ T-cell effector activity and peripheral CD8+ T-cell memory in the respiratory tract. *Nat Med* Vol. 8, No. 1, pp. 54-60.

Chang, J., Srikiatkhachorn, A., and Braciale, T.J. (2001). Visualization and characterization of respiratory syncytial virus F-specific CD8(+) T cells during experimental virus infection. *J Immunol* Vol. 167, No. 8, pp. 4254-4260.

Chanock, R., Roizman, B., and Myers, R. (1957). Recovery from infants with respiratory illness of a virus related to chimpanzee coryza agent (CCA). I. Isolation, properties and characterization. *Am J Hyg* Vol. 66, No. 3, pp. 281-290.

Chanock, R.M. (1956). Association of a new type of cytopathogenic myxovirus with infantile croup. *J Exp Med* Vol. 104, No. 4, pp. 555-576.

Cheng, X., Zhou, H., Tang, R.S., Munoz, M.G., and Jin, H. (2001). Chimeric subgroup A respiratory syncytial virus with the glycoproteins substituted by those of subgroup B and RSV without the M2-2 gene are attenuated in African green monkeys. *Virology* Vol. 283, No. 1, pp. 59-68.

Coates, H.V., and Chanock, R.M. (1962). Experimental infection with respiratory syncytial virus in several species of animals. *Am J Hyg* Vol. 76, No. pp. 302-312.

Collins, P.L., Crowe, J.E., Jr., Knipe, D.M., and Howley, P.M. (2006). Respiratory Syncytial Virus and Metapneumovirus. In Fields Virology (Lippincott, Williams, & Wilkins).

Collins, P.L., Hill, M.G., Camargo, E., Grosfeld, H., Chanock, R.M., and Murphy, B.R. (1995). Production of infectious human respiratory syncytial virus from cloned cDNA confirms an essential role for the transcription elongation factor from the 5' proximal open reading frame of the M2 mRNA in gene expression and provides a capability for vaccine development. *Proc Natl Acad Sci USA* Vol. 92, No. 25, pp. 11563-11567.

Collins, P.L., and Murphy, B.R. (2005). New generation live vaccines against human respiratory syncytial virus designed by reverse genetics. *Proc Am Thorac Soc* Vol. 2, No. 2, pp. 166-173.

Crowe, J.E., Jr. (1998). Immune responses of infants to infection with respiratory viruses and live attenuated respiratory virus candidate vaccines. *Vaccine* Vol. 16, No. 14-15, pp. 1423-1432.

Crowe, J.E., Jr. (2001a). Influence of maternal antibodies on neonatal immunization against respiratory viruses. *Clin Inf Dis* Vol. 33, No. 10, pp. 1720-1727.

Crowe, J.E., Jr. (2001b). Respiratory syncytial virus vaccine development. *Vaccine* Vol. 20 Suppl 1, No. pp. S32-37.

Crowe, J.E., Jr. (2001c). Respiratory syncytial virus vaccine development. *Vaccine* Vol. 20 Suppl 1, No. pp. S32-S37.

Crowe, J.E., Jr., Firestone, C.Y., and Murphy, B.R. (2001). Passively acquired antibodies suppress humoral but not cell-mediated immunity in mice immunized with live attenuated respiratory syncytial virus vaccines. *J Immunol* Vol. 167, No. 7, pp. 3910-3918.

Crowe, J.E., Jr., and Williams, J.V. (2003). Immunology of viral respiratory tract infection in infancy. *Paediatr Respir Rev* Vol. 4, No. 2, pp. 112-119.

Delgado, M.F., Coviello, S., Monsalvo, A.C., Melendi, G.A., Hernandez, J.Z., Batalle, J.P., Diaz, L., Trento, A., Chang, H.Y., Mitzner, W., Ravetch, J., Melero, J.A., Irusta, P.M., and Polack, F.P. (2009). Lack of antibody affinity maturation due to poor Toll-like receptor stimulation leads to enhanced respiratory syncytial virus disease. *Nat Med* Vol. 15, No. 1, pp. 34-41.

DeVincenzo, J.P. (2007). A new direction in understanding the pathogenesis of respiratory syncytial virus bronchiolitis: how real infants suffer. *J Infect Dis* Vol. 195, No. 8, pp. 1084-1086.

Domachowske, J.B., Bonville, C.A., Easton, A.J., and Rosenberg, H.F. (2002). Differential expression of proinflammatory cytokine genes in vivo in response to pathogenic and nonpathogenic pneumovirus infections. *J Infect Dis* Vol. 186, No. 1, pp. 8-14.

Durham, P.J., and Hassard, L.E. (1990). Prevalence of antibodies to infectious bovine rhinotracheitis, parainfluenza 3, bovine respiratory syncytial, and bovine viral diarrhea viruses in cattle in Saskatchewan and Alberta. *Can Vet J* Vol. 31, No. 12, pp. 815-820.

Elazhary, M.A., Silim, A., and Morin, M. (1982). A natural outbreak of bovine respiratory disease caused by bovine respiratory syncytial virus. *Cornell Vet* Vol. 72, No. 3, pp. 325-333.

Ellis, J., West, K., Konoby, C., Leard, T., Gallo, G., Conlon, J., and Fitzgerald, N. (2001). Efficacy of an inactivated respiratory syncytial virus vaccine in calves. *J Am Vet Med Assoc* Vol. 218, No. 12, pp. 1973-1980.

Ellis, J.A., Gow, S.P., and Goji, N. (2010). Response to experimentally induced infection with bovine respiratory syncytial virus following intranasal vaccination of seropositive and seronegative calves. *J Am Vet Med Assoc* Vol. 236, No. 9, pp. 991-999.

Ellis, J.A., Hassard, L.E., and Morley, P.S. (1995). Bovine respiratory syncytial virus-specific immune responses in calves after inoculation with commercially available vaccines. *J Am Vet Med Assoc* Vol. 206, No. 3, pp. 354-361.

Ellis, J.A., West, K.H., Waldner, C., and Rhodes, C. (2005). Efficacy of a saponin-adjuvanted inactivated respiratory syncytial virus vaccine in calves. *Can Vet J* Vol. 46, No. 2, pp. 155-162.

Fulton, R.B., Meyerholz, D.K., and Varga, S.M. (2010). Foxp3+ CD4 regulatory T cells limit pulmonary immunopathology by modulating the CD8 T cell response during respiratory syncytial virus infection. *J Immunol* Vol. 185, No. 4, pp. 2382-2392.

Gans, H.A., Maldonado, Y., Yasukawa, L.L., Beeler, J., Audet, S., Rinki, M.M., DeHovitz, R., and Arvin, A.M. (1999). IL-12, IFN-gamma, and T cell proliferation to measles in immunized infants. *J Immunol* Vol. 162, No. 9, pp. 5569-5575.

Garofalo, R.P., Patti, J., Hintz, K.A., Hill, V., Ogra, P.L., and Welliver, R.C. (2001). Macrophage inflammatory protein-1alpha (not T helper type 2 cytokines) is associated with severe forms of respiratory syncytial virus bronchiolitis. *J Infect Dis* Vol. 184, No. 4, pp. 393-399.

Gaunt, E.R., Jansen, R.R., Poovorawan, Y., Templeton, K.E., Toms, G.L., and Simmonds, P. (2011). Molecular epidemiology and evolution of human respiratory syncytial virus and human metapneumovirus. *PLoS ONE* Vol. 6, No. 3, pp. e17427.

Gershwin, L.J., Gunther, R.A., Anderson, M.L., Woolums, A.R., McArthur-Vaughan, K., Randel, K.E., Boyle, G.A., Friebertshauser, K.E., and McInturff, P.S. (2000). Bovine respiratory syncytial virus-specific IgE is associated with interleukin-2 and -4, and interferon-gamma expression in pulmonary lymph of experimentally infected calves. *Am J Vet Res* Vol. 61, No. 3, pp. 291-298.

Gershwin, L.J., Schelegle, E.S., Gunther, R.A., Anderson, M.L., Woolums, A.R., Larochelle, D.R., Boyle, G.A., Friebertshauser, K.E., and Singer, R.S. (1998). A bovine model of vaccine enhanced respiratory syncytial virus pathophysiology. *Vaccine* Vol. 16, No. 11-12, pp. 1225-1236.

Gonzalez, P.A., Prado, C.E., Leiva, E.D., Carreno, L.J., Bueno, S.M., Riedel, C.A., and Kalergis, A.M. (2008). Respiratory syncytial virus impairs T cell activation by preventing synapse assembly with dendritic cells. *Proc Natl Acad Sci USA* Vol. 105, No. 39, pp. 14999-15004.

Graham, B.S. (2011). Biological challenges and technological opportunities for respiratory syncytial virus vaccine development. *Immunol Rev* Vol. 239, No. 1, pp. 149-166.

Graham, B.S., Bunton, L.A., Wright, P.F., and Karzon, D.T. (1991). Role of T lymphocyte subsets in the pathogenesis of primary infection and rechallenge with respiratory syncytial virus in mice. *J Clin Invest* Vol. 88, No. 3, pp. 1026-1033.

Graham, B.S., Henderson, G.S., Tang, Y.W., Lu, X., Neuzil, K.M., and Colley, D.G. (1993). Priming immunization determines T helper cytokine mRNA expression patterns in lungs of mice challenged with respiratory syncytial virus. *J Immunol* Vol. 151, No. 4, pp. 2032-2040.

Group, I.-R.S. (1998). Palivizumab, a Humanized Respiratory Syncytial Virus Monoclonal Antibody, Reduces Hospitalization From Respiratory Syncytial Virus Infection in High-risk Infants. *Pediatrics* Vol. 102, No. 3, pp. 531-537.

Harmeyer, S.S., Murray, J., Imrie, C., Wiseman, A., and Salt, J.S. (2006). Efficacy of a live bovine respiratory syncytial virus vaccine in seropositive calves. *Vet Rec* Vol. 159, No. 14, pp. 456-457.

Hatta, M., Gao, P., Halfmann, P., and Kawaoka, Y. (2001). Molecular basis for high virulence of Hong Kong H5N1 influenza A viruses. *Science* Vol. 293, No. 5536, pp. 1840-1842.

Hay, A.J., Gregory, V., Douglas, A.R., and Lin, Y.P. (2001). The evolution of human influenza viruses. *Philos Trans R Soc Lond B Biol Sci* Vol. 356, No. 1416, pp. 1861-1870.

Herlocher, M.L., Ewasyshyn, M., Sambhara, S., Gharaee-Kermani, M., Cho, D., Lai, J., Klein, M., and Maassab, H.F. (1999). Immunological properties of plaque purified strains of live attenuated respiratory syncytial virus (RSV) for human vaccine. *Vaccine* Vol. 17, No. 2, pp. 172-181.

Howley, P.M., Munger, K., Werness, B.A., Phelps, W.C., and Schlegel, R. (1989). Molecular mechanisms of transformation by the human papillomaviruses. *Princess Takamatsu Symp* Vol. 20, No. pp. 199-206.

Hussell, T., and Openshaw, P.J. (1998). Intracellular IFN-gamma expression in natural killer cells precedes lung CD8+ T cell recruitment during respiratory syncytial virus infection. *J Gen Virol* Vol. 79 (Pt 11), No. pp. 2593-2601.

Jelonek, M.T., Maskrey, J.L., Steimer, K.S., Potts, B.J., Higgins, K.W., and Keller, M.A. (1996). Maternal monoclonal antibody to the V3 loop alters specificity of the response to a human immunodeficiency virus vaccine. *J Infect Dis* Vol. 174, No. 4, pp. 866-869.

Jenkins, G.M., Rambaut, A., Pybus, O.G., and Holmes, E.C. (2002). Rates of molecular evolution in RNA viruses: a quantitative phylogenetic analysis. *J Mol Evol* Vol. 54, No. 2, pp. 156-165.

Jennings, G.T., and Bachmann, M.F. (2008). The coming of age of virus-like particle vaccines. *Biol Chem* Vol., No. pp.

Jin, H., Cheng, X., Traina-Dorge, V.L., Park, H.J., Zhou, H., Soike, K., and Kemble, G. (2003). Evaluation of recombinant respiratory syncytial virus gene deletion mutants in

African green monkeys for their potential as live attenuated vaccine candidates. *Vaccine* Vol. 21, No. 25-26, pp. 3647-3652.

Jin, H., Clarke, D., Zhou, H.Z., Cheng, X., Coelingh, K., Bryant, M., and Li, S. (1998). Recombinant human respiratory syncytial virus (RSV) from cDNA and construction of subgroup A and B chimeric RSV. *Virology* Vol. 251, No. 1, pp. 206-214.

Johnson, J.E., Gonzales, R.A., Olson, S.J., Wright, P.F., and Graham, B.S. (2007). The histopathology of fatal untreated human respiratory syncytial virus infection. *Mod Pathol* Vol. 20, No. 1, pp. 108-119.

Johnson, P.R., Jr., Olmsted, R.A., Prince, G.A., Murphy, B.R., Alling, D.W., Walsh, E.E., and Collins, P.L. (1987). Antigenic relatedness between glycoproteins of human respiratory syncytial virus subgroups A and B: evaluation of the contributions of F and G glycoproteins to immunity. *J Virol* Vol. 61, No. 10, pp. 3163-3166.

Johnson, T.R., Teng, M.N., Collins, P.L., and Graham, B.S. (2004a). Respiratory syncytial virus (RSV) G glycoprotein is not necessary for vaccine-enhanced disease induced by immunization with formalin-inactivated RSV. *J Virol* Vol. 78, No. 11, pp. 6024-6032.

Johnson, T.R., Varga, S.M., Braciale, T.J., and Graham, B.S. (2004b). Vbeta14(+) T cells mediate the vaccine-enhanced disease induced by immunization with respiratory syncytial virus (RSV) G glycoprotein but not with formalin-inactivated RSV. *J Virol* Vol. 78, No. 16, pp. 8753-8760.

Jolly, S., Detilleux, J., and Desmecht, D. (2004). Extensive mast cell degranulation in bovine respiratory syncytial virus-associated paroxystic respiratory distress syndrome. *Vet Immunol Immunopathol* Vol. 97, No. 3-4, pp. 125-136.

Kalina, W.V., Woolums, A.R., Berghaus, R.D., and Gershwin, L.J. (2004). Formalin-inactivated bovine RSV vaccine enhances a Th2 mediated immune response in infected cattle. *Vaccine* Vol. 22, No. 11-12, pp. 1465-1474.

Kalina, W.V., Woolums, A.R., and Gershwin, L.J. (2005). Formalin-inactivated bovine RSV vaccine influences antibody levels in bronchoalveolar lavage fluid and disease outcome in experimentally infected calves. *Vaccine* Vol. 23, No. 37, pp. 4625-4630.

Kang, S.M., Yoo, D.G., Lipatov, A.S., Song, J.M., Davis, C.T., Quan, F.S., Chen, L.M., Donis, R.O., and Compans, R.W. (2009). Induction of long-term protective immune responses by influenza H5N1 virus-like particles. *PLoS ONE* Vol. 4, No. 3, pp. e4667.

Kapikian, A.Z., Mitchell, R.H., Chanock, R.M., Shvedoff, R.A., and Stewart, C.E. (1969). An epidemiologic study of altered clinical reactivity to respiratory syncytial (RS) virus infection in children previously vaccinated with an inactivated RS virus vaccine. *Am J Epidemiol* Vol. 89, No. 4, pp. 405-421.

Karlsson, M.C., Wernersson, S., Diaz de Stahl, T., Gustavsson, S., and Heyman, B. (1999). Efficient IgG-mediated suppression of primary antibody responses in Fcgamma receptor-deficient mice. *Proc Natl Acad Sci USA* Vol. 96, No. 5, pp. 2244-2249.

Karron, R.A., Wright, P.F., Belshe, R.B., Thumar, B., Casey, R., Newman, F., Polack, F.P., Randolph, V.B., Deatly, A., Hackell, J., Gruber, W., Murphy, B.R., and Collins, P.L. (2005). Identification of a recombinant live attenuated respiratory syncytial virus vaccine candidate that is highly attenuated in infants. *J Infect Dis* Vol. 191, No. 7, pp. 1093-1104.

Kim, H.W., Canchola, J.G., Brandt, C.D., Pyles, G., Chanock, R.M., Jensen, K., and Parrott, R.H. (1969). Respiratory syncytial virus disease in infants despite prior administration of antigenic inactivated vaccine. *Am J Epidemiol* Vol. 89, No. 4, pp. 422-434.

Kimman, T.G., Sol, J., Westenbrink, F., and Straver, P.J. (1989a). A severe outbreak of respiratory tract disease associated with bovine respiratory syncytial virus probably enhanced by vaccination with modified live vaccine. *Vet Q* Vol. 11, No. 4, pp. 250-253.

Kimman, T.G., Terpstra, G.K., Daha, M.R., and Westenbrink, F. (1989b). Pathogenesis of naturally acquired bovine respiratory syncytial virus infection in calves: evidence for the involvement of complement and mast cell mediators. *Am J Vet Res* Vol. 50, No. 5, pp. 694-700.

Kimman, T.G., Westenbrink, F., and Straver, P.J. (1989c). Priming for local and systemic antibody memory responses to bovine respiratory syncytial virus: effect of amount of virus, virus replication, route of administration and maternal antibodies. *Vet Immunol Immunopathol* Vol. 22, No. 2, pp. 145-160.

Kneyber, M.C., and Kimpen, J.L. (2004). Advances in respiratory syncytial virus vaccine development. *Curr Opin Investig Drugs* Vol. 5, No. 2, pp. 163-170.

Krempl, C.D., Lamirande, E.W., and Collins, P.L. (2005). Complete sequence of the RNA genome of pneumonia virus of mice (PVM). *Virus Genes* Vol. 30, No. 2, pp. 237-249.

Kurikka, S., Olander, R.M., Eskola, J., and Kayhty, H. (1996). Passively acquired anti-tetanus and anti-Haemophilus antibodies and the response to Haemophilus influenzae type b-tetanus toxoid conjugate vaccine in infancy. *Pediatr Infect Dis J* Vol. 15, No. 6, pp. 530-535.

Le Nouen, C., Hillyer, P., Winter, C.C., McCarty, T., Rabin, R.L., Collins, P.L., and Buchholz, U.J. (2011). Low CCR7-Mediated Migration of Human Monocyte Derived Dendritic Cells in Response to Human Respiratory Syncytial Virus and Human Metapneumovirus. *PLoS pathogens* Vol. 7, No. 6, pp. e1002105.

Le Nouen, C., Munir, S., Losq, S., Winter, C.C., McCarty, T., Stephany, D.A., Holmes, K.L., Bukreyev, A., Rabin, R.L., Collins, P.L., and Buchholz, U.J. (2009). Infection and maturation of monocyte-derived human dendritic cells by human respiratory syncytial virus, human metapneumovirus, and human parainfluenza virus type 3. *Virology* Vol. 385, No. 1, pp. 169-182.

Lee, S., Miller, S.A., Wright, D.W., Rock, M.T., and Crowe, J.E., Jr. (2007). Tissue-specific regulation of CD8+ T-lymphocyte immunodominance in respiratory syncytial virus infection. *J Virol* Vol. 81, No. 5, pp. 2349-2358.

Legg, J.P., Hussain, I.R., Warner, J.A., Johnston, S.L., and Warner, J.O. (2003). Type 1 and type 2 cytokine imbalance in acute respiratory syncytial virus bronchiolitis. *Am J Respir Crit Care Med* Vol. 168, No. 6, pp. 633-639.

Lehmann, M., Meyer, M.F., Monazahian, M., Tillmann, H.L., Manns, M.P., and Wedemeyer, H. (2004). High rate of spontaneous clearance of acute hepatitis C virus genotype 3 infection. *J Med Virol* Vol. 73, No. 3, pp. 387-391.

Lindell, D.M., Morris, S.B., White, M.P., Kallal, L.E., Lundy, P.K., Hamouda, T., Baker, J.R., Jr., and Lukacs, N.W. (2011). A Novel Inactivated Intranasal Respiratory Syncytial Virus Vaccine Promotes Viral Clearance without Th2 Associated Vaccine-Enhanced Disease. *PLoS ONE* Vol. 6, No. 7, pp. e21823.

Lugo, R.A., and Nahata, M.C. (1993). Pathogenesis and treatment of bronchiolitis. *Clin Pharm* Vol. 12, No. 2, pp. 95-116.

Lukacs, N.W., Moore, M.L., Rudd, B.D., Berlin, A.A., Collins, R.D., Olson, S.J., Ho, S.B., and Peebles, R.S., Jr. (2006). Differential immune responses and pulmonary pathophysiology are induced by two different strains of respiratory syncytial virus. *Am J Pathol* Vol. 169, No. 3, pp. 977-986.

Lukacs, N.W., Smit, J.J., Mukherjee, S., Morris, S.B., Nunez, G., and Lindell, D.M. (2010). Respiratory virus-induced TLR7 activation controls IL-17-associated increased mucus via IL-23 regulation. *J Immunol* Vol. 185, No. 4, pp. 2231-2239.

Luongo, C., Yang, L., Winter, C.C., Spann, K.M., Murphy, B.R., Collins, P.L., and Buchholz, U.J. (2009). Codon stabilization analysis of the "248" temperature sensitive mutation for increased phenotypic stability of respiratory syncytial virus vaccine candidates. *Vaccine* Vol. 27, No. 41, pp. 5667-5676.

Mapletoft, J.W., Oumouna, M., Kovacs-Nolan, J., Latimer, L., Mutwiri, G., Babiuk, L.A., and van Drunen Littel-van den Hurk, S. (2008). Intranasal immunization of mice with a formalin-inactivated bovine respiratory syncytial virus vaccine co-formulated with CpG oligodeoxynucleotides and polyphosphazenes results in enhanced protection. *J Gen Virol* Vol. 89, No. Pt 1, pp. 250-260.

Matheson, J.W., Rich, F.J., Cohet, C., Grimwood, K., Huang, Q.S., Penny, D., Hendy, M.D., and Kirman, J.R. (2006). Distinct patterns of evolution between respiratory syncytial virus subgroups A and B from New Zealand isolates collected over thirty-seven years. *J Med Virol* Vol. 78, No. 10, pp. 1354-1364.

McLellan, J.S., Yang, Y., Graham, B.S., and Kwong, P.D. (2011). Structure of respiratory syncytial virus fusion glycoprotein in the postfusion conformation reveals preservation of neutralizing epitopes. *J Virol* Vol. 85, No. 15, pp. 7788-7796.

McNulty, M.S., Bryson, D.G., and Allan, G.M. (1983). Experimental respiratory syncytial virus pneumonia in young calves: microbiologic and immunofluorescent findings. *Am J Vet Res* Vol. 44, No. 9, pp. 1656-1659.

Meissner, H.C., and Long, S.S. (2003). Revised indications for the use of palivizumab and respiratory syncytial virus immune globulin intravenous for the prevention of respiratory syncytial virus infections. *Pediatrics* Vol. 112, No. 6 Pt 1, pp. 1447-1452.

Mellow, T.E., Murphy, P.C., Carson, J.L., Noah, T.L., Zhang, L., and Pickles, R.J. (2004). The effect of respiratory synctial virus on chemokine release by differentiated airway epithelium. *ExpLung Res* Vol. 30, No. 1, pp. 43-57.

Miller, E.K., Edwards, K.M., Weinberg, G.A., Iwane, M.K., Griffin, M.R., Hall, C.B., Zhu, Y., Szilagyi, P.G., Morin, L.L., Heil, L.H., Lu, X., and Williams, J.V. (2009). A novel group of rhinoviruses is associated with asthma hospitalizations. *J Allergy Clin Immunol* Vol. 123, No. 1, pp. 98-104 e101.

Moghaddam, A., Olszewska, W., Wang, B., Tregoning, J.S., Helson, R., Sattentau, Q.J., and Openshaw, P.J. (2006). A potential molecular mechanism for hypersensitivity caused by formalin-inactivated vaccines. *Nat Med* Vol. 12, No. 8, pp. 905-907.

Mohanty, S.B., Rockemann, D.D., Davidson, J.P., Sharabrin, O.I., and Forst, S.M. (1981). Effect of vaccinal serum antibodies on bovine respiratory syncytial viral infection in calves. *Am J Vet Res* Vol. 42, No. 5, pp. 881-883.

Mok, H., Lee, S., Utley, T.J., Shepherd, B.E., Polosukhin, V.V., Collier, M.L., Davis, N.L., Johnston, R.E., and Crowe, J.E., Jr. (2007). Venezuelan equine encephalitis virus replicon particles encoding respiratory syncytial virus surface glycoproteins induce protective mucosal responses in mice and cotton rats. *J Virol* Vol. 81, No. 24, pp. 13710-13722.

Moore, M.L., Chi, M.H., Luongo, C., Lukacs, N.W., Polosukhin, V.V., Huckabee, M.M., Newcomb, D.C., Buchholz, U.J., Crowe, J.E., Jr., Goleniewska, K., Williams, J.V., Collins, P.L., and Peebles, R.S., Jr. (2009a). A chimeric A2 strain of respiratory syncytial virus (RSV) with the fusion protein of RSV strain line 19 exhibits enhanced viral load, mucus, and airway dysfunction. *J Virol* Vol. 83, No. 9, pp. 4185-4194.

Moore, M.L., Newcomb, D.C., Parekh, V.V., Van Kaer, L., Collins, R.D., Zhou, W., Goleniewska, K., Chi, M.H., Mitchell, D., Boyce, J.A., Durbin, J.E., Sturkie, C., and Peebles, R.S., Jr. (2009b). STAT1 negatively regulates lung basophil IL-4 expression induced by respiratory syncytial virus infection. *J Immunol* Vol. 183, No. 3, pp. 2016-2026.

Moore, M.L., and Peebles, R.S., Jr. (2006). Respiratory syncytial virus disease mechanisms implicated by human, animal model, and in vitro data facilitate vaccine strategies and new therapeutics. *Pharmacol Ther* Vol., No. pp.

Mukherjee, S., Lindell, D.M., Berlin, A.A., Morris, S.B., Shanley, T.P., Hershenson, M.B., and Lukacs, N.W. (2011). IL-17-induced pulmonary pathogenesis during respiratory viral infection and exacerbation of allergic disease. *Am J Pathol* Vol. 179, No. 1, pp. 248-258.

Munir, S., Hillyer, P., Le Nouen, C., Buchholz, U.J., Rabin, R.L., Collins, P.L., and Bukreyev, A. (2011). Respiratory syncytial virus interferon antagonist NS1 protein suppresses and skews the human T lymphocyte response. *PLoS pathogens* Vol. 7, No. 4, pp. e1001336.

Murawski, M.R., McGinnes, L.W., Finberg, R.W., Kurt-Jones, E.A., Massare, M.J., Smith, G., Heaton, P.M., Fraire, A.E., and Morrison, T.G. (2009). Newcastle Disease Virus-Like Particles Containing Respiratory Syncytial Virus (RSV) G protein Induced Protection in BALB/c Mice With No Evidence of Immunopathology. *J Virol* Vol., No. pp.

Murphy, B.R., Graham, B.S., Prince, G.A., Walsh, E.E., Chanock, R.M., Karzon, D.T., and Wright, P.F. (1986a). Serum and nasal-wash immunoglobulin G and A antibody response of infants and children to respiratory syncytial virus F and G glycoproteins following primary infection. *J Clin Microbiol* Vol. 23, No. 6, pp. 1009-1014.

Murphy, B.R., Prince, G.A., Walsh, E.E., Kim, H.W., Parrott, R.H., Hemming, V.G., Rodriguez, W.J., and Chanock, R.M. (1986b). Dissociation between serum neutralizing and glycoprotein antibody responses of infants and children who received inactivated respiratory syncytial virus vaccine. *J Clin Microbiol* Vol. 24, No. 2, pp. 197-202.

Murphy, B.R., and Walsh, E.E. (1988). Formalin-inactivated respiratory syncytial virus vaccine induces antibodies to the fusion glycoprotein that are deficient in fusion-inhibiting activity. *J Clin Microbiol* Vol. 26, No. 8, pp. 1595-1597.

Neuzil, K.M., Johnson, J.E., Tang, Y.W., Prieels, J.P., Slaoui, M., Gar, N., and Graham, B.S. (1997). Adjuvants influence the quantitative and qualitative immune response in BALB/c mice immunized with respiratory syncytial virus FG subunit vaccine. *Vaccine* Vol. 15, No. 5, pp. 525-532.

Nohynek, H., Gustafsson, L., Capeding, M.R., Kayhty, H., Olander, R.M., Pascualk, L., and Ruutu, P. (1999). Effect of transplacentally acquired tetanus antibodies on the antibody responses to Haemophilus influenzae type b-tetanus toxoid conjugate and tetanus toxoid vaccines in Filipino infants. *Pediatr Infect Dis J* Vol. 18, No. 1, pp. 25-30.

Olivier, A., Gallup, J., de Macedo, M.M., Varga, S.M., and Ackermann, M. (2009). Human respiratory syncytial virus A2 strain replicates and induces innate immune responses by respiratory epithelia of neonatal lambs. *Intl J Exp Pathol* Vol. 90, No. 4, pp. 431-438.

Olson, M.R., and Varga, S.M. (2007). CD8 T cells inhibit respiratory syncytial virus (RSV) vaccine-enhanced disease. *J Immunol* Vol. 179, No. 8, pp. 5415-5424.

Openshaw, P.J., and Tregoning, J.S. (2005). Immune responses and disease enhancement during respiratory syncytial virus infection. *Clin Micro Rev* Vol. 18, No. 3, pp. 541-555.

Oumouna, M., Mapletoft, J.W., Karvonen, B.C., Babiuk, L.A., and van Drunen Littel-van den Hurk, S. (2005). Formulation with CpG oligodeoxynucleotides prevents induction of pulmonary immunopathology following priming with formalin-inactivated or commercial killed bovine respiratory syncytial virus vaccine. *J Virol* Vol. 79, No. 4, pp. 2024-2032.

Pabst, H.F., Spady, D.W., Carson, M.M., Krezolek, M.P., Barreto, L., and Wittes, R.C. (1999). Cell-mediated and antibody immune responses to AIK-C and Connaught monovalent measles vaccine given to 6 month old infants. *Vaccine* Vol. 17, No. 15-16, pp. 1910-1918.

Parveen, S., Broor, S., Kapoor, S.K., Fowler, K., and Sullender, W.M. (2006). Genetic diversity among respiratory syncytial viruses that have caused repeated infections in children from rural India. *J Med Virol* Vol. 78, No. 5, pp. 659-665.

Peebles, R.S., Jr., Sheller, J.R., Collins, R.D., Jarzecka, A.K., Mitchell, D.B., Parker, R.A., and Graham, B.S. (2001). Respiratory syncytial virus infection does not increase allergen-induced type 2 cytokine production, yet increases airway hyperresponsiveness in mice. *J Med Virol* Vol. 63, No. 2, pp. 178-188.

Percopo, C.M., Qiu, Z., Phipps, S., Foster, P.S., Domachowske, J.B., and Rosenberg, H.F. (2009). Pulmonary eosinophils and their role in immunopathologic responses to formalin-inactivated pneumonia virus of mice. *J Immunol* Vol. 183, No. 1, pp. 604-612.

Peret, T.C., Hall, C.B., Hammond, G.W., Piedra, P.A., Storch, G.A., Sullender, W.M., Tsou, C., and Anderson, L.J. (2000). Circulation patterns of group A and B human respiratory syncytial virus genotypes in 5 communities in North America. *J Infect Dis* Vol. 181, No. 6, pp. 1891-1896.

Peret, T.C., Hall, C.B., Schnabel, K.C., Golub, J.A., and Anderson, L.J. (1998). Circulation patterns of genetically distinct group A and B strains of human respiratory syncytial virus in a community. *J Gen Virol* Vol. 79 (Pt 9), No. pp. 2221-2229.

Pirie, H.M., Petrie, L., Allan, E.M., and Pringle, C.R. (1981). Acute fatal pneumonia in calves due to respiratory syncytial virus. *Vet Rec* Vol. 109, No. 4, pp. 87.

Polack, F.P., and Karron, R.A. (2004). The future of respiratory syncytial virus vaccine development. *Pediatr Infect Dis J* Vol. 23, No. 1 Suppl, pp. S65-73.

Polack, F.P., Teng, M.N., Collins, P.L., Prince, G.A., Exner, M., Regele, H., Lirman, D.D., Rabold, R., Hoffman, S.J., Karp, C.L., Kleeberger, S.R., Wills-Karp, M., and Karron, R.A. (2002). A role for immune complexes in enhanced respiratory syncytial virus disease. *J Exp Med* Vol. 196, No. 6, pp. 859-865.

Preston, F.M., Beier, P.L., and Pope, J.H. (1992). Infectious respiratory syncytial virus (RSV) effectively inhibits the proliferative T cell response to inactivated RSV in vitro. *J Infect Dis* Vol. 165, No. 5, pp. 819-825.

Preston, F.M., Beier, P.L., and Pope, J.H. (1995). Identification of the respiratory syncytial virus-induced immunosuppressive factor produced by human peripheral blood mononuclear cells in vitro as interferon-alpha. *J Infect Dis* Vol. 172, No. 4, pp. 919-926.

Prince, G.A., Hemming, V.G., Horswood, R.L., Baron, P.A., Murphy, B.R., and Chanock, R.M. (1990). Mechanism of antibody-mediated viral clearance in immunotherapy of respiratory syncytial virus infection of cotton rats. *J Virol* Vol. 64, No. 6, pp. 3091-3092.

Prince, G.A., Horswood, R.L., Berndt, J., Suffin, S.C., and Chanock, R.M. (1979). Respiratory syncytial virus infection in inbred mice. *Infect Immun* Vol. 26, No. 2, pp. 764-766.

Prince, G.A., Horswood, R.L., and Chanock, R.M. (1985). Quantitative aspects of passive immunity to respiratory syncytial virus infection in infant cotton rats. *J Virol* Vol. 55, No. 3, pp. 517-520.

Prince, G.A., Jenson, A.B., Hemming, V.G., Murphy, B.R., Walsh, E.E., Horswood, R.L., and Chanock, R.M. (1986). Enhancement of respiratory syncytial virus pulmonary pathology in cotton rats by prior intramuscular inoculation of formalin-inactiva ted virus. *J Virol* Vol. 57, No. 3, pp. 721-728.

Prince, G.A., Jenson, A.B., Horswood, R.L., Camargo, E., and Chanock, R.M. (1978). The pathogenesis of respiratory syncytial virus infection in cotton rats. *Am J Pathol* Vol. 93, No. 3, pp. 771-791.

Prince, G.A., and Porter, D.D. (1976). The pathogenesis of respiratory syncytial virus infection in infant ferrets. *Am J Pathol* Vol. 82, No. 2, pp. 339-352.

Quan, F.S., Sailaja, G., Skountzou, I., Huang, C., Vzorov, A., Compans, R.W., and Kang, S.M. (2007). Immunogenicity of virus-like particles containing modified human immunodeficiency virus envelope proteins. *Vaccine* Vol. 25, No. 19, pp. 3841-3850.

Roberts, N.J., Jr., Prill, A.H., and Mann, T.N. (1986). Interleukin 1 and interleukin 1 inhibitor production by human macrophages exposed to influenza virus or respiratory syncytial virus. Respiratory syncytial virus is a potent inducer of inhibitor activity. *J Exp Med* Vol. 163, No. 3, pp. 511-519.

Roman, M., Calhoun, W.J., Hinton, K.L., Avendano, L.F., Simon, V., Escobar, A.M., Gaggero, A., and Diaz, P.V. (1997). Respiratory syncytial virus infection in infants is associated with predominant Th-2-like response. *Am J Respir Crit Care Med* Vol. 156, No. 1, pp. 190-195.

Rosenberg, H.F., Bonville, C.A., Easton, A.J., and Domachowske, J.B. (2005). The pneumonia virus of mice infection model for severe respiratory syncytial virus infection: identifying novel targets for therapeutic intervention. *Pharmacol Ther* Vol. 105, No. 1, pp. 1-6.

Ruckwardt, T.J., Luongo, C., Malloy, A.M., Liu, J., Chen, M., Collins, P.L., and Graham, B.S. (2010). Responses against a subdominant CD8+ T cell epitope protect against immunopathology caused by a dominant epitope. *J Immunol* Vol. 185, No. 8, pp. 4673-4680.

Schickli, J.H., Dubovsky, F., and Tang, R.S. (2009). Challenges in developing a pediatric RSV vaccine. *Hum Vaccin* Vol. 5, No. 9, pp. 582-591.

Schreiber, P., Matheise, J.P., Dessy, F., Heimann, M., Letesson, J.J., Coppe, P., and Collard, A. (2000). High mortality rate associated with bovine respiratory syncytial virus (BRSV) infection in Belgian white blue calves previously vaccinated with an inactivated BRSV vaccine. *J Vet Med B* Vol. 47, No. 7, pp. 535-550.

Scott, P.D., Ochola, R., Ngama, M., Okiro, E.A., James, N.D., Medley, G.F., and Cane, P.A. (2006). Molecular analysis of respiratory syncytial virus reinfections in infants from coastal Kenya. *J Infect Dis* Vol. 193, No. 1, pp. 59-67.

Scott, P.D., Ochola, R., Sande, C., Ngama, M., Okiro, E.A., Medley, G.F., Nokes, D.J., and Cane, P.A. (2007). Comparison of strain-specific antibody responses during primary and secondary infections with respiratory syncytial virus. *J Med Virol* Vol. 79, No. 12, pp. 1943-1950.

Shay, D.K., Holman, R.C., Newman, R.D., Liu, L.L., Stout, J.W., and Anderson, L.J. (1999). Bronchiolitis-associated hospitalizations among US children, 1980-1996. *JAMA*

Shinoff, J.J., O'Brien, K.L., Thumar, B., Shaw, J.B., Reid, R., Hua, W., Santosham, M., and Karron, R.A. (2008). Young infants can develop protective levels of neutralizing antibody after infection with respiratory syncytial virus. *J Infect Dis* Vol. 198, No. 7, pp. 1007-1015.

Shirey, K.A., Pletneva, L.M., Puche, A.C., Keegan, A.D., Prince, G.A., Blanco, J.C., and Vogel, S.N. (2010). Control of RSV-induced lung injury by alternatively activated macrophages is IL-4R alpha-, TLR4-, and IFN-beta-dependent. *Mucosal Immunol* Vol. 3, No. 3, pp. 291-300.

Siegrist, C.A. (2003). Mechanisms by which maternal antibodies influence infant vaccine responses: review of hypotheses and definition of main determinants. *Vaccine* Vol. 21, No. 24, pp. 3406-3412.

Simoes, E.A., Hayward, A.R., Ponnuraj, E.M., Straumanis, J.P., Stenmark, K.R., Wilson, H.L., and Babu, P.G. (1999). Respiratory syncytial virus infects the Bonnet monkey, Macaca radiata. *Pediatr Dev Pathol* Vol. 2, No. 4, pp. 316-326.

Sow, F.B., Gallup, J.M., Olivier, A., Krishnan, S., Patera, A.C., Suzich, J., and Ackermann, M.R. (2011). Respiratory syncytial virus is associated with an inflammatory response in lungs and architectural remodeling of lung-draining lymph nodes of newborn lambs. *Am J Physiol Lung Cell Mol Physiol* Vol. 300, No. 1, pp. L12-24.

Srikiatkhachorn, A., and Braciale, T.J. (1997). Virus-specific CD8+ T lymphocytes downregulate T helper cell type 2 cytokine secretion and pulmonary eosinophilia during experimental murine respiratory syncytial virus infection. *J Exp Med* Vol. 186, No. 3, pp. 421-432.

Stensballe, L.G., Ravn, H., Kristensen, K., Meakins, T., Aaby, P., and Simoes, E.A. (2009). Seasonal variation of maternally derived respiratory syncytial virus antibodies and association with infant hospitalizations for respiratory syncytial virus. *J Pediatr* Vol. 154, No. 2, pp. 296-298.

Stokes, K.L., Chi, M.H., Sakamoto, K., Newcomb, D.C., Currier, M.G., Huckabee, M.M., Lee, S., Goleniewska, K., Pretto, C., Williams, J.V., Hotard, A., Sherrill, T.P., Peebles, R.S., Jr., and Moore, M.L. (2011). Differential pathogenesis of respiratory syncytial virus clinical isolates in BALB/c mice. *J Virol* Vol. 85, No. 12, pp. 5782-5793.

Sullender, W.M. (2000). Respiratory syncytial virus genetic and antigenic diversity. *Clin Microbiol Rev* Vol. 13, No. 1, pp. 1-15, table.

Sullender, W.M., Mufson, M.A., Prince, G.A., Anderson, L.J., and Wertz, G.W. (1998). Antigenic and genetic diversity among the attachment proteins of group A respiratory syncytial viruses that have caused repeat infections in children. *J Infect Dis* Vol. 178, No. 4, pp. 925-932.

Tekkanat, K.K., Maassab, H., Miller, A., Berlin, A.A., Kunkel, S.L., and Lukacs, N.W. (2002). RANTES (CCL5) production during primary respiratory syncytial virus infection exacerbates airway disease. *Eur J Immunol* Vol. 32, No. 11, pp. 3276-3284.

Tekkanat, K.K., Maassab, H.F., Cho, D.S., Lai, J.J., John, A., Berlin, A., Kaplan, M.H., and Lukacs, N.W. (2001). IL-13-induced airway hyperreactivity during respiratory syncytial virus infection is STAT6 dependent. *J Immunol* Vol. 166, No. 5, pp. 3542-3548.

Teng, M.N., Whitehead, S.S., Bermingham, A., St Claire, M., Elkins, W.R., Murphy, B.R., and Collins, P.L. (2000). Recombinant respiratory syncytial virus that does not express the NS1 or M2-2 protein is highly attenuated and immunogenic in chimpanzees. *J Virol* Vol. 74, No. 19, pp. 9317-9321.

Thompson, W.W., Shay, D.K., Weintraub, E., Brammer, L., Cox, N., Anderson, L.J., and Fukuda, K. (2003). Mortality associated with influenza and respiratory syncytial virus in the United States. *JAMA* Vol. 289, No. 2, pp. 179-186.

Tumpey, T.M., Basler, C.F., Aguilar, P.V., Zeng, H., Solorzano, A., Swayne, D.E., Cox, N.J., Katz, J.M., Taubenberger, J.K., Palese, P., and Garcia-Sastre, A. (2005). Characterization of the reconstructed 1918 Spanish influenza pandemic virus. *Science* Vol. 310, No. 5745, pp. 77-80.

Van Donkersgoed, J., Janzen, E.D., Townsend, H.G., and Durham, P.J. (1990a). Five field trials on the efficacy of a bovine respiratory syncytial virus vaccine. *Can Vet J* Vol. 31, No. 2, pp. 93-100.

Van Donkersgoed, J., Janzen, E.D., Townsend, H.G., and Durham, P.J. (1990b). Five field trials on the efficacy of a bovine respiratory syncytial virus vaccine. *Can Vet J* Vol. 31, No. 2, pp. 93-100.

Vangeel, I., Antonis, A.F., Fluess, M., Riegler, L., Peters, A.R., and Harmeyer, S.S. (2007a). Efficacy of a modified live intranasal bovine respiratory syncytial virus vaccine in 3-week-old calves experimentally challenged with BRSV. *Vet J* Vol. 174, No. 3, pp. 627-635.

Vangeel, I., Antonis, A.F., Fluess, M., Riegler, L., Peters, A.R., and Harmeyer, S.S. (2007b). Efficacy of a modified live intranasal bovine respiratory syncytial virus vaccine in 3-week-old calves experimentally challenged with BRSV. *Vet J* Vol. 174, No. 3, pp. 627-635.

Vangeel, I., Ioannou, F., Riegler, L., Salt, J.S., and Harmeyer, S.S. (2009). Efficacy of an intranasal modified live bovine respiratory syncytial virus and temperature-sensitive parainfluenza type 3 virus vaccine in 3-week-old calves experimentally challenged with PI3V. *Vet J* Vol. 179, No. 1, pp. 101-108.

Verhoeff, J., and van Nieuwstadt, A.P. (1984). Prevention of bovine respiratory syncytial virus infection and clinical disease by vaccination. *Vet Rec* Vol. 115, No. 19, pp. 488-492.

Villenave, R., O'Donoghue, D., Thavagnanam, S., Touzelet, O., Skibinski, G., Heaney, L.G., McKaigue, J.P., Coyle, P.V., Shields, M.D., and Power, U.F. (2011). Differential cytopathogenesis of respiratory syncytial virus prototypic and clinical isolates in primary pediatric bronchial epithelial cells. *Virol J* Vol. 8, No. pp. 43.

Villenave, R., Touzelet, O., Thavagnanam, S., Sarlang, S., Parker, J., Skibinski, G., Heaney, L.G., McKaigue, J.P., Coyle, P.V., Shields, M.D., and Power, U.F. (2010). Cytopathogenesis of Sendai virus in well-differentiated primary pediatric bronchial epithelial cells. *J Virol* Vol. 84, No. 22, pp. 11718-11728.

Viuff, B., Tjornehoj, K., Larsen, L.E., Rontved, C.M., Uttenthal, A., Ronsholt, L., and Alexandersen, S. (2002). Replication and clearance of respiratory syncytial virus: apoptosis is an important pathway of virus clearance after experimental infection with bovine respiratory syncytial virus. *Am J Pathol* Vol. 161, No. 6, pp. 2195-2207.

Wagner, D.K., Muelenaer, P., Henderson, F.W., Snyder, M.H., Reimer, C.B., Walsh, E.E., Anderson, L.J., Nelson, D.L., and Murphy, B.R. (1989). Serum immunoglobulin G antibody subclass response to respiratory syncytial virus F and G glycoproteins after first, second, and third infections. *J Clin Microbiol* Vol. 27, No. 3, pp. 589-592.

Walsh, E.E. (1993). Mucosal immunization with a subunit respiratory syncytial virus vaccine in mice. *Vaccine* Vol. 11, No. 11, pp. 1135-1138.

Weitkamp, J.H., Lafleur, B.J., Greenberg, H.B., and Crowe, J.E., Jr. (2005). Natural evolution of a human virus-specific antibody gene repertoire by somatic hypermutation requires both hotspot-directed and randomly-directed processes. *Hum Immunol* Vol. 66, No. 6, pp. 666-676.

Welliver, R.C., Kaul, T.N., Putnam, T.I., Sun, M., Riddlesberger, K., and Ogra, P.L. (1980). The antibody response to primary and secondary infection with respiratory syncytial virus: kinetics of class-specific responses. *J Pediatr* Vol. 96, No. 5, pp. 808-813.

Welliver, T.P., Garofalo, R.P., Hosakote, Y., Hintz, K.H., Avendano, L., Sanchez, K., Velozo, L., Jafri, H., Chavez-Bueno, S., Ogra, P.L., McKinney, L., Reed, J.L., and Welliver, R.C., Sr. (2007). Severe human lower respiratory tract illness caused by respiratory syncytial virus and influenza virus is characterized by the absence of pulmonary cytotoxic lymphocyte responses. *J Infect Dis* Vol. 195, No. 8, pp. 1126-1136.

West, K., Petrie, L., Haines, D.M., Konoby, C., Clark, E.G., Martin, K., and Ellis, J.A. (1999a). The effect of formalin-inactivated vaccine on respiratory disease associated with bovine respiratory syncytial virus infection in calves. *Vaccine* Vol. 17, No. 7-8, pp. 809-820.

West, K., Petrie, L., Konoby, C., Haines, D.M., Cortese, V., and Ellis, J.A. (1999b). The efficacy of modified-live bovine respiratory syncytial virus vaccines in experimentally infected calves. *Vaccine* Vol. 18, No. 9-10, pp. 907-919.

Whitehead, S.S., Hill, M.G., Firestone, C.Y., St Claire, M., Elkins, W.R., Murphy, B.R., and Collins, P.L. (1999). Replacement of the F and G proteins of respiratory syncytial virus (RSV) subgroup A with those of subgroup B generates chimeric live attenuated RSV subgroup B vaccine candidates. *J Virol* Vol. 73, No. 12, pp. 9773-9780.

Williams, J.V., Weitkamp, J.H., Blum, D.L., Lafleur, B.J., and Crowe, J.E., Jr. (2009). The human neonatal B cell response to respiratory syncytial virus uses a biased antibody variable gene repertoire that lacks somatic mutations. *Mol Immunol* Vol., No. pp.

Woolums, A.R., Singer, R.S., Boyle, G.A., and Gershwin, L.J. (1999). Interferon gamma production during bovine respiratory syncytial virus (BRSV) infection is diminished in calves vaccinated with formalin-inactivated BRSV. *Vaccine* Vol. 17, No. 11-12, pp. 1293-1297.

Wright, P.F., Gruber, W.C., Peters, M., Reed, G., Zhu, Y., Robinson, F., Coleman-Dockery, S., and Graham, B.S. (2002). Illness severity, viral shedding, and antibody responses in infants hospitalized with bronchiolitis caused by respiratory syncytial virus. *J Infect Dis* Vol. 185, No. 8, pp. 1011-1018.

Wright, P.F., Karron, R.A., Belshe, R.B., Shi, J.R., Randolph, V.B., Collins, P.L., O'Shea, A.F., Gruber, W.C., and Murphy, B.R. (2007). The absence of enhanced disease with wild type respiratory syncytial virus infection occurring after receipt of live, attenuated, respiratory syncytial virus vaccines. *Vaccine* Vol. 25, No. 42, pp. 7372-7378.

Wright, P.F., Karron, R.A., Belshe, R.B., Thompson, J., Crowe, J.E., Jr., Boyce, T.G., Halburnt, L.L., Reed, G.W., Whitehead, S.S., Anderson, E.L., Wittek, A.E., Casey, R., Eichelberger, M., Thumar, B., Randolph, V.B., Udem, S.A., Chanock, R.M., and Murphy, B.R. (2000). Evaluation of a live, cold-passaged, temperature-sensitive, respiratory syncytial virus vaccine candidate in infancy. *J Infect Dis* Vol. 182, No. 5, pp. 1331-1342.

Xue, W., Ellis, J., Mattick, D., Smith, L., Brady, R., and Trigo, E. (2010). Immunogenicity of a modified-live virus vaccine against bovine viral diarrhea virus types 1 and 2, infectious bovine rhinotracheitis virus, bovine parainfluenza-3 virus, and bovine respiratory syncytial virus when administered intranasally in young calves. *Vaccine* Vol. 28, No. 22, pp. 3784-3792.

Yu, X., Tsibane, T., McGraw, P.A., House, F.S., Keefer, C.J., Hicar, M.D., Tumpey, T.M., Pappas, C., Perrone, L.A., Martinez, O., Stevens, J., Wilson, I.A., Aguilar, P.V., Altschuler, E.L., Basler, C.F., and Crowe, J.E., Jr. (2008). Neutralizing antibodies derived from the B cells of 1918 influenza pandemic survivors. *Nature* Vol. 455, No. 7212, pp. 532-536.

Zhang, L., Peeples, M.E., Boucher, R.C., Collins, P.L., and Pickles, R.J. (2002). Respiratory syncytial virus infection of human airway epithelial cells is polarized, specific to ciliated cells, and without obvious cytopathology. *J Virol* Vol. 76, No. 11, pp. 5654-5666.

Zlateva, K.T., Lemey, P., Moes, E., Vandamme, A.M., and Van Ranst, M. (2005). Genetic variability and molecular evolution of the human respiratory syncytial virus subgroup B attachment G protein. *J Virol* Vol. 79, No. 14, pp. 9157-9167.

4

Structural and Functional Aspects of the Small Hydrophobic (SH) Protein in the Human Respiratory Syncytial Virus

Siok Wan Gan and Jaume Torres
School of Biological Sciences, Nanyang Technological University
Singapore

1. Introduction

hRSV is the leading cause of respiratory disease in infants, elderly, and immunocompromised populations worldwide (Falsey et al., 2005; Nair et al., 2010). Most individuals are infected at a young age, before 3 years old (Glezen et al., 1986). In fact, RSV infection is the most common cause of hospitalization in children 5 years old and below. When severe infection occurs, respiratory airways and pulmonary development are affected. However, the viral determinants of disease severity are not well defined, as little is known about its molecular mechanism of pathogenesis.

Disease caused by hRSV infection is unique in the sense that repeated infections throughout life can take place even though genetic diversity is not extreme, and antigenic sites are highly conserved between strains (Glezen et al., 1986). It is likely that natural RSV infection only confers imperfect immunity against subsequent infections; the virus probably has evolved to evade the natural immune system so that the durability of antibody response for life-long immunity is poor.

Although the virus was identified half a century ago, there are still no licensed vaccines against infection, and current vaccine-based antiviral therapies are not effective. Reviews describing efforts in the development of antiviral vaccines have been published over the years, e.g. (Collins & Murphy, 2006) and recently (Murata, 2009; Chang, 2011). In the initial trial of RSV vaccine with formalin-inactivated RSV (FI-RSV) during the 1960s, the vaccine proved to be poorly protective and actually enhanced the severity of RSV disease (Kapikian et al., 1969). This failure significantly increased safety concerns surrounding RSV vaccine development. The several hurdles in the development of a pediatric RSV vaccine, and the use of attenuated viruses, subunit particles, peptides, virus-like particles, and live viral vectors as vaccine candidates, which show potential for further development, have been discussed elsewhere, e.g., (Chang, 2011).

In general, currently available prophylactic and therapeutic methods are limited (Murata, 2009; Olszewska & Openshaw, 2009; Weisman, 2009; Chang, 2011). For example, a humanized monoclonal antibody, palivizumab (S. Johnson et al., 1997) targeting hRSV F glycoprotein, a trimeric fusion protein, is licensed for use as prophylactic therapy for the high-risk pediatric population. The drug ribavirin is the only antiviral therapy for patients with hRSV infection, although not recommended in most cases for its unsatisfactory clinical efficacy and safety concerns (Vujovic & Mills, 2001). In addition to the approved monoclonal antibody palivizumab (Group, 1998), several small molecule inhibitors, e.g., disulfonated stilbenes (Razinkov et al., 2001), benzotriazoles (Cianci et al., 2004), benzimidazoles (Andries et al., 2003), and triphenol compounds (McKimm-Breschkin, 2000) that target F protein are also potent inhibitors of hRSV infectivity.

hRSV is a member of the Paramyxoviridae family of nonsegmented negative strand RNA viruses, and encodes 11 proteins, 9 of which are structural. Amongst these, the genome of hRSV encodes three membrane proteins that are accessible on the surface of the virion: fusion (F), attachment (G), and small hydrophobic (SH) protein. Protein G and F are key factors during virus entry, attachment and fusion (Lamb, 1993; Krusat & Streckert, 1997), and are the only hRSV proteins that induce neutralizing antibodies (Walsh et al., 1987; Connors et al., 1991).

Based on the reactive patterns to monoclonal antibodies, hRSV can be divided into two antigenic subgroups, A and B (P. R. Johnson et al., 1987), which co-circulate in human populations. Although antibodies against both F and G proteins were found in the serum of hRSV infected patients, they only provide temporary protection . Thus, the combination of low immunoprotection and lack of suitable antivirals leads logically towards the search and characterization of new drug targets for the effective treatments of hRSV infection.

2. SH protein

2.1 Topology, polymorphism and localization

In contrast to F and G proteins, little is known about the specific functions played by SH protein in hRSV infection and replication. The SH protein is the smallest transmembrane (TM) surface glycoprotein encoded by hRSV (Murphy et al., 1986; Collins & Mottet, 1993), with 64 to 65 amino acids, depending on the viral strain, A or B, respectively (Collins et al., 1990). Biochemical studies have shown that the SH protein is a type II integral membrane protein with a single TM domain (Fig. 1), where the C-terminus is confirmed to be oriented extracellularly (Collins & Mottet, 1993). The TMHMM algorithm, based on the Hidden Markov Model (Krogh et al., 2001) indicates that the TM domain spans residues 20 to 42 (Fig. 1, red line). This has been confirmed experimentally by us using a synthetic peptide corresponding to the TM domain of SH protein, SH-TM (residue 18-43), which when inserted into supported lipid bilayers was protected from hydrogen/deuterium (H/D) exchange and was α-helical (Gan et al., 2008).

During infection, the majority of the SH protein accumulates at lipid-raft structures of the Golgi complex, the endoplasmic reticulum (ER), and the cell surface (Rixon et al., 2004). Lipid rafts are enriched in cholesterol and sphingolipids and form a platform for various protein-protein interactions necessary during signal transduction events (Dykstra et al., 2003), protein trafficking (Helms & Zurzolo, 2004), and also virus entry, assembly, and budding (Suzuki & Suzuki, 2006). Indeed, hRSV has been shown to utilize lipid rafts, and in particular caveolae, a caveolin-1 enriched subdomain (Werling et al., 1999; Brown et al., 2002), to gain entry and in the assembly of virus particles. Only a very low amount of SH protein is associated with the viral envelope (Rixon et al., 2004).

Several forms of SH protein are present during infection, which vary in their glycosylation status (Olmsted & Collins, 1989): two non-glycosylated forms, a full length 7.5 kDa (SH_0) form, a truncated 4.5 kDa species (SH_t), an N-linked glycosylated form (SH_g), and a polylactosaminoglycan-modified form (SH_p). All these, except the truncated SH_t, are incorporated at the surface of the infected cells, where the non-glycosylated SH_0 appears to be the most abundant form (Collins & Mottet, 1993). In addition to these modifications, the tyrosine residues of SH protein are phosphorylated during infection, and this modification affects cellular distribution (Rixon et al., 2005).

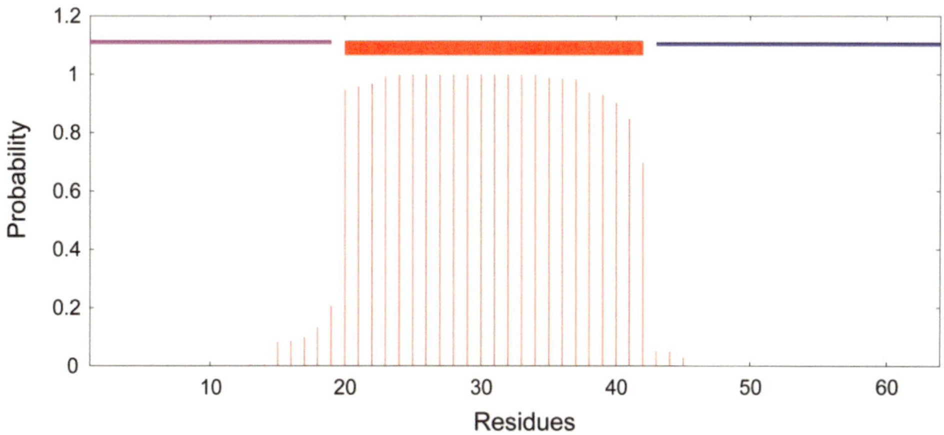

MENTSITIEFSSKFWPYFTLIHMITTIISLLIIISIMIAILNKLCEYNVFHNKTFEELPRARVNT

TM

Fig. 1. Prediction of TM helices for SH protein by TMHMM (Krogh et al., 2001) (http://www.cbs.dtu.dk/services/TMHMM/). Only one TM α-helix is predicted (thick red line). The blue line represents residues inside the cell, whereas the magenta line indicates residues outside the cell, although this prediction turns out to be wrong (see text).

2.2 The role of SH protein

The function of SH protein in RSV replication cycle remains unclear. SH has no crucial role in viral survival in *in vitro* cell culture systems (Bukreyev et al., 1997), but it is essential for effective infection in animal models: mouse and chimpanzee (Bukreyev et al., 1997; Whitehead et al., 1999). This suggests a potential role for SH in immune evasion or in immunomodulation. Interestingly, a vaccine based on the use of live attenuated virus carrying a deletion of the SH gene, rA2cpts248/404/1030/ΔSH, showed significant improvement of disease symptoms and protection against re-infection when compared to another version, cpts248/404, which only carried mutations at other two genes, L and M (Karron et al., 2005).

Some studies suggest an ancillary role for SH protein in virus-mediated cell fusion (Heminway et al., 1994; Techaarpornkul et al., 2001). More recently, it has been shown that SH protein from simian virus 5 (SV5) (He et al., 2001), parainfluenza virus 5 (PIV 5) (Fuentes et al., 2007), Mump virus (MuV) (Wilson et al., 2006), and hRSV (Fuentes et al., 2007), all members of the *paramyxoviridae* family, inhibit apoptosis in several mammalian cell lines.

While promotion of apoptosis helps release the virus from the cell, it is possible that inhibition of apoptosis in host cells during infection gives an advantage to the virus in replication. For RSV and PIV 5, SH protein is necessary for the inhibition of tumor necrosis factor alpha (TNF-α)-induced apoptosis (Y. Lin et al., 2003; Fuentes et al., 2007). However, this is also the case in A549 cells, which are insensitive to TNF-α induced cell death (Fuentes et al., 2007). This suggests that this effect is not uniquely mediated by a TNF-α pathway.

In addition to the above, SH increases membrane permeability to low-molecular-weight compounds, as shown when expressed in *Escherichia coli* (Perez et al., 1997). Thus, SH protein has been suggested to belong to the viroporin class, a group of small, highly hydrophobic virus proteins that can oligomerize and form pores (Gonzalez & Carrasco, 2003). Support for this hypothesis was gained when we confirmed that the synthetic peptide corresponding to the predicted TM domain of SH protein (SH-TM) forms pentameric cation-selective ion channels in model planar lipid bilayers (Gan et al., 2008).

Ion leakage may lead to dissipation of membrane potential and disruption of cell homeostasis, but the consequences of these are not clear. Further studies on hRSV infected cells should gain insight into the significance of SH viroporin activity in the hRSV life cycle. One possible indication may be derived from experiments in MDBK and L929 cells, where SH from PIV5 or from RSV A or B subgroups has a protective role against the cytopathic effect (CPE) produced by PIV5 (He et al., 2001; Y. Lin et al., 2003; Wilson et al., 2006). Similarly, the SH protein from PIV5 could be substituted by SH from mumps virus (Wilson et al., 2006), even though these two SH proteins have no sequence homology. These data argue against a mechanism mediated by a specific protein-protein interaction with an unknown protein, and for a possible functional role of a membrane permeabilizing pentameric structure that would be common to all these species.

2.3 Interaction of SH with viral and host proteins

Extensive protein-protein interactions have been observed between the three membrane proteins on the RSV envelope, F, G, and SH (Feldman et al., 2001; Techaarpornkul et al., 2001; Low et al., 2008) and these interactions have an effect on fusion activity of hRSV on the host (Heminway et al., 1994; Techaarpornkul et al., 2001). In cells transiently expressing hRSV membrane proteins, the presence of G and SH proteins enhanced fusion activity mediated by F protein (Heminway et al., 1994). However, using virus-infected cells the presence of G protein alone enhanced F-mediated fusion activity (Techaarpornkul et al., 2001), whereas SH protein in the absence of G protein inhibited it, suggesting a possible interaction between SH and G (Techaarpornkul et al., 2001).

Protein complexes F-G and G-SH have been detected on the surface of infected cells using immunoprecipitation (Low et al., 2008) and heparin agarose affinity chromatography (Feldman et al., 2001). Direct evidence of the existence of an F-SH complex has never been reported. A trimeric complex F-G-SH was not detected on the surface of hRSV infected Hep-2 line cells (Low et al., 2008), but it was present in Vero cell lines co-transfected with F, G, and SH proteins (Feldman et al., 2001), suggesting that this hypothetical ternary interaction may be short lived, or takes place in very specific conditions. These three proteins not only form hetero-oligomers, but also homo-oligomers: F forms trimers (Calder et al., 2000), G forms tetramers (Escribano-Romero et al., 2004), and SH forms pentamers (Collins & Mottet,

1993; Rixon et al., 2005; Gan et al., 2008). Thus, a complicated regulatory network of interactions may exist which probably includes both homo- and hetero-oligomeric forms.

In addition to interactions with viral proteins, the fact that SH proteins of RSV and PIV 5 are necessary for the inhibition of tumor necrosis factor alpha (TNF-α)-induced apoptosis (Y. Lin et al., 2003; Fuentes et al., 2007) also suggests a possible interaction with host proteins, although this has not been confirmed experimentally.

2.4 Oligomerization of SH protein

Hetero- or homo-dimerization at the TM domain is very common in membrane proteins, e.g. homo- and hetero-dimeric integrins (X. Lin et al., 2006), or trimeric viral fusion proteins (Lamb et al., 1999). Tetramers and above suggest pore or channel formation, e.g., in influenza A M2 (a tetrameric proton channel) (Kovacs & Cross, 1997), CorA (a pentameric divalent cation transporter) (Eshaghi et al., 2006), and MscL (a hexameric mechanosensitive channel) (Sukharev et al., 1997). SH protein can be cross-linked with disuccinimidyl suberate and dithiobis-(succinimidyl)-propionate, to produce higher oligomers, from dimers to pentamers (Collins & Mottet, 1993; Rixon et al., 2005).

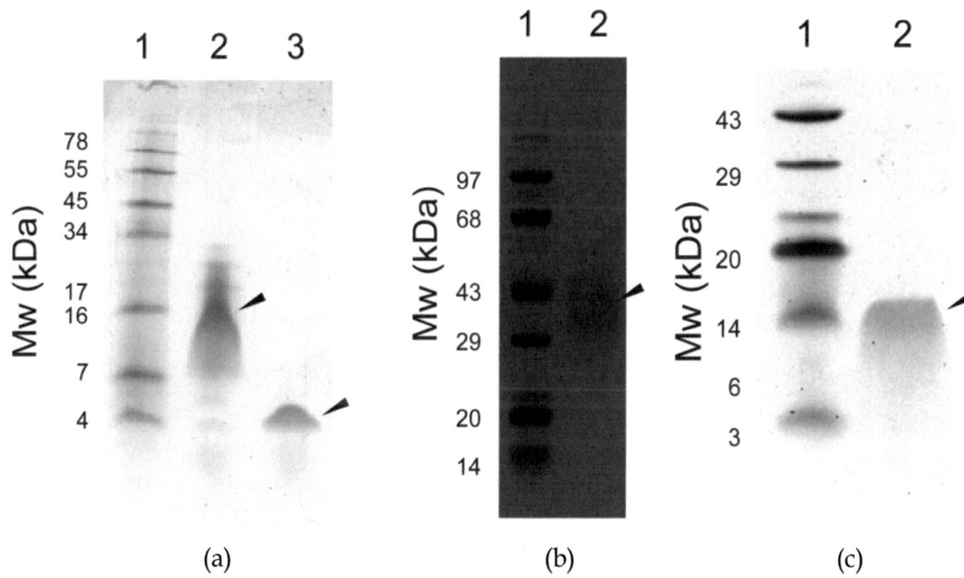

Fig. 2. PAGE analysis of SH protein and SH-TM in SDS ad PFO. (a) SDS-PAGE of SH protein and SH-TM. Lane 1, protein markers; lane 2, SH protein (expected M.W. 7,808 Da); lane 3, SH-TM (expected M.W. 2,983 Da); (b) PFO-PAGE of SH protein. Lane 1, protein markers; lane 2, SH protein; (c) PFO-PAGE of SH-TM. Lane 1 is protein markers and lane 2 is SH-TM.

We have studied SH protein oligomerization using a purified recombinant form corresponding to subgroup A. The protein was successfully over-expressed in *E. coli* and purified by RP-HPLC to high purity. One of the methods that can be used to study oligomerization is SDS-PAGE electrophoresis, which can maintain native oligomeric size in some cases, e.g., glycophorin A and phospholamban (Lemmon et al., 1992; Simmerman et al., 1996). Usually, however, SDS destabilizes oligomer formation, induces non-specific oligomer formation, or results in anomalous migration (Rath et al., 2009). Thus, in the presence of SDS, SH protein migrated as a diffused band with a molecular weight (~ 17 kDa) consistent with either dimers, or slow monomers (Fig. 2A, lane 2). In contrast, the TM domain of SH protein, SH-TM (residue 18-43), formed only monomers (~3 kDa) in SDS-PAGE (Fig. 2A, lane 3). This indicates that SDS destabilizes possible SH protein oligomers. In contrast to SDS, perfluoro-octanoic acid (PFO) is a milder detergent that protects weak interactions and maintains native oligomeric size (Ramjeesingh et al., 1999). In presence of PFO, SH protein produced a band consistent with a higher molecular weight (~35-40 kDa) compatible with pentamers (Fig. 2B, lane 2). Consistently, the TM domain, SH-TM (residues 18-43), also formed pentamers (~ 15 kDa) in PFO-PAGE (Fig. 2C, lane 2), confirming that the TM domain of SH protein is the main driving force for SH protein pentamerization.

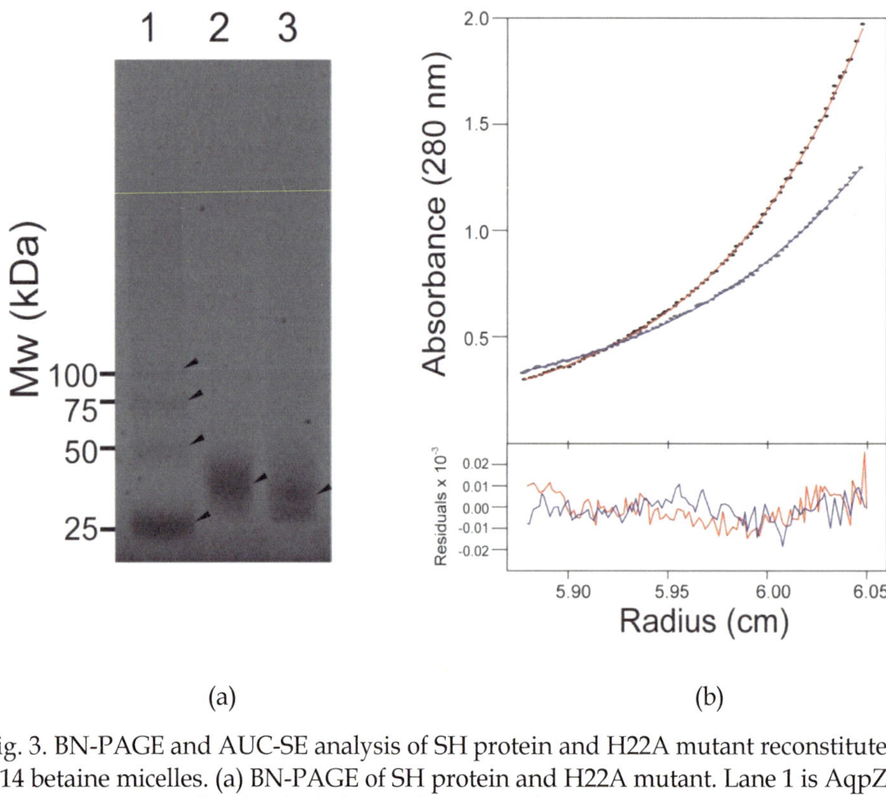

Fig. 3. BN-PAGE and AUC-SE analysis of SH protein and H22A mutant reconstituted in C14 betaine micelles. (a) BN-PAGE of SH protein and H22A mutant. Lane 1 is AqpZ (monomeric size 25 kDa), which forms oligomers of several sizes in these conditions was used as protein markers; lane 2 is SH protein (expected MW 7808 Da), and lane 3 is H22A mutant (expected MW 7742 Da); (b) Representative traces of a global fit analysis of SH protein to a monomer-pentamer self-association model (red line), and H22A mutant to a monomer-tetramer model (blue line). The data shown were collected with 80 μM protein solubilized in 5 mM C14 betaine micelles, centrifuged at 24,000 rpm. The data is shown as black filled circles. The residuals of the fit are shown below.

As both SDS and PFO are anionic charge detergents, we also studied SH oligomerization in C14 betaine, a zwitterionic detergent. This was assessed in both Blue Native-PAGE (BN-PAGE) and in analytical ultracentrifugation sedimentation equilibrium (AUC-SE) experiments (Fig. 3). In the presence of C14 betaine, SH protein migrates as a single band in BN-PAGE, between monomeric and dimeric AqpZ (i.e., between 25 and 50 kDa), consistent with an SH pentamer (~40 kDa) (Fig. 3A, lane 2). The AUC-SE data for SH protein reconstituted into C14 betaine micelles was also best fitted to a monomer-pentamer model (Fig. 3B, red line). Therefore, the above studies point unequivocally to a pentameric form for SH. Recent electron microscopy studies using a >80 residue long construct containing SH protein have produced ambiguous results that could be assigned to a pentamer or a hexamer (Carter et al., 2010).

The energetics of the interaction between SH monomers was also obtained from AUC-SE data. These studies provide dissociation constant and distribution of oligomeric species over a wide range of concentrations for a reversibly associating system in solution. The calculated standard free energy ($\Delta G°$) was -16.3 kcal/mol, i.e., 78% to 88% of SH protein forms pentamers in these conditions. For comparison, SARS-CoV E protein, also a small membrane protein of 76 amino acids with a single α-helical TM domain (Torres et al., 2006), associates forming pentamers with standard free energy of -9.45 kcal/mol, therefore SH protein has a higher propensity for pentamerization.

2.5 His22 mutation destabilizes the pentameric form of SH protein

The pentameric structure of SH-TM has been modeled by combining evolutionary conservation data in global search molecular dynamics (GSMD) simulations and orientational restrains derived from infrared linear dichroism analysis of an isotopically labeled SH-TM peptide in lipid bilayers (Gan et al., 2008). In this model, His22 was located facing the lumen or inter-helical region of the pentamer. This is reminiscent of a similar residue (His37) found at the TM domain of Influenza A M2 proton channel. In M2, this histidine residue is located in a lumenal orientation, and it has been shown to be important for the tetramerization of M2 (Howard et al., 2002), as well as an essential residue involved in proton transport.

Consistent with this lumenal or interfacial location, a H22A mutant in C14 betaine migrated faster than wild type (WT) SH protein, likely as tetramers (Fig. 3A, lane 3). Also, AUC-SE data in C14 betaine micelles could not be fitted to a monomer-pentamer equilibrium model, but it could be fitted to a monomer-tetramer model (Fig. 3B, blue line). The standard free energy of association was -12.83 kcal/mol. Indeed, histidine is a good candidate to mediate TM α-helix association; the polar Nδ and Nε atoms of the imidazole ring are capable of being both hydrogen bond donor and acceptor.

2.6 SH protein as a viroporin

Viroporin is a general term applied to small hydrophobic proteins encoded by viruses that increase membrane permeability (Gonzalez & Carrasco, 2003). Generally, these proteins are 60-120 amino acids long with one or two α-helical TM domains. They oligomerize in membranes to form pores, allowing passage of ions or small molecules across the lipid bilayer. It has been suggested that viroporins acts as a virulence factor during infection. They are not essential for virus replication but their presence enhances virus growth. Forming an ion channel may be one of the strategies for viruses to survive in the host system. The channel activity of viroporins leads to the dissipation of the membrane potential and disruption of cells homeostasis, leading to gradually damage of cells as infection progresses. To date, more than ten viroporins have been identified from various viruses, and influenza A virus M2 proton channel is probably the best studied example (Zhou et al., 2001; Schnell & Chou, 2008; Stouffer et al., 2008). Structural and *in vivo* electrophysiological studies of viroporins are lacking, partially due to the difficulty in expression and purification of the hydrophobic membrane proteins. Nonetheless, structures of the SARS-CoV E protein (Pervushin et al., 2009), the HCV p7 protein(Cook & Opella, 2009), and the HIV-1 Vpu proteins (Park et al., 2003; Sharpe et al., 2006) have been studied by NMR methods. Channel activities for these proteins have been confirmed using black lipid membranes (BLM) and can be blocked by hexamethylene amiloride (HMA) (Ewart et al., 2002; Premkumar et al., 2004; Pervushin et al., 2009), whereas we have shown that SARS-CoV E protein also displays channel activity in a mammalian whole-cell patch clamp set-up (Pervushin et al., 2009).

In the case of SH protein, both SH-TM (residues 18-43) (Gan et al., 2008) and full-length SH protein have channel activity when reconstituted in BLMs (Fig. 4A). More direct evidence for channel activity is provided using whole-cell patch clamp experiments of SH protein-transfected HEK293 cell lines. In these experiments, expression of full-length SH gene was monitored by GFP, and the fluorescence intensity was correlated with expression level of SH protein (Marshall et al., 1995). The full-length SH protein displayed channel activity when transiently expressed in HEK293 cells (Fig. 4B). When placed in bath solution with neutral pH, the transfected cells produced significant higher channel activity than the controls, the cells transfected with vector alone (Fig. 4B, left panel). Molecular modeling of the α-helical region of SH protein shows several polar residues lining the lumen of the pore, including charged residues: His22, Lys43, and His51. The pK_a for lysine and histidine are about 11.1 and 6, respectively. Therefore, histidines are most likely contributing to changes in SH channel activity if the pH of the bath solution was changed from neutral to acidic pH.

We have shown in a BLM experiment that SH-TM which contains His22 was acid sensitive (Gan et al., 2008). To test the effect of acidification on channel activity for the full-length SH protein, the bath solution were changed to pH 5.5 after a stable conductance were recorded in neutral pH. In contrast to the control, in which no changes were observed upon pH changes (Fig. 4B, right panel), the SH channel responded more actively in acidic solution. Larger outward current was detected upon exposure of SH channel to acidic solution, therefore we have shown that SH channel activity is pH dependent. Whether residue His22 or His51 is involved in the pH regulation, and the role of the channel activity in virus life cycle, requires further investigation.

Recently, studies have indicated that SH protein can inhibit apoptosis in several mammalian cell lines by blocking the tumor necrosis factor alpha (TNF-α)-mediated apoptotic signaling pathway (Fuentes et al., 2007). However, ion channels may also control apoptosis in cells (Szabo et al., 2004; Lang et al., 2005; Burg et al., 2006; Madan et al., 2008). Disruption of cells homeostasis is a common sign of apoptosis, leading to plasma membrane depolarization associated with intracellular cation overload and cell volume decreases due to anion and water efflux (Burg et al., 2006). In fact, the viroporin of Sindbis virus 6K, murine hepatitisvirus E protein, Influenza A M2 protein, HCV p7 protein, poliovirus 2b and 3A protein have been reported to manipulate apoptosis of infected cells (Neznanov et al., 2001; Campanella et al., 2004; Madan et al., 2008). While promotion of apoptosis helps to release the virus, inhibition of apoptosis in host cells during infection gives an advantage to the virus to replicate. In future, drugs that block ion channel of several viroporins, such as amantadine, rimantadine, and HMA could be tested on SH ion channel to obtain further understanding of the channel properties of SH protein.

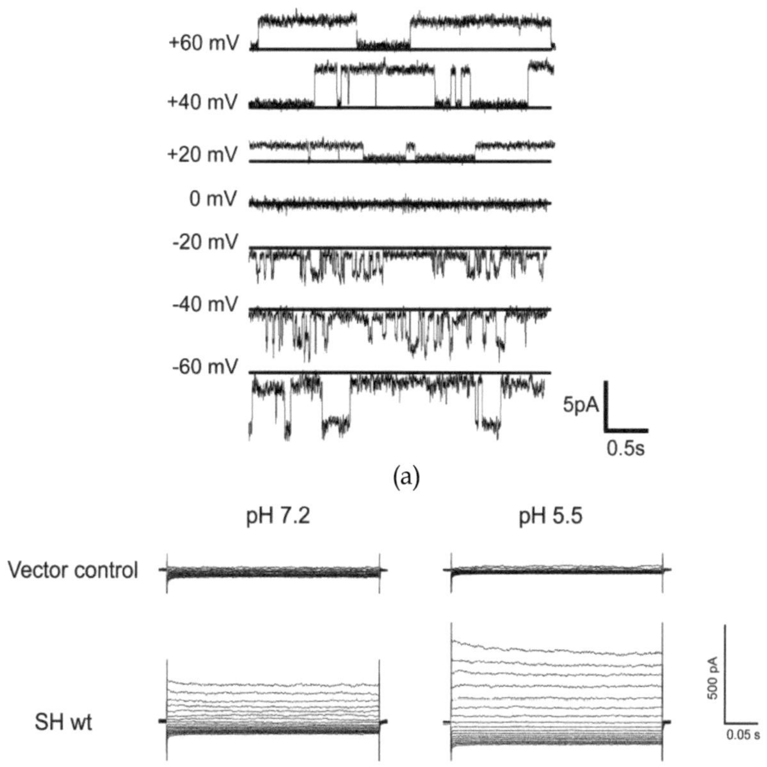

Fig. 4. SH is a viroporin. (a) Single channel elicited by SH protein when inserted into BLMs, recorded in 300 mM KCl, 5 mM Hepes, pH 5.5 buffer solution; (b) Traces of currents evoked in HEK-292 cells transfected with a vector carrying SH protein or vector alone, in neutral or acidic pH bath solutions.

2.7 Secondary structure of SH protein using attenuated total reflection fourier transform infrared (ATR-FTIR) spectroscopy

The amide I region in the infrared spectrum (Fig. 5A) can be assigned to different secondary structure elements (Byler & Susi, 1986). Full length SH protein shows a major peak centered at 1653 cm^{-1} and a shoulder centered at 1632 cm^{-1} indicating a mixture of α-helix and β-strand (Fig. 5A, upper panel). For SH-TM, a narrow band centered at 1654 cm^{-1} indicates a large fraction of α-helix (Fig. 5A, middle panel). For a synthetic peptide that consists of the last 20 C-terminal residues (SH-C20) the spectrum is centered at 1635 cm^{-1}, indicating a majority of β-strand structure (Fig. 5A, bottom panel). A quantification of the α-helix present in full length SH protein produced ~40 residues whereas only ~20 were present in the TM domain alone. This suggests that some α-helix is present in the extramembrane domain.

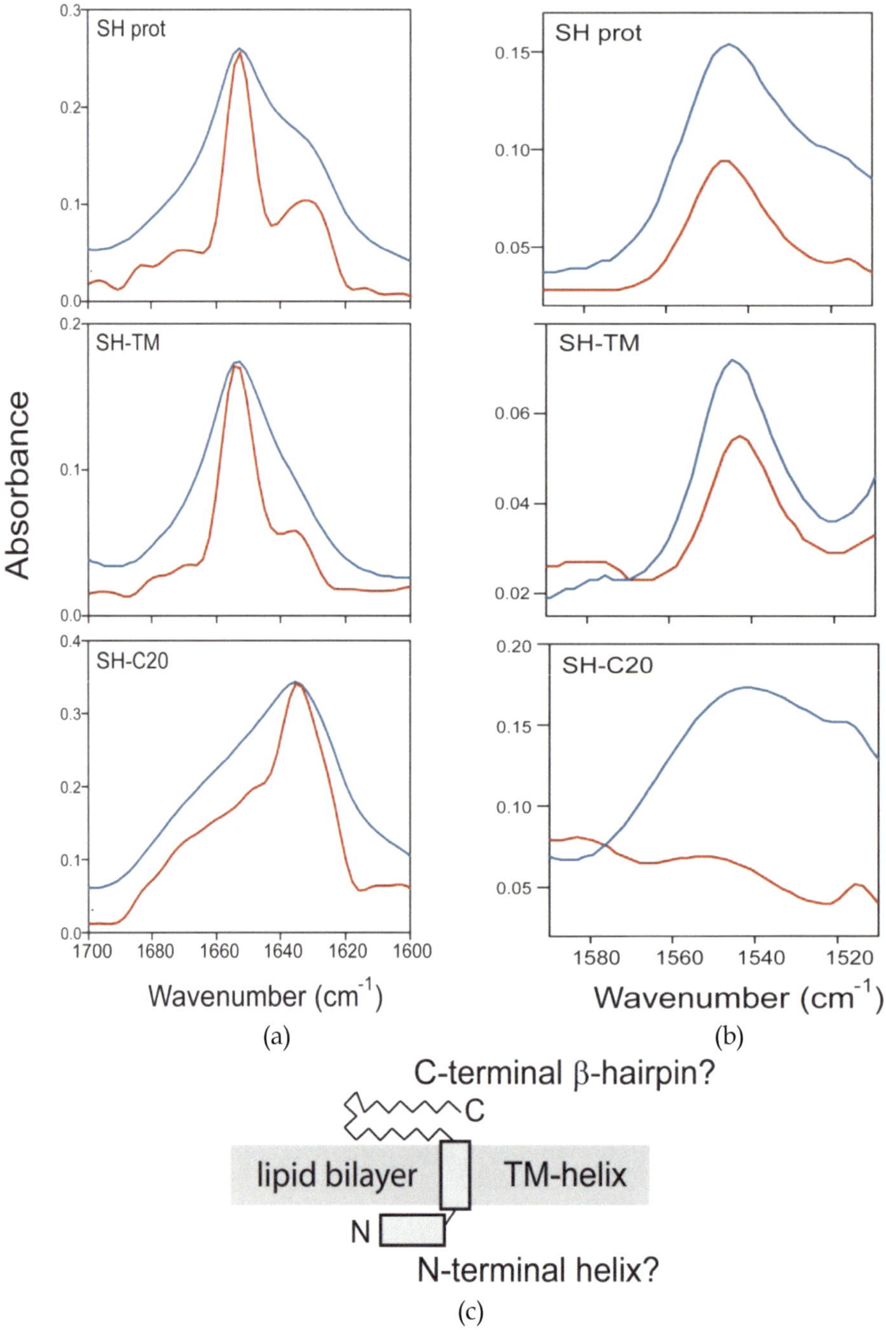

Fig. 5. ATR-FTIR spectra and H/D exchange of SH protein and fragments. (a) Amide I region corresponding to SH protein, SH-TM, and SH-C20. Lines for original spectrum (blue) and Fourier self deconvolved spectrum (red) are shown; (b) Amide II region of the same samples before (blue) and after (red) 1 hour exposure to D_2O (Torres et al., 2006); (c) Sketch representing the main features of SH according to the data in (A-B).

The amide II band in the infrared spectrum, due to peptide backbone N-H bending vibration, is used to monitor protein hydrogen-deuterium (H/D) exchange kinetics. Upon H/D exchange, the frequency of amide II downshifts from ~1545 to ~1450 cm^{-1} (~100 cm^{-1}). Thus, amide exchange can be measured following the decrease in intensity of the unexchanged amide II. H/D exchange can be used to determine the number of residues embedded in the bilayer. The spectra of the amide II band of SH protein, SH-TM, and SH-C20 recorded in H_2O and after one hour exposure to D_2O (Fig. 5B) shows 45%, 80% and 11% of protected residues, respectively. These results suggest that the only embedded fraction corresponds to TM α-helix whereas SH-C20 is not inserted into the membrane. A preliminary sketch of the pentameric model and its secondary structural elements is shown in Fig. 5C.

2.8 Effects of SH, SH-TM and SH-C20 on lipid order

ATR-FTIR is a most suitable tool to study lipid-protein interactions because lipids absorb in many regions of the infrared spectrum. Further, lipid orientational order parameter determination and lipid phase information can be obtained because the frequencies of methylene stretching change upon gel-to-liquid crystal phase transition. The lipid methylene C-H stretching transition dipole is oriented perpendicular to the long axis of an all-*trans* fatty acid chain, therefore measuring linear dichroism of lipid methylene stretching vibrations can be used to probe the orientation of lipid bilayers when deposited on a germanium trapezoid. The order parameter S_L (Tamm & Tatulian, 1997) is calculated for lipid bilayer deposited on the surface of a germanium trapezoid, with electric field components for the evanescent field (Arkin et al., 1997). Thus, a decrease in the dichroic ratio, R_L, corresponds to an increase in the acyl chain order parameter, S_L. Lipid-protein interactions of SH protein, SH-TM, and SH-C20 were investigated in supported DMPC and POPC bilayers (Fig. 6) using both lipid methylene symmetric (~2851 cm^{-1}) and antisymmetric (~2919 cm^{-1}) stretching vibrations to calculate R_L and S_L. The measured values of R_L for DMPC bilayers were 1.14 (S_L = 0.59) for symmetric, and 1.20 (S_L =0.55) for antisymmetric vibrations. These values are in good agreement with published data (Hubner & Mantsch, 1991), indicating well-ordered lipid bilayers.

The frequency of the lipid methylene C-H stretching bands of DMPC (T_m = 23°C) indicated that the membranes were in the gel phase (Tamm & Tatulian, 1997). Therefore, spectra for SH protein and SH-TM were recorded also in POPC (T_m = -2°C), which should form a fluid liquid crystal phase due to the presence of unsaturated bonds in the *sn*-2 chain of the POPC acyl chain. This was evident from the shift in the lipid symmetric stretching vibration, from 2851 to 2853 cm^{-1}, and the anti-symmetric methylene stretching vibration, from 2919 to 2923 cm^{-1} (Tamm & Tatulian, 1997). The values of R_L for POPC bilayers measured in our system were 1.31 (S_L = 0.38) and 1.32 (S_L = 0.37) for symmetric and antisymmetric vibrations, respectively. These values are lower than those of DMPC.

In the presence of protein, for simplicity, only lipid methylene symmetric vibrations were measured. Although no changes in lipid order parameter were observed after SH protein was reconstituted in DMPC (R_L = 1.14 and S_L = 0.59), disorder was observed in POPC (R_L = 1.46 and S_L = 0.23). In contrast, SH-TM increased the order of the acyl chains in both DMPC

(R_L = 1.07 and S_L = 0.69) and POPC (R_L = 1.27 and S_L = 0.43). Interaction of SH-C20 was measured only in DMPC, where a 20% increase in disorder was observed (R_L = 1.27 and S_L = 0.43). Thus, this short β-structure forming peptide (Fig. 5C) is able to destabilize membranes.

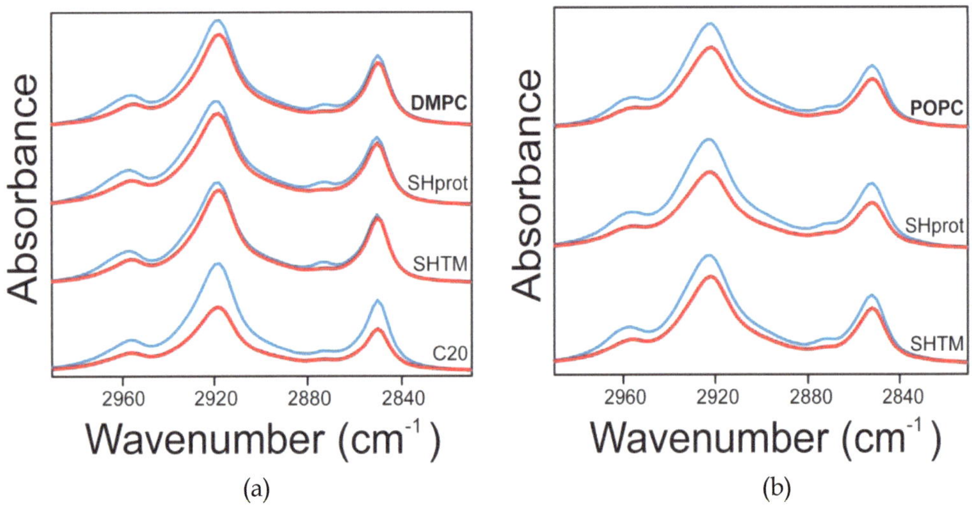

Fig. 6. Polarized ATR-FTIR spectra of the lipid methylene stretching vibrations. Supported DMPC (a) and POPC (b) lipid bilayers in the absence or presence of SH protein, SH-TM, and SH-C20. Blue and red lines correspond to parallel and perpendicular polarizations, respectively.

2.9 Detection of an intra-helical hydrogen bond in SH-TM

During our attempts to measure the dichroism of labeled SH-TM, we observed that the $^{13}C=^{18}O$ isotope label at L31 was shifted to a lower frequency, from 1592 cm^{-1} to 1576 cm^{-1} (Gan et al., 2008). According to the harmonic oscillator model, downshift of a vibrational frequency can occur if the reduced mass is increased, or the strength of a bond is weakened. This data is consistent with the presence of an intra-helical hydrogen bond between the hydroxyl side chain of Ser35 and the backbone carbonyl oxygen from Leu31 (Fig. 7B). Indeed, when Ser35 was replaced by alanine, the frequency of the $^{13}C=^{18}O$ isotope label at L31 reverted to its expected range, at 1589 cm^{-1} (Fig. 7A). This indicates that an intra-helical hydrogen bond exists in the TM domain of SH protein, which weakens the carbonyl bond, resulting in the downshift observed.

There is a high tendency for serine or threonine residues in α-helices to form intrahelical hydrogen bonds to carbonyl oxygen at position *i*-4 (Baker & Hubbard, 1984), which could induce a kink in the α-helix that may be important for functionality (Ballesteros et al., 2000). Indeed, viral ion channels display certain degree of structural flexibility, as seen in the influenza A virus M2 protein (Li et al., 2007) and SARS-CoV E protein (Parthasarathy et al., 2008).

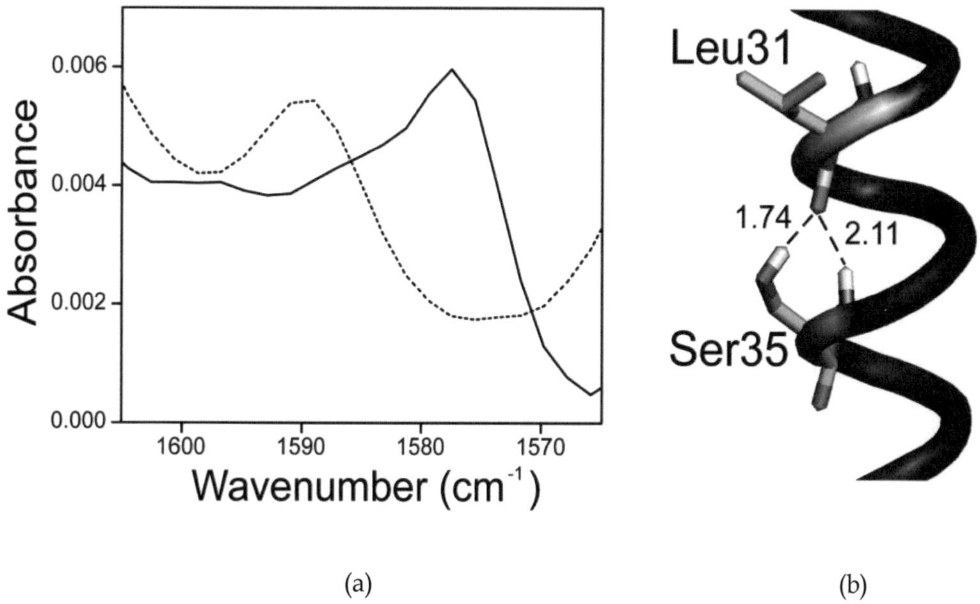

Fig. 7. Hydrogen bonding in SH-TM detected by FTIR. (a) Infrared spectra of SH-TM labeled at L31 $^{13}C=^{18}O$ (solid line) and for a S35A mutant (broken line); (b) Schematic representation of the proposed hydrogen bond between Ser35 side chain and Leu31 backbone C=O.

2.10 Structural determination of SH protein in detergent micelles by solution NMR

The HSQC spectrum of ^{15}N labeled SH protein was tested in three detergents: DPC (medium-chain, zwitterionic), DHPC (short-chain, zwitterionic), and SDS (anionic) (Fig. 8). Although SDS is a harsh detergent, well-resolved spectra of membrane proteins have been recorded (Howell et al., 2005; Franzin et al., 2007; Teriete et al., 2007). In contrast, DPC and DHPC have a headgroup that closely mimics that of phosphatidylcholine, the most abundant headgroup in natural membranes, successfully used in KcsA (Yu et al., 2005), human phospholamban (Oxenoid & Chou, 2005), diacylglycerol kinase (Van Horn et al., 2009), Rv1761c from Mycobacterium tuberculosis (Page et al., 2009), influenza A M2 (Schnell & Chou, 2008) or HIV Vpu (Park et al., 2003).

For SH protein, $^{1}H/^{15}N$-HSQC spectra showed limited peak dispersion, resonances not well-resolved, and overlapping peaks (Fig. 8). Only about 50% of the peaks could be observed in SDS and DHPC, whereas DPC appeared to be the best detergent with about 75% of peaks observed. Sample heterogeneity was observed in all three detergents, evidenced by the double resonance observed for the tryptophan indole side chain, Nε-Hε, at around 10.0-10.5 ^{1}H ppm (see the inserts of Fig. 8). As only one tryptophan residue is present in SH protein, only one peak should be observed. This indicates the presence of two backbone conformations, or two different rotameric states of the tryptophan indole side chain.

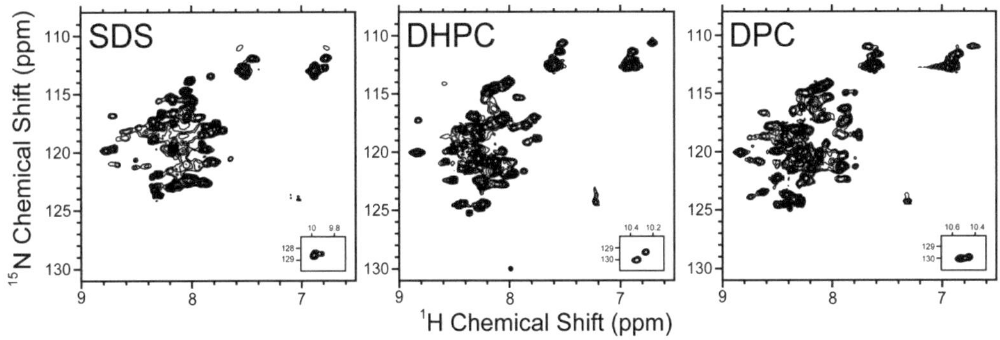

Fig. 8. Effect of different micellar environments on SH protein shown by $^{1}H/^{15}N$-HSQC spectra. The detergents SDS (left), DHPC (middle), and DPC (right) were used to obtain the spectra. In each graph, the resonance of Trp15 side chain is shown in the insert.

3. Summary and conclusions

Viral respiratory diseases pose serious threats to human health and effective antiviral agents are limited. Specifically, hRSV is one of the main agents responsible to widespread infection causing millions of clinical cases each year. Vaccines, antibodies and small drugs are being sought, but effective treatments are not yet available. The discovery of proteins known as 'viroporins' in many viruses has opened a potentially effective field for antiviral therapy. In hRSV, biochemical and biophysical studies have shown that SH protein has the characteristics of a viroporin, and this chapter has described biophysical properties of this purified protein that ultimately may help elucidate its role in RSV infection.

A first step in the characterization of a protein is its successful expression and purification. Both the full length and the TM domain of SH protein assemble as homopentamers, with His22 having a stabilizing role. The study of SH protein by solution NMR methods is in progress, and it shows good potential, especially in DPC micelles and in bicelles, although at present dual conformations are observed. Other lower resolution techniques, such as FTIR, have provided data that allow to obtain a preliminary model of full length SH protein, based on H/D exchange, β-structure in the last 20 amino acids, and the higher than expected helical content in the full length protein, when compared to the TM domain. The C-terminal β-structure has a destabilizing effect on membranes and may fold as a β-hairpin. FTIR of isotopically labeled TM domain has detected an intra-helical hydrogen bond between the backbone carbonyl oxygen of Leu31 and the side chain of Ser35 in the TM domain that could be important for channel activity. Conductance studies of SH protein provide compelling evidence that SH behaves as an ion channel, where histidine side chains may have an important regulatory role. The involvement of histidine as a pH sensor has been observed in other ion channels. In influenza A M2, His 37 is responsible for pH sensitivity (Schnell & Chou, 2008; Stouffer et al., 2008), and other examples of histidine regulated pH sensitive ion channels exist, for example the bacterial potassium channel KscA (His25) (Takeuchi et al., 2007), the potassium channel ROMK1 (four histidine residues are involved) (Chanchevalap et al., 2000), the potassium channel TASK1 (His98) (Yuill et al., 2007), potassium channel TREK-1 (His126) or TREK-2 (His151) (Sandoz et al., 2009). Therefore, the hypothesis that the TM histidine in SH protein (His22) has a regulatory role is worth exploring.

SH protein has been associated with fusion activity during infection, and with membrane permeabilization, and the structural features observed seem to reflect these functions.

Finally, channel activity in other viroporins can be blocked, e.g., the influenza A virus M2 proton channel blocked by amantadine and rimantadine (Wang et al., 1994; Chizhmakov et al., 1996), the amiloride derivative hexamethylene amiloride (HMA) inhibits ion channel activity of HIV-1 Vpu proteins (Ewart et al., 2002), SARS-CoV E protein (Pervushin et al., 2009), and HCV p7 protein (Premkumar et al., 2004). At present, there are no drugs reported that can block SH channel activity. The discovery of such compounds is important both for antiviral therapy and to understand the biology of SH protein.

4. Acknowledgement

This work has been funded by the Singapore National Research Foundation Grant (NRF-CRP4-2008-02) [to J.T.]. We also thank Edward Tan and Ye Hong for collecting some of the NMR HSQC data shown.

5. References

Andries, K., Moeremans, M., Gevers, T., Willebrords, R., Sommen, C., Lacrampe, J., Janssens, F. & Wyde, P.R. 2003. Substituted benzimidazoles with nanomolar activity against respiratory syncytial virus. *Antiviral Res*, Vol. 60, pp. 209-219.

Arkin, I.T., MacKenzie, K.R. & Brunger, A.T. 1997. Site-directed dichroism as a method for obtaining rotational and orientational constraints for oriented polymers. *J Am Chem Soc*, Vol. 119, pp. 8973-8980.

Baker, E.N. & Hubbard, R.E. 1984. Hydrogen bonding in globular proteins 78. *Prog Biophys Mol Biol*, Vol. 44, pp. 97-179.

Ballesteros, J.A., Deupi, X., Olivella, M., Haaksma, E.E. & Pardo, L. 2000. Serine and threonine residues bend alpha-helices in the chi(1) = g(-) conformation. *Biophys J*, Vol. 79, pp. 2754-2760.

Brown, G., Aitken, J., Rixon, H.W. & Sugrue, R.J. 2002. Caveolin-1 is incorporated into mature respiratory syncytial virus particles during virus assembly on the surface of virus-infected cells. *J Gen Virol*, Vol. 83, pp. 611-621.

Bukreyev, A., Whitehead, S.S., Murphy, B.R. & Collins, P.L. 1997. Recombinant respiratory syncytial virus from which the entire SH gene has been deleted grows efficiently in cell culture and exhibits site-specific attenuation in the respiratory tract of the mouse. *J Virol*, Vol. 71, pp. 8973-8982.

Burg, E.D., Remillard, C.V. & Yuan, J.X.J. 2006. K+ channels in apoptosis. *J Membr Biol*, Vol. 209, pp. 3-20.

Byler, D.M. & Susi, H. 1986. Examination of the secondary structure of proteins by deconvolved FTIR spectra. *Biopolymers*, Vol. 25, pp. 469-487.

Calder, L.J., Gonzalez-Reyes, L., Garcia-Barreno, B., Wharton, S.A., Skehel, J.J., Wiley, D.C. & Melero, J.A. 2000. Electron microscopy of the human respiratory syncytial virus fusion protein and complexes that it forms with monoclonal antibodies. *Virology*, Vol. 271, pp. 122-131.

Campanella, M., de Jong, A.S., Lanke, K.W., Melchers, W.J., Willems, P.H., Pinton, P., Rizzuto, R. & van Kuppeveld, F.J. 2004. The coxsackievirus 2B protein suppresses apoptotic host cell responses by manipulating intracellular Ca2+ homeostasis. *J Biol Chem*, Vol. 279, pp. 18440-18450.

Carter, S.D., Dent, K.C., Atkins, E., Foster, T.L., Verow, M., Gorny, P., Harris, M., Hiscox, J.A., Ranson, N.A., Griffin, S. & Barr, J.N. 2010. Direct visualization of the small hydrophobic protein of human respiratory syncytial virus reveals the structural basis for membrane permeability. *FEBS Lett*, Vol. 584, pp. 2786-2790.

Chanchevalap, S., Yang, Z., Cui, N., Qu, Z., Zhu, G., Liu, C., Giwa, L.R., Abdulkadir, L. & Jiang, C. 2000. Involvement of histidine residues in proton sensing of ROMK1 channel. *J Biol Chem*, Vol. 275, pp. 7811-7817.

Chang, J. 2011. Current progress on development of respiratory syncytial virus vaccine. *BMB Reports*, Vol. 44, pp. 232-237.

Chizhmakov, I.V., Geraghty, F.M., Ogden, D.C., Hayhurst, A., Antoniou, M. & Hay, A.J. 1996. Selective proton permeability and pH regulation of the influenza virus M2 channel expressed in mouse erythroleukaemia cells. *J Physiol*, Vol. 494 (Pt 2), pp. 329-336.

Cianci, C., Yu, K.L., Combrink, K., Sin, N., Pearce, B., Wang, A., Civiello, R., Voss, S., Luo, G., Kadow, K., Genovesi, E.V., Venables, B., Gulgeze, H., Trehan, A., James, J., Lamb, L., Medina, I., Roach, J., Yang, Z., Zadjura, L., Colonno, R., Clark, J., Meanwell, N. & Krystal, M. 2004. Orally active fusion inhibitor of respiratory syncytial virus. *Antimicrob Agents Chemother*, Vol. 48, pp. 413-422.

Collins, P.L. & Mottet, G. 1993. Membrane orientation and oligomerization of the small hydrophobic protein of human respiratory syncytial virus. *J Gen Virol*, Vol. 74 (Pt 7), pp. 1445-1450.

Collins, P.L. & Murphy, B.R. 2006. Vaccines against Human Respiratory Syncytial Virus. In *Perspectives in Medical Virology*, pp. 233-278.

Collins, P.L., Olmsted, R.A. & Johnson, P.R. 1990. The small hydrophobic protein of human respiratory syncytial virus: comparison between antigenic subgroups A and B. *J Gen Virol*, Vol. 71 (Pt 7), pp. 1571-1576.

Connors, M., Collins, P.L., Firestone, C.Y. & Murphy, B.R. 1991. Respiratory syncytial virus (RSV) F, G, M2 (22K), and N proteins each induce resistance to RSV challenge, but resistance induced by M2 and N proteins is relatively short-lived. *J Virol*, Vol. 65, pp. 1634-1637.

Cook, G.A. & Opella, S.J. 2009. NMR studies of p7 protein from hepatitis C virus. *Eur Biophys J*, Vol. 39, pp. 1097-1104

Dykstra, M., Cherukuri, A., Sohn, H.W., Tzeng, S.J. & Pierce, S.K. 2003. Location is everything: lipid rafts and immune cell signaling. *Annu Rev Immunol*, Vol. 21, pp. 457-481.

Escribano-Romero, E., Rawling, J., Garcia-Barreno, B. & Melero, J.A. 2004. The soluble form of human respiratory syncytial virus attachment protein differs from the membrane-bound form in its oligomeric state but is still capable of binding to cell surface proteoglycans. *J Virol*, Vol. 78, pp. 3524-3532.

Eshaghi, S., Niegowski, D., Kohl, A., Martinez Molina, D., Lesley, S.A. & Nordlund, P. 2006. Crystal structure of a divalent metal ion transporter CorA at 2.9 angstrom resolution. *Science*, Vol. 313, pp. 354-357.

Ewart, G.D., Mills, K., Cox, G.B. & Gage, P.W. 2002. Amiloride derivatives block ion channel activity and enhancement of virus-like particle budding caused by HIV-1 protein Vpu. *Eur Biophysical Journal*, Vol. 31, pp. 26-35.

Falsey, A.R., Hennessey, P.A., Formica, M.A., Cox, C. & Walsh, E.E. 2005. Respiratory syncytial virus infection in elderly and high-risk adults. *N Engl J Med*, Vol. 352, pp. 1749-1759.

Feldman, S.A., Crim, R.L., Audet, S.A. & Beeler, J.A. 2001. Human respiratory syncytial virus surface glycoproteins F, G and SH form an oligomeric complex. *Arch Virol*, Vol. 146, pp. 2369-2383.

Franzin, C.M., Teriete, P. & Marassi, F.M. 2007. Structural similarity of a membrane protein in micelles and membranes. *J Am Chem Soc*, Vol. 129, pp. 8078-8079.

Fuentes, S., Tran, K.C., Luthra, P., Teng, M.N. & He, B. 2007. Function of the respiratory syncytial virus small hydrophobic protein. *Journal of Virology*, Vol. 81, pp. 8361-8366.

Gan, S.W., Ng, L., Lin, X., Gong, X. & Torres, J. 2008. Structure and ion channel activity of the human respiratory syncytial virus (hRSV) small hydrophobic protein transmembrane domain. *Protein Sci*, Vol. 17, pp. 813-820.

Glezen, W.P., Taber, L.H., Frank, A.L. & Kasel, J.A. 1986. Risk of primary infection and reinfection with respiratory syncytial virus. *American Journal of Diseases of Children*, Vol. 140, pp. 543-546.

Gonzalez, M.E. & Carrasco, L. 2003. Viroporins. *FEBS Letters*, Vol. 552, pp. 28-34.

Group, T.I.-R.S. 1998. Palivizumab, a humanized respiratory syncytial virus monoclonal antibody, reduces hospitalization from respiratory syncytial virus infection in high-risk infants. The IMpact-RSV Study Group. *Pediatrics*, Vol. 102, pp. 531-537.

He, B., Lin, G.Y., Durbin, J.E., Durbin, R.K. & Lamb, R.A. 2001. The SH integral membrane protein of the paramyxovirus simian virus 5 is required to block apoptosis in MDBK cells. *J Virol*, Vol. 75, pp. 4068-4079.

Helms, J.B. & Zurzolo, C. 2004. Lipids as targeting signals: lipid rafts and intracellular trafficking. *Traffic*, Vol. 5, pp. 247-254.

Heminway, B.R., Yu, Y., Tanaka, Y., Perrine, K.G., Gustafson, E., Bernstein, J.M. & Galinski, M.S. 1994. Analysis of respiratory syncytial virus F, G, and SH proteins in cell fusion. *Virology*, Vol. 200, pp. 801-805.

Howard, K.P., Lear, J.D. & DeGrado, W.F. 2002. Sequence determinants of the energetics of folding of a transmembrane four-helix-bundle protein. *Proc Natl Acad Sci U S A*, Vol. 99, pp. 8568-8572.

Howell, S.C., Mesleh, M.F. & Opella, S.J. 2005. NMR structure determination of a membrane protein with two transmembrane helices in micelles: MerF of the bacterial mercury detoxification system. *Biochemistry*, Vol. 44, pp. 5196-5206.

Hubner, W. & Mantsch, H.H. 1991. Orientation of specifically 13C=O labeled phosphatidylcholine multilayers from polarized attenuated total reflection FT-IR spectroscopy. *Biophys J*, Vol. 59, pp. 1261-1272.

Johnson, P.R., Spriggs, M.K., Olmsted, R.A. & Collins, P.L. 1987. The G glycoprotein of human respiratory syncytial viruses of subgroups A and B: extensive sequence divergence between antigenically related proteins. *Proc Nat Acad Sci USA*, Vol. 84, pp. 5625-5629.

Johnson, S., Oliver, C., Prince, G.A., Hemming, V.G., Pfarr, D.S., Wang, S.C., Dormitzcr, M., O'Grady, J., Koenig, S., Tamura, J.K., Woods, R., Bansal, G., Couchenour, D., Tsao, E., Hall, W.C. & Young, J.F. 1997. Development of a humanized monoclonal antibody (MEDI-493) with potent in vitro and in vivo activity against respiratory syncytial virus. *J Infect Dis*, Vol. 176, pp. 1215-1224.

Kapikian, A.Z., Mitchell, R.H., Chanock, R.M., Shvedoff, R.A. & Stewart, C.E. 1969. An epidemiologic study of altered clinical reactivity to Respiratory Syncytial (RS) virus infection in children previously vaccinated with an inactivated RS virus vaccine. *Am J Epidemiol*, Vol. 89, pp. 405-421.

Karron, R.A., Wright, P.F., Belshe, R.B., Thumar, B., Casey, R., Newman, F., Polack, F.P., Randolph, V.B., Deatly, A., Hackell, J., Gruber, W., Murphy, B.R. & Collins, P.L. 2005. Identification of a recombinant live attenuated respiratory syncytial virus vaccine candidate that is highly attenuated in infants. *J Infect Dis*, Vol. 191, pp. 1093-1104.

Kovacs, F.A. & Cross, T.A. 1997. Transmembrane four-helix bundle of influenza A M2 protein channel: structural implications from helix tilt and orientation. *Biophys J*, Vol. 73, pp. 2511-2517.

Krogh, A., Larsson, B., von Heijne, G. & Sonnhammer, E.L.L. 2001. Predicting transmembrane protein topology with a hidden Markov model: Application to complete genomes. *J Mol Biol*, Vol. 305, pp. 567-580.

Krusat, T. & Streckert, H.J. 1997. Heparin-dependent attachment of respiratory syncytial virus (RSV) to host cells. *Arch Virol*, Vol. 142, pp. 1247-1254.

Lamb, R.A. 1993. Paramyxovirus fusion: a hypothesis for changes. *Virology*, Vol. 197, pp. 1-11.

Lamb, R.A., Joshi, S.B. & Dutch, R.E. 1999. The paramyxovirus fusion protein forms an extremely stable core trimer: structural parallels to influenza virus haemagglutinin and HIV-1 gp41. *Mol Membr Biol*, Vol. 16, pp. 11-19.

Lang, F., Foller, M., Lang, K.S., Lang, P.A., Ritter, M., Gulbins, E., Vereninov, A. & Huber, S.M. 2005. Ion channels in cell proliferation and apoptotic cell death. *J Membr Biol*, Vol. 205, pp. 147-157.

Lemmon, M.A., Flanagan, J.M., Treutlein, H.R., Zhang, J. & Engelman, D.M. 1992. Sequence specificity in the dimerization of transmembrane alpha-helices. *Biochemistry*, Vol. 31, pp. 12719-12725.

Li, C., Qin, H., Gao, F.P. & Cross, T.A. 2007. Solid-state NMR characterization of conformational plasticity within the transmembrane domain of the influenza A M2 proton channel. *Biochim Biophys Acta*, Vol. 1768, pp. 3162-3170.

Lin, X., Tan, S.M., Law, S.K.A. & Torres, J. 2006. Two types of transmembrane homomeric interactions in the integrin receptor family are evolutionarily conserved. *Proteins*, Vol. 63, pp. 16-23.

Lin, Y., Bright, A.C., Rothermel, T.A. & He, B. 2003. Induction of apoptosis by paramyxovirus simian virus 5 lacking a small hydrophobic gene. *J Virol*, Vol. 77, pp. 3371-3383.

Low, K.W., Tan, T., Ng, K., Tan, B.H. & Sugrue, R.J. 2008. The RSV F and G glycoproteins interact to form a complex on the surface of infected cells. *Biochem Biophys Res Commun*, Vol. 366, pp. 308-313.

Madan, V., Castello, A. & Carrasco, L. 2008. Viroporins from RNA viruses induce caspase-dependent apoptosis. *Cell Microbiol*, Vol. 10, pp. 437-451.

Marshall, J., Molloy, R., Moss, G.W., Howe, J.R. & Hughes, T.E. 1995. The jellyfish green fluorescent protein: a new tool for studying ion channel expression and function. *Neuron*, Vol. 14, pp. 211-215.

McKimm-Breschkin, J. 2000. VP-14637 ViroPharma. *Curr Opin Investig Drugs*, Vol. 1, pp. 425-427.

Murata, Y. 2009. Respiratory Syncytial Virus Vaccine Development. *Clinics in Laboratory Medicine*, Vol. 29, pp. 725-739.

Murphy, B.R., Alling, D.W., Snyder, M.H., Walsh, E.E., Prince, G.A., Chanock, R.M., Hemming, V.G., Rodriguez, W.J., Kim, H.W., Graham, B.S. & et al. 1986. Effect of age and preexisting antibody on serum antibody response of infants and children to the F and G glycoproteins during respiratory syncytial virus infection. *J Clin Microbiol*, Vol. 24, pp. 894-898.

Nair, H., Nokes, D.J., Gessner, B.D., Dherani, M., Madhi, S.A., Singleton, R.J., O'Brien, K.L., Roca, A., Wright, P.F., Bruce, N., Chandran, A., Theodoratou, E., Sutanto, A., Sedyaningsih, E.R., Ngama, M., Munywoki, P.K., Kartasasmita, C., Simoes, E.A., Rudan, I., Weber, M.W. & Campbell, H. 2010. Global burden of acute lower respiratory infections due to respiratory syncytial virus in young children: a systematic review and meta-analysis. *Lancet*, Vol. 375, pp. 1545-1555.

Neznanov, N., Kondratova, A., Chumakov, K.M., Angres, B., Zhumabayeva, B., Agol, V.I. & Gudkov, A.V. 2001. Poliovirus protein 3A inhibits tumor necrosis factor (TNF)-induced apoptosis by eliminating the TNF receptor from the cell surface. *J Virol*, Vol. 75, pp. 10409-10420.

Olmsted, R.A. & Collins, P.L. 1989. The 1A protein of respiratory syncytial virus is an integral membrane protein present as multiple, structurally distinct species. *J Virol*, Vol. 63, pp. 2019-2029.

Olszewska, W. & Openshaw, P. 2009. Emerging drugs for respiratory syncytial virus infection. *Expert Opinion on Emerging Drugs*, Vol. 14, pp. 207-217.

Oxenoid, K. & Chou, J.J. 2005. The structure of phospholamban pentamer reveals a channel-like architecture in membranes. *Proc Natl Acad Sci U S A*, Vol. 102, pp. 10870-10875.

Page, R.C., Lee, S., Moore, J.D., Opella, S.J. & Cross, T.A. 2009. Backbone structure of a small helical integral membrane protein: A unique structural characterization. *Protein Sci*, Vol. 18, pp. 134-146.

Park, S.H., Mrse, A.A., Nevzorov, A.A., Mesleh, M.F., Oblatt-Montal, M., Montal, M. & Opella, S.J. 2003. Three-dimensional structure of the channel-forming trans-membrane domain of virus protein "u" (Vpu) from HIV-1. *J Mol Biol*, Vol. 333, pp. 409-424.

Parthasarathy, K., Ng, L., Lin, X., Liu, D.X., Pervushin, K., Gong, X. & Torres, J. 2008. Structural flexibility of the pentameric SARS coronavirus envelope protein ion channel. *Biophys J*, Vol. 95, pp. L39-41.

Perez, M., Garcia-Barreno, B., Melero, J.A., Carrasco, L. & Guinea, R. 1997. Membrane permeability changes induced in Escherichia coli by the SH protein of human respiratory syncytial virus. *Virology*, Vol. 235, pp. 342-351.

Pervushin, K., Tan, E., Parthasarathy, K., Lin, X., Jiang, F.L., Yu, D., Vararattanavech, A., Soong, T.W., Liu, D.X. & Torres, J. 2009. Structure and inhibition of the SARS coronavirus envelope protein ion channel. *PLoS Pathog*, Vol. 5, pp. e1000511.

Premkumar, A., Wilson, L., Ewart, G.D. & Gage, P.W. 2004. Cation-selective ion channels formed by p7 of hepatitis C virus are blocked by hexamethylene amiloride. *FEBS Lett*, Vol. 557, pp. 99-103.

Ramjeesingh, M., Huan, L.J., Garami, E. & Bear, C.E. 1999. Novel method for evaluation of the oligomeric structure of membrane proteins. *Biochem J*, Vol. 342 (Pt 1), pp. 119-123.

Rath, A., Glibowicka, M., Nadeau, V.G., Chen, G. & Deber, C.M. 2009. Detergent binding explains anomalous SDS-PAGE migration of membrane proteins. *Proc Natl Acad Sci U S A*, Vol. 106, pp. 1760-1765.

Razinkov, V., Gazumyan, A., Nikitenko, A., Ellestad, G. & Krishnamurthy, G. 2001. RFI-641 inhibits entry of respiratory syncytial virus via interactions with fusion protein. *Chem Biol*, Vol. 8, pp. 645-659.

Rixon, H.W.M., Brown, G., Aitken, J., McDonald, T., Graham, S. & Sugrue, R.J. 2004. The small hydrophobic (SH) protein accumulates within lipid-raft structures of the Golgi complex during respiratory syncytial virus infection. *J Gen Virol*, Vol. 85, pp. 1153-1165.

Rixon, H.W.M., Brown, G., Murray, J.T. & Sugrue, R.J. 2005. The respiratory syncytial virus small hydrophobic protein is phosphorylated via a mitogen-activated protein kinase p38-dependent tyrosine kinase activity during virus infection. *J Gen Virol*, Vol. 86, pp. 375-384.

Sandoz, G., Douguet, D., Chatelain, F., Lazdunski, M. & Lesage, F. 2009. Extracellular acidification exerts opposite actions on TREK1 and TREK2 potassium channels via a single conserved histidine residue. *Proc Natl Acad Sci U S A*, Vol. 106, pp. 14628-14633.

Schnell, J.R. & Chou, J.J. 2008. Structure and mechanism of the M2 proton channel of influenza A virus. *Nature*, Vol. 451, pp. 591-595.

Sharpe, S., Yau, W.M. & Tycko, R. 2006. Structure and dynamics of the HIV-1 Vpu transmembrane domain revealed by solid-state NMR with magic-angle spinning. *Biochemistry*, Vol. 45, pp. 918-933.

Simmerman, H.K., Kobayashi, Y.M., Autry, J.M. & Jones, L.R. 1996. A leucine zipper stabilizes the pentameric membrane domain of phospholamban and forms a coiled-coil pore structure. *J Biol Chem*, Vol. 271, pp. 5941-5946.

Stouffer, A.L., Acharya, R., Salom, D., Levine, A.S., Di Costanzo, L., Soto, C.S., Tereshko, V., Nanda, V., Stayrook, S. & DeGrado, W.F. 2008. Structural basis for the function and inhibition of an influenza virus proton channel. *Nature*, Vol. 451, pp. 596-599.

Sukharev, S.I., Blount, P., Martinac, B. & Kung, C. 1997. Mechanosensitive channels of Escherichia coli: the MscL gene, protein, and activities. *Annu Rev Physiol*, Vol. 59, pp. 633-657.

Suzuki, T. & Suzuki, Y. 2006. Virus infection and lipid rafts. *Biol Pharm Bull*, Vol. 29, pp. 1538-1541.

Szabo, I., Adams, C. & Gulbins, E. 2004. Ion channels and membrane rafts in apoptosis. *Pfluegers Arch Eur J Physiol*, Vol. 448, pp. 304-312.

Takeuchi, K., Takahashi, H., Kawano, S. & Shimada, I. 2007. Identification and characterization of the slowly exchanging pH-dependent conformational rearrangement in KcsA. *J Biol Chem*, Vol. 282, pp. 15179-15186.

Tamm, L.K. & Tatulian, S.A. 1997. Infrared spectroscopy of proteins and peptides in lipid bilayers. *Q Rev Biophys*, Vol. 30, pp. 365-429.

Techaarpornkul, S., Barretto, N. & Peeples, M.E. 2001. Functional analysis of recombinant respiratory syncytial virus deletion mutants lacking the small hydrophobic and/or attachment glycoprotein gene. *J Virol*, Vol. 75, pp. 6825-6834.

Teriete, P., Franzin, C.M., Choi, J. & Marassi, F.M. 2007. Structure of the Na,K-ATPase regulatory protein FXYD1 in micelles. *Biochemistry*, Vol. 46, pp. 6774-6783.

Torres, J., Parthasarathy, K., Lin, X., Saravanan, R., Kukol, A. & Liu, D.X. 2006. Model of a putative pore: the pentameric α-helical bundle of SARS coronavirus E protein in lipid bilayers. *Biophys J*, Vol. 91, pp. 938-947.

Van Horn, W.D., Kim, H.J., Ellis, C.D., Hadziselimovic, A., Sulistijo, E.S., Karra, M.D., Tian, C., Sonnichsen, F.D. & Sanders, C.R. 2009. Solution nuclear magnetic resonance structure of membrane-integral diacylglycerol kinase. *Science*, Vol. 324, pp. 1726-1729.

Vujovic, O. & Mills, J. 2001. Preventive and therapeutic strategies for respiratory syncytial virus infection. *Curr Opin Pharmacol*, Vol. 1, pp. 497-503.

Walsh, E.E., Hall, C.B. & Briselli, M. 1987. Immunization with glycoprotein subunits of respiratory syncytial virus to protect cotton rats against viral infection. *J Infect Dis*, Vol. 155, pp. 1198-1204.

Wang, C., Lamb, R.A. & Pinto, L.H. 1994. Direct measurement of the influenza A virus M2 protein ion channel activity in mammalian cells. *Virology*, Vol. 205, pp. 133-140.

Weisman, L.E. 2009. Respiratory syncytial virus (RSV) prevention and treatment: Past, present, and future. *Card Hemat Ag in Med Chem*, Vol. 7, pp. 223-233.

Werling, D., Hope, J.C., Chaplin, P., Collins, R.A., Taylor, G. & Howard, C.J. 1999. Involvement of caveolae in the uptake of respiratory syncytial virus antigen by dendritic cells. *J Leukoc Biol*, Vol. 66, pp. 50-58.

Whitehead, S.S., Bukreyev, A., Teng, M.N., Firestone, C.Y., St Claire, M., Elkins, W.R., Collins, P.L. & Murphy, B.R. 1999. Recombinant respiratory syncytial virus bearing a deletion of either the NS2 or SH gene is attenuated in chimpanzees. *J Virol*, Vol. 73, pp. 3438-3442.

Wilson, R.L., Fuentes, S.M., Wang, P., Taddeo, E.C., Klatt, A., Henderson, A.J. & He, B. 2006. Function of small hydrophobic proteins of paramyxovirus. *J Virol*, Vol. 80, pp. 1700-1709.

Yu, L., Sun, C., Song, D., Shen, J., Xu, N., Gunasekera, A., Hajduk, P.J. & Olejniczak, E.T. 2005. Nuclear magnetic resonance structural studies of a potassium channel-charybdotoxin complex. *Biochemistry*, Vol. 44, pp. 15834-15841.

Yuill, K.H., Stansfeld, P.J., Ashmole, I., Sutcliffe, M.J. & Stanfield, P.R. 2007. The selectivity, voltage-dependence and acid sensitivity of the tandem pore potassium channel TASK-1: contributions of the pore domains. *Pflugers Arch*, Vol. 455, pp. 333-348.

Zhou, F.X., Merianos, H.J., Brunger, A.T. & Engelman, D.M. 2001. Polar residues drive association of polyleucine transmembrane helices. *Proc Nat Acad Sci USA*, Vol. 98, pp. 2250-2255.

5

Cellular and Molecular Characteristics of RSV-Induced Disease in Humans

Olivier Touzelet and Ultan F. Power
Queen's University Belfast, Northern Ireland
UK

1. Introduction

Respiratory syncytial virus is associated with a large spectrum of illnesses ranging from mild upper respiratory tract (URT) disease to severe lower respiratory tract (LRT) disease. All infections start initially in the upper respiratory tract (URTI), where the virus replicates primarily in the nasopharynx (Brandenburg, 2000; Collins and Graham, 2008). The incubation period is thought to be 4 to 5 days before the onset of symptoms, which are characterised by a runny nose/nasal congestion, a non-productive cough, ear pain, sinus pain and sometimes a low-grade fever (Brandenburg, 2000; Freymuth *et al*, 2001; Rietveld, 2003). In most cases the infection induces mild illnesses of the upper airways, such as rhinitis, pharyngitis or otitis media. However, in some cases (mainly children < 2 years of age) the infection progresses within 1 to 3 days to the lower respiratory tract (LRTI) (Brandenburg, 2000; Graham *et al*, 2002; Tregoning and Schwarze, 2010) and may lead to mild or severe LRT diseases (tracheobronchitis or croup, bronchitis, bronchiolitis or pneumonia). The mechanisms by which RSV spreads to the LRT remain unknown but aspiration of nasopharyngeal secretions loaded with progeny virus is a plausible explanation (Brandenburg, 2000; Freymuth *et al*, 2001; Rietveld, 2003).

In two surveillance studies collating clinical data on RSV over a 20-year period, RSV-LRTI was identified in 37.8% children (2 weeks to 5 years-old, Fischer *et al*, 1997) and 26% healthy adults (18 to 60 years, Hall *et al*, 2001) were diagnosed with a RSV symptomatic infection. Moreover, Fischer *et al* (1997) observed that between 0 and 12 months of age almost half of the children diagnosed with RSV infection developed LRT disease, with a peak at 60% for infants aged between 3 to 6 months. For yet unknown reasons, several factors pre-dispose to severe forms of RSV-LRTI, including young age (< 3 weeks to 3 months), old age (> 65 years), premature birth (<34 weeks of gestation) and underlying medical conditions (bronchopulmonary dysplasia, congenital heart disease and congenital or acquired immunodeficiencies) (Brandenburg, 2000; Collins and Graham, 2008).

There are currently three types of severe disease associated with a RSV-LRTI: bronchitis, which is a disease limited to the large airways (bronchus), bronchiolitis, which involves the small conducting airways (bronchioles), and pneumonia, which implicates the involvement of the alveolar compartment (Tregoning and Schwarze, 2010). These illnesses are often characterised by dyspnea (breathing discomfort/difficulties), tachypnea (rapid breathing, >20 breaths/min), chest retractions, polypnea (increase of breathing frequency, bronchial obstruction), wheezing (bronchiolar involvement) and rales/ronchi (crepitations, alveolar involvement) (Freymuth *et al*, 2001; Rietveld, 2003). Thus, in a 13-year prospective study in infants and children in the United states, RSV was detected in 43%, 25%, 11% and 10% of paediatric hospitalisations for bronchiolitis, pneumonia, bronchitis and croup, respectively (Collins and Graham, 2008). RSV-LRTI can vary from mild to severe, the latter requiring admission to the intensive care unit (ICU) since the patients often need respiration support. Furthermore, Wang *et al* (1995) observed that among children hospitalised with RSV-LRTIs, 0.9% were associated with fatal cases. However, the mechanisms leading to either an URTI or a LRTI upon RSV infection are still not well understood and require further investigation.

In order to facilitate a better understanding of severe RSV-induced diseases, this chapter will review the histopathology of RSV fatal cases, the cellular responses to infection and the factors associated with the severity of the illness in humans.

2. Histopathology of fatal RSV cases

Since its isolation in 1956 several reports have investigated the histopathology associated with fatal cases of RSV in children (Aherne *et al*, 1970; Downham *et al*, 1975; Ebbert *et al*, 2005; Johnson *et al*, 2007; Kurlandsky *et al*, 1988; Neilson *et al*, 1990; Padman *et al*, 1985; Welliver *et al*, 2007) and adults (Levenson *et al*, 1987), starting with the autopsies of the two unfortunate recipients of the first-ever RSV vaccine candidate. Undertaken in the late sixties, this first human RSV vaccine field trial was based on a formalin-inactivated alum-precipitated whole virus (FI-RSV). However, instead of inducing protective immunity, FI-RSV primed the vast majority of vaccinees for exacerbated disease upon exposure to natural RSV infection, leading to the deaths of two of the vaccinated infants. The autopsies of these infants revealed a prominent neutrophilic and lymphocytic pulmonary infiltration, with some evidence of eosinophilia (Graham *et al*, 2002; Prince *et al*, 2001). These observations were further perpetuated by similar findings in animal models of RSV infection (cotton rats, BALB/c mice, monkeys), which led to the general belief of an immunopathogenic nature of RSV disease.

In this section we will comprehensively review the histopathological observations in children and adults in 3 parts: the damage and cytopathic effects caused to the lungs, the site of RSV infection and the type and site of cell infiltrates.

2.1 Damage and cytopathic effects to the lungs

Bronchiolitis and pneumonia are most commonly associated with severe forms of RSV-LRTI and, not surprisingly, are also the most frequent diseases linked with a fatal outcome. As stated above, they involve different areas of the lower respiratory tract and, therefore, their histopathological characteristics are distinct.

2.1.1 Bronchiolitis

In a study involving 22 children, Aherne *et al* (1970) described the hallmarks of each disease when associated with RSV. The earliest lesion of acute bronchiolitis is the necrosis of the bronchiolar epithelium, principally the destruction of ciliated cells, followed by the peri-bronchiolar infiltration of lymphocytes, macrophages and some plasma cells. Markers of apoptosis, such as caspase 3 (Welliver *et al*, 2007) and Fas (Reed *et al*, 2008), were clearly evident in bronchiolar epithelium cells of children who died from fatal RSV LRTI compared with uninfected paediatric lung tissue. However, alveoli are usually not involved in the bronchiolitis inflammatory process.

The submucosa and adventitial tissues become oedematous and congested but typically there is no damage to elastic fibres or muscle. The secretion of mucus is enhanced and a thick plug forms in the bronchiolar lumina composed of epithelial cell debris, fibrin and inflammatory cells (Fig. 1) (Downham *et al*, 1975). The occlusion of the bronchioles may lead to various degrees of mechanical lesions, the most severe being the complete collapse of the alveoli that the affected bronchiole supplies. At later stages, two types of cells can be seen that are thought to be involved in the regeneration of the bronchiolar epithelium: undifferentiated pleomorphic cells lining small bronchioles, varying in thickness and showing occasional mitotic activity; and more occasionally, elongated basophilic cells spreading over recently denuded lamina propria. In a comparable study of fatal RSV-LRTI in children (1 to 14 months old) Neilson *et al* (1990) similarly reported the occasional uneven proliferation of epithelial cells with protrusion into the bronchiolar lumen, creating a polypoid appearance.

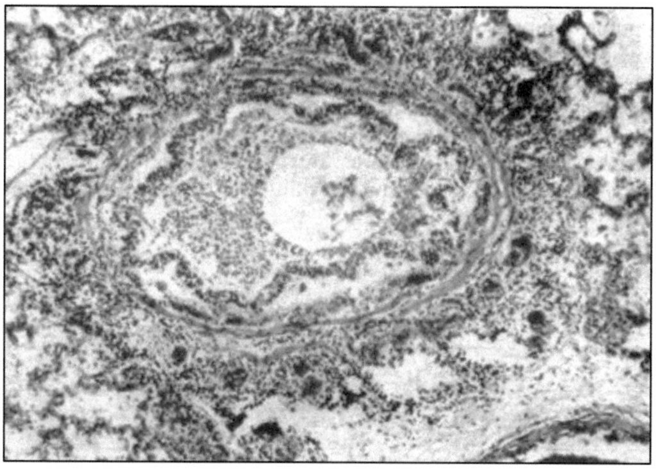

Fig. 1. Histological appearance of lungs of children deceased from a severe RSV bronchiolitis. Varying degrees of peribronchiolar lymphocytic infiltration can be observed alongside a necrosis of the bronchiolar epithelium. The small bronchioles are often plugged with mucus and cell debris. Magnification x 112. Reproduced from [Role of respiratory viruses in childhood mortality, Downham *et al*, 1 (5952), 235-239, 1975] with permission from BMJ Publishing Group Ltd.

2.1.2 Pneumonia

The most thorough description of fatal pneumonia associated with RSV was published in 2007 by Johnson *et al* (2007). In their histopathology report of autopsy tissues from 4 children, they noted extensive damage to the lungs, from medium and small bronchioles to the alveoli. As outlined in an earlier study of fatal pneumonia in infants (Aherne *et al*, 1970), Johnson *et al* (2007) observed widespread destruction of bronchial and bronchiolar epithelium resulting in occlusion of the airways by cell debris (sloughed epithelial cells), fibrin, a minor component of mucin and inflammatory cells (mostly macrophages).

Conversely, Welliver *et al* (2007) were unable to stain for mucus in their autopsy slides. In addition, the small bronchioles were surrounded by fibrotic tissue (excess connective tissue) and the mucosa was often hyperplastic (Kurlandsky *et al*, 1988).

Similar to bronchiolitis, occasional marked uneven proliferation and metaplasia of the bronchiolar epithelium could be detected. These resulted in papillary protusions, which are likely to contribute to airway narrowing. This feature was seen in other comparable studies of infant cases (Aherne *et al*, 1970; Neilson *et al*, 1990) and also in an elderly woman (Levenson *et al*, 1987).

One patient in the Johnson *et al* (2007) study showed multiple syncytia lining the bronchiolar epithelium, an observation that had been previously reported in children (Neilson *et al*, 1990). However, if occasional intra-bronchiolar and intra-alveolar syncytia can be seen in fatal RSV pneumonitis in children (Welliver *et al*, 2007), multiple giant nucleated cells are not a common occurrence associated with RSV pneumonitis. Giant cell pneumonia is the typical disease syndrome of immunosuppressed patients, such as subjects with immunodeficiency diseases or recipients of organ transplant (bone-marrow, lung) (Graham *et al*, 2002). Indeed, several patients in the study by Neilson *et al* (1990) had underlying conditions associated with various degrees of immunodeficiency, which may explain their observations. However, there were no reported underlying conditions that could justify this pattern in the study by Johnson *et al* (2007).

As for bronchiolitis, pneumonia is characterised by a massive bronchiolar inflammation and a peri-bronchiolar infiltration of inflammatory cells, deep to the muscularis layer. The pattern of inflammatory infiltrate around an airway appears to be determined by the distribution of arterioles adjacent to the airway. Sometimes, the infiltrates around the bronchovascular bundle can be so dense that they resemble hyperplastic node follicles, also called bronchiolar-associated lymphoid tissue (BALT), which in turn are responsible for the congestion of the arterioles. Occasionally, BALT nodules projected into the bronchiolar lumens, thereby participating in the narrowing of the airways (Johnson *et al*, 2007).

One of the hallmarks of pneumonitis is the diffuse alveolar damage caused by RSV. This is characterised in children and adults by the proliferation of type II pneumocytes, in order to regenerate destroyed type I pneumocytes, but also interstitial and intra-alveolar fibrosis (Aherne *et al*, 1970; Kurlansky *et al*, 1988; Levenson *et al*, 1987). In addition, an extensive interstitial infiltration occurs, leading to a marked capillary congestion, and is often accompanied by intra-alveolar leakage of fibrin and inflammatory cells (macrophages and occasional neutrophils). Due to a lack of aeration, alveolar parenchyma necrosis and intra-alveolar haemorrhage can be observed in severe cases of pneumonitis, along with oedema and the apparition of a thick hyaline membrane lining the alveoli (Aherne *et al*, 1970; Johnson *et al*, 2007). This latter feature was also observed in elderly patients (Levenson *et al*, 1987).

The observations described above are further supported by Downham *et al* (1975), who corroborated the histopathology described for either bronchiolitis or pneumonia. In this study, they assessed the histological changes in the lungs of 13 children without knowledge of the virus findings. The 2 categories of pathological changes in patients that were later diagnosed with a RSV infection were: 1/ varying degrees of peribronchiolar lymphocytic infiltration, necrosis of bronchiolar epithelium, plugging of the small bronchioles by mucus and cell debris; 2/ lymphocytic infiltration of alveolar walls and interstitial lung tissue, sometimes associated with a minor degree of peribronchiolar lymphocytic infiltration (Fig. 2). Indeed, the type 1 and 2 patterns showed striking similarities with the histopathology of fatal RSV bronchiolitis and pneumonia cases, respectively.

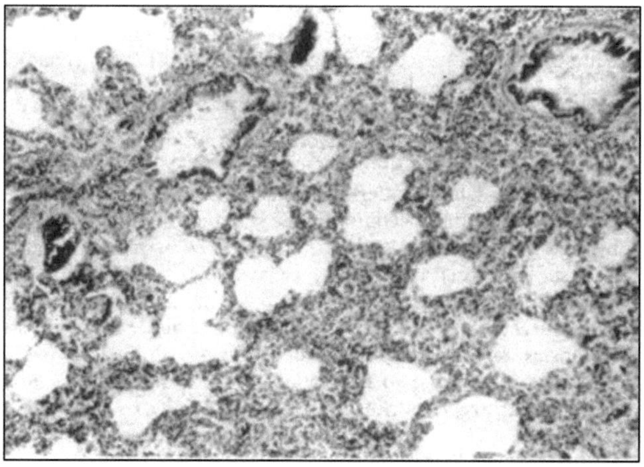

Fig. 2. Histological appearance of lungs of a child that died following severe RSV pneumonia. Cell infiltration of alveolar walls and interstitial lung tissue is clearly identifiable and is associated with a peribronchiolar infiltration. Magnification x 84 Reproduced from [Role of respiratory viruses in childhood mortality, Downham *et al*, 1 (5952), 235-239, 1975] with permission from BMJ Publishing Group Ltd.

2.2 Site of RSV infection in the lungs

In fatal cases of RSV disease, infection was highly restricted to the superficial cells of the respiratory epithelium (Johnson *et al*, 2007; Neilson *et al*, 1990; Welliver *et al*, 2007). In the URT RSV initially replicates in the ciliated cells of the nasopharynx, while in the LRT ciliated cells of the large and small airways and type I pneumocytes in the alveoli are the major targets (Collins and Graham, 2008; Graham *et al*, 2002). This is consistent with the early loss of cilia/ciliated cells observed by Aherne *et al* (1970) in both bronchiolitis and pneumonitis illnesses. This was elegantly demonstrated in 2 recent studies of young children (1 to 15 month-old) who died of "atypical pneumonia" (Johnson *et al*, 2007) or of a severe LRTI (Welliver *et al*, 2007) due to RSV. Although Welliver *et al* (2007) did not mention the type of disease, the histopathological aspects pointed towards a severe form of pneumonitis. In these publications Johnson *et al* (2007) and Welliver *et al* (2007) detected extensive RSV-positive staining in the bronchial and bronchiolar epithelium of all cases (Fig 3a and b), but also in the alveolar epithelium of most patients (Fig. 3a). As expected, Johnson *et al* (2007) observed RSV-positive staining in ciliated cells but also, surprisingly, in non-ciliated cells. As suggested previously (Aherne *et al*, 1970), this may be due to a loss of cilia following RSV infection.

They also noted that the infection was restricted to the superficial epithelium, as basal cells routinely stained negative. Evidence from the infection of well differentiated human airway epithelial cells (WD-HAE) by RSV indicates that progeny virus release is polarised, forcing the virus to the apical surface (Villenave *et al*, unpublished observations; Zhang *et al*, 2002). Coupled with this, the tight junctions are likely to restrict access of the released virus to the basal layers. Interestingly, when Zhang *et al* (2002) damaged their WD-HAE cultures so that some basal cells were exposed, there was still very little RSV infection of these cells, implying that they somehow have an innate protection from RSV. In addition, Johnson *et al* (2007) further identified the infected alveolar cells as being predominantly type I pneumocytes but also some cuboidal cells thought to be reparative type II pneumocytes. At this level, RSV antigens were detected in a continuous linear fashion along the alveolar surfaces. Similarly, they found that the smallest airways often had circumferential staining, while the larger airways showed a patchy RSV immunostaining, often localised in clusters of 3 to 5 cells.

Several histopathology reports described RSV antigens in giant multinucleated cells (Johnson *et al*, 2007; Kurlansky *et al*, 1988; Neilson *et al*, 1990; Welliver *et al*, 2007) when these syncytia were observable, and also within the material obstructing the lumen of the bronchioli and alveoli (Johnson *et al*, 2007). More specifically, this material was composed of cell debris, infiltrating alveolar macrophages (Johnson *et al*, 2007) and sloughed bronchiolar and alveolar cells (Neilson *et al*, 1990). The positive staining of macrophages for RSV antigens may have resulted from phagocytosed antigen or the infection of these cells by RSV. Indeed, there is evidence suggesting that RSV can infect and replicate in a human macrophage-like cell line (Zhao *et al*, 2007) and in human monocyte-derived macrophages (Spann *et al*, 2004).

Finally, cytoplasmic inclusions have also been observed, both in children (Neilson *et al*, 1990; Aherne *et al*, 1970) and adults (Levenson *et al*, 1987), although this is not a systematic feature in RSV subjects (Johnson *et al*, 2007). These inclusions can be granular, basophilic and peripherally located (Neilson *et al*, 19990) or homogenous eosinophilic and paranuclear in location (Levenson *et al*, 1987; Neilson *et al*, 1990). They can vary markedly in size and are occasionally surrounded by halos. These inclusions are found in the cytoplasm of bronchial, brionchiolar and alveolar epithelial cells, as well as within syncytia and sloughed intra-bronchiolar and intra-alveolar cells (Aherne *et al*, 1970; Levenson *et al*, 1987; Neilson *et al*, 1990). However, it is still unclear what these inclusions are or to what extent they are involved in the pathology.

Interestingly, Welliver *et al* (2007) compared histopathology findings between RSV and influenza fatal cases and showed that viral antigen was more extensively present in RSV subjects and that damage to the bronchiolar epithelium was also greater. This might suggest an association between viral load and disease severity, as was hypothesised previously (DeVincenzo *et al*, 2005). On the other hand, a closer examination of images from various reports shows vast areas of intact virus-infected cells, especially in the bronchiolar epithelium, implying that the infection might not be the only phenomenon involved in the cytopathic effects (Welliver *et al*, 2007). The uneven distribution of the damage across the lungs, another characteristic associated with RSV fatal cases, further reinforces this impression. For instance, Johnson *et al* (2007) described diffuse pulmonary oedema in areas uninvolved with pneumonitis and Bronchiolitis and Aherne *et al* (1970) found that the severity of the pathological changes varies widely from one region to another. It is also important to note that while the infection can be patchy, the damage to the bronchiolar epithelium and alveoli is often widespread, as is the infiltration of immune cells, such as macrophages and neutrophils. This theory of an immune-mediated disease is supported, at least partly, by work on *ex vivo* models of human WD-PBECS. These models showed limited gross cytopathic effects following RSV infection (mainly restricted to the ciliated cells) (Henderson *et al*, 1978; Zhang *et al*, 2002; Villenave *et al*,- unpublished observations), although increased epithelial cell sloughing was observed compared to uninfected controls.

However, the extent of sloughing and damage *in vivo* is unlikely to explain the widespread sloughing of epithelial and type I/II penumocytes observed in autopsy cases (Aherne *et al*, 1970; Johnson *et al*, 2007; Welliver al, 2007).

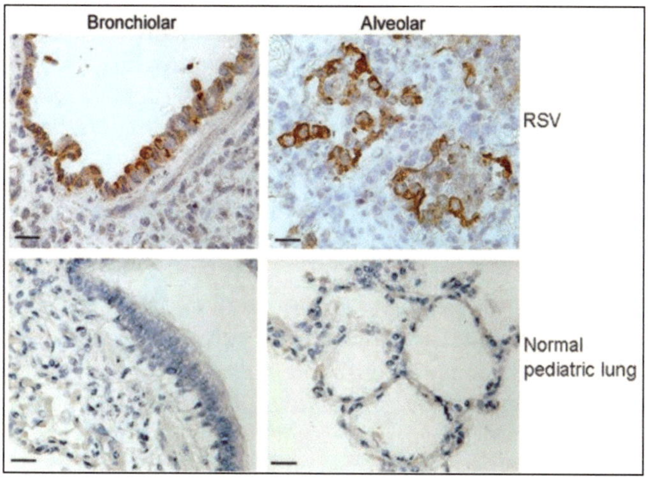

(a)

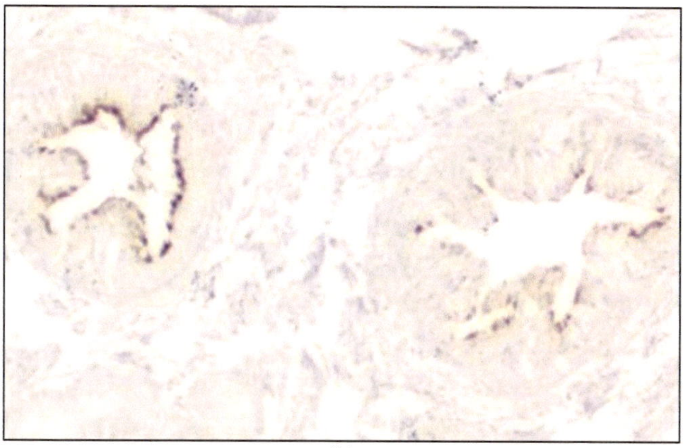

(b)

Fig. 3. Immunohistochemical staining for respiratory syncytial virus (RSV) antigen in bronchiolar and alveolar tissues from infants with lower respiratory tract infection (LRTI). (a) Autopsy tissues were obtained from human infants with fatal cases of LRTI caused by RSV. Normal infant lung tissue (from an infant that died of asphyxia) is stained as a control. Brown stain indicates the presence of viral antigen. Original magnification x 40. (Welliver *et al*, Severe human lower respiratory tract illness caused by respiratory syncytial virus and influenza virus is characterized by the absence of pulmonary cytotoxic lymphocyte responses, The Journal of Infectious Diseases, 2007, 195, 8, 1126-36, by permission of Oxford University Press) (b) Medium-sized muscular bronchioles demonstrate RSV antigen circumferentially and restricted to the apical epithelium. Dark purple stain indicates RSV antigen. Original magnification x 25. Reprinted by permission from Macmillan Publishers Ltd: [Modern Pathology] (Johnson *et al*, The histopathology of fatal untreated human respiratory syncytial virus infection, 20 (1), 108–119), copyright (2007).

2.3 Inflammation and cell infiltration

2.3.1 Bronchiolitis versus pneumonia

One of the common aspects of fatal RSV bronchiolitis and pneunmonia is the massive infiltration of multiple inflammatory cell types into the airways. The main cells composing the infiltrates included macrophages, lymphocytes, neutrophils and, to a lesser extent, eosinophils, or subsets of these populations. However, their proportions among the infiltrate and, more importantly, the areas of infiltration differ depending on the form of the disease and the strength of the immune system at the time of death.

The inflammatory cells are centred on the bronchial arteries and arterioles, consistent with their migration out of the bloodstream. They are also massively detected in the sub-muscularis layer of the peri-bronchiolar tissue (Fig. 4), indicating their migration from the arteries/arterioles towards the airways (Johnson *et al*, 2007). Therefore, due to the distribution of the pulmonary arteries, which are surrounding large and medium-sized bronchiolar branches, the inflammatory infiltrate appears symmetrical and circumferential around medium bronchioles and larger airways. On the other hand, because of the diminution of blood vessels converging in the smallest airways, such as terminal bronchioles, the inflammation is often asymmetrical and densely localised between arterioles and the most proximal bronchiole. Overall, the pattern of the inflammatory infiltrate around an airway appears to be determined by the distribution of the blood vessels (arteries and arterioles) adjacent to the airway (Johnson *et al*, 2007).

In the case of pneumonitis, the inflammation is equally important at the alveolar level. In numerous reports of fatal pneumonitis, infiltrating cells are extensively seen in the alveolar interstitium (interstitial pneumonitis) (Fig. 2) and/or within the intra-alveolar exudate (intra-alveolar pneumonia). These observations were consistent in children (Aherne *et al*, 1970; Downham *et al*, 1975; Johnson *et al*, 2007; Kurlansky, 1988; Neilson *et al*, 1990; Welliver *et al*, 2007), adults (Levenson *et al*, 1987) and immunocompromised hosts (Hertz *et al*, 1989; Padman *et al*, 1985)

Irrespective of whether there is a bronchiolar or alveolar inflammation, the main cells migrating from the blood stream towards the airways are mononuclear cells, with a predominance of macrophages followed by lymphocytes. Their distribution is diffuse around the bronchiolar lumen (submuscular area) and within the alveolar parenchyma, and they are a component of the airway plug.

2.3.2 Mononuclear cells

In fatal cases of RSV, macrophages ($CD68^+$ cells) were detected in great abundance around the bronchioles and in the bronchiolar exudate, the alveolar interstitium (interstitial pneumonia) and/or within the alveolar lumen (intra-alveolar pneumonia) (Johnson *et al*, 2007, Welliver *et al*, 2007). Thus, despite their submuscular localisation in the case of an acute bronchiolitis (Fig. 5a), macrophages are able to migrate through the smooth muscle towards the bronchiolar lumen. This ability to migrate is illustrated by Johnson *et al* (2007) who observed inflammatory cells moving through gaps across the muscularis (Fig. 5b) and detected the presence of macrophages within the bronchiolar epithelium. On the other hand, at the alveolar level, infiltrated macrophages represent either alveolar macrophages that migrated inside the alveolar space or macrophages that were recruited from the surrounding arterioles/capillaries. Finally, macrophages were also found to be an important component of the follicule-like expanded BALT (Johnson *et al*, 2007).

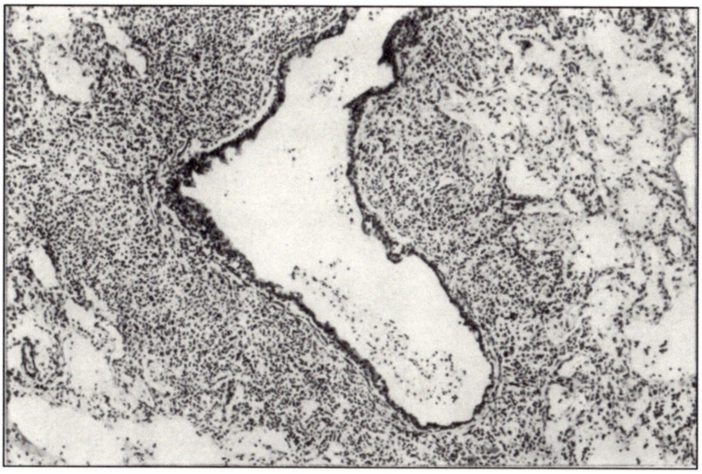

Fig. 4. The peribronchiolar lymphoid infiltration in acute bronchiolitis. Note also the epithelial irregularity. H.E. x 60. Reproduced from [Pathological changes in virus infections of the lower respiratory tract in children, Aherne *et al*, 23 (1), 7-18, 1970] with permission from BMJ Publishing Group Ltd.

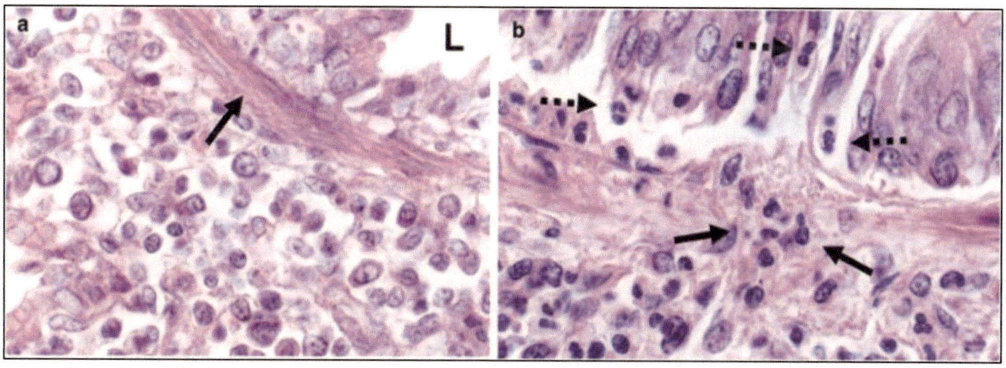

Fig. 5. Relative segregation of mononuclear cells and polymorphonuclear leukocytes in airway. (a) Peribronchiolar mononuclear inflammatory infiltrate is primarily submuscular, and is peripheral to the smooth muscle (arrow). L indicates the airway lumen. (b) While neutrophils are commonly found in BAL, the predominant cells in the peribronchiolar tissues are mononuclear. Neutrophils can sometimes be found migrating across gaps in the muscularis (arrow) towards the airway lumen and interspersed within the epithelium (dashed arrow). Original magnification x 250 (a and b). Reprinted by permission from Macmillan Publishers Ltd: [Modern Pathology] (Johnson *et al*, The histopathology of fatal untreated human respiratory syncytial virus infection, 20 (1), 108–119), copyright (2007).

T Lymphocytes (CD3+) are also among the mononuclear cells involved in the inflammation process. Their distribution within the lung tissue is similar to macrophages - diffuse, peribronchiolar and in the alveolar interstitium (Welliver *et al*, 2007; Johnson *et al*, 2007). Lymphocytes have also been found in the basal part of the bronchiolar epithelium (Johnson *et al*, 2007) suggesting that, like macrophages, they can probably migrate through gaps of the muscularis. However, the extent of lymphocytic peri-bronchial and interstitial infiltration varies between studies, and there are discrepancies in the literature about their presence within the bronchiolar or alveolar lumens (Welliver *et al*, 2007; Johnson *et al*, 2007 Padman *et al*, 1985; Aherne *et al*, 1970). It is not clear whether these discrepancies reflect technical variations or actual pathological differences in different individuals, for example due to underlying medical conditions, or the extent of disease at the time of death.

Independent of the extent of lymphocyte infiltration, detailed investigation of lymphocyte subsets indicated that $CD3^+CD8^+$ T cells were predominant over $CD3^+CD4^+$ T cells within the lung tissue. Furthermore, Johnson *et al* (2007) specifically observed that the presence of $CD8^+$ T cells was often associated with virus-infected areas, which is consistent with a putative role in virus clearance. However, Welliver *et al* (2007) failed to detect granzyme in lung tissue suggesting that these $CD8^+$ T cells might not be fully activated or functional (granzyme being an effector molecule secreted by cytotoxic T cells to kill infected cells). They also failed to detect NK cells ($CD56^+$), another cell type involved with cytotoxic responses to viruses. Interestingly, Johnson *et al* (2007) observed that many of the $CD3^+$ T cells were actually CD4 and CD8 negative (double negative, DN), a population suspected to be T-regulatory cells (DN Tregs) or NK T cells, but whose role remains to be elucidated. Overall, these findings suggest that T lymphocyte activation and cytotoxic activity may be abstent or compromised in the lungs at the time when infants are experiencing their most severe symptoms.

In 1970, Aherne *et al* observed that plasma cells were a component of the peri-bronchiolar and peri-alveolar inflammatory response in fatal cases of bronchiolitis and pneumonitis in children. This observation was recently corroborated by Welliver *et al* (2007) and Johnson *et al* (2007), using infant autopsy tissues. More specifically, large populations of $CD20^+$ B cells were detected within the BALT follicules and nodules partially obstructing the airways (Johnson *et al*, 2007) (Fig. 6a), the alveolar interstitium and the perivascular areas, compared to a control group (infants that died of hypoxia) (Reed *et al*, 2009) (Fig 6b). Indeed, this was concomitant with strong IgA-, IgG- and, to a lesser extent, IgM-positive staining within the cytoplasm of cells localised in the alveolar, bronchiolar and perivascular spaces (Fig. 7), identifying these cells as plasmocytes (Reed *et al*, 2009). IgA and IgG staining was particularly strong in the alveolar interstitium and exudate, and in the sub-muscularis layer of the peribonchiolar area. IgA also appeared to be strongly deposited on bronchiolar epithelium, which correlates with its essential involvement in mucosal immunity. Because a vigorous B cell response was observed, while in the same study $CD4^+$ T cells were rarely detected, Reed *et al* suggested (2009) the possibility of a T-independent B lymphocyte antibody production. This hypothesis was supported by the perivascular, bronchiolar and alveolar expression of factors known to be involved in T cell-independent B cell activation, Ig production and class-switch recombination. These factors were identified as vasoactive intestinal peptide (VIP), B cell-activating factor (BAFF) and a proliferation-inducing ligand (APRIL). The up-regulation of the APRIL and BAFF receptors on lymphocytes having plasmocyte morphological characteristics, compared to an age-matched control group, further supported this concept (BAFF-R, transmembrane activator calcium modulator and cyclophylin ligand interactor [TACI] and B cells maturation antigen [BCMA]).

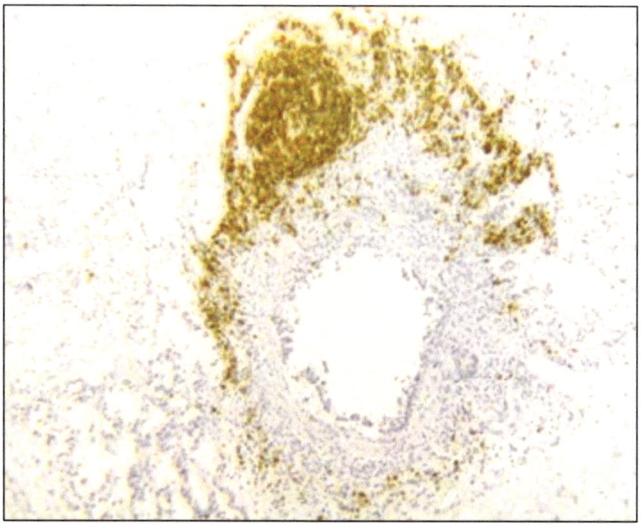

(a)

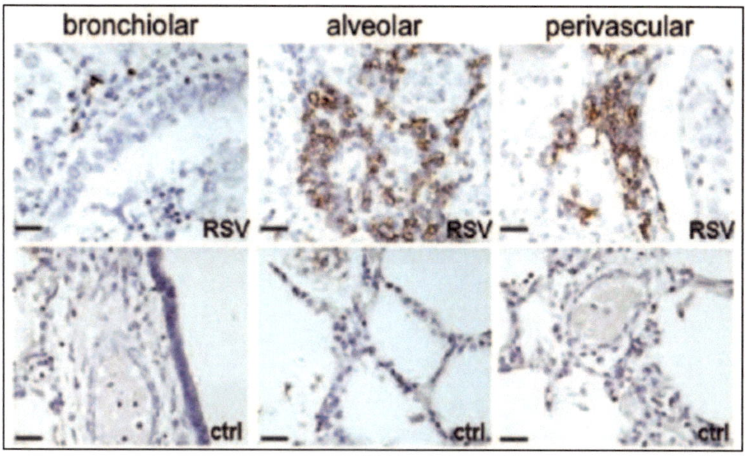

(b)

Fig. 6. B cell distribution within the lungs of children who died of severe LRTI. (a) Peribronchial lymphoid aggregates are primarily composed of CD20+ B lymphocytes (in brown), presumably part of the BALT. During the response to RSV infection, some areas appear to develop the appearance of a hyperplastic lymph node follicle. Original magnification x 25. Reprinted by permission from Macmillan Publishers Ltd: [Modern Pathology] (Johnson *et al*, The histopathology of fatal untreated human respiratory syncytial virus infection, 20 (1), 108–119), copyright (2007). (b) CD20+ lymphocytes were detected at autopsy from infants who died of acute RSV LRI (RSV) or asphyxia (ctrl). Original magnification, x40. Representative fields from bronchiolar (left), alveolar (middle), and perivascular (right) spaces are shown. CD20+ cells were detected by immunohistochemistry analysis in formalin-fixed, paraffin-embedded lung tissue. (Reed *et al*, Innate immune signals modulate antiviral and polyreactive antibody responses during severe respiratory syncytial virus infection, The Journal of Infectious Diseases, 2007, 199, 8, 1128-38, by permission of Oxford University Press)

It is important to keep in mind that most of these conclusions regarding lymphocyte subsets associated with RSV LRTI are drawn from only 3 reports and a relatively small number of infants (Johnson *et al*, 2007; Reed *et al*, 2009; Welliver *et al*, 2007). Also, several of the children included in these studies had underlying conditions that are often associated with an immunodeficient status (Down's syndrome, heart disease) (Tregoning and Schwarze, 2010). Therefore, while these publications are of huge relevance for the understanding of RSV pathology, the particular background of these children suggests that generalising these observations to entire populations may be premature and that further studies are warranted.

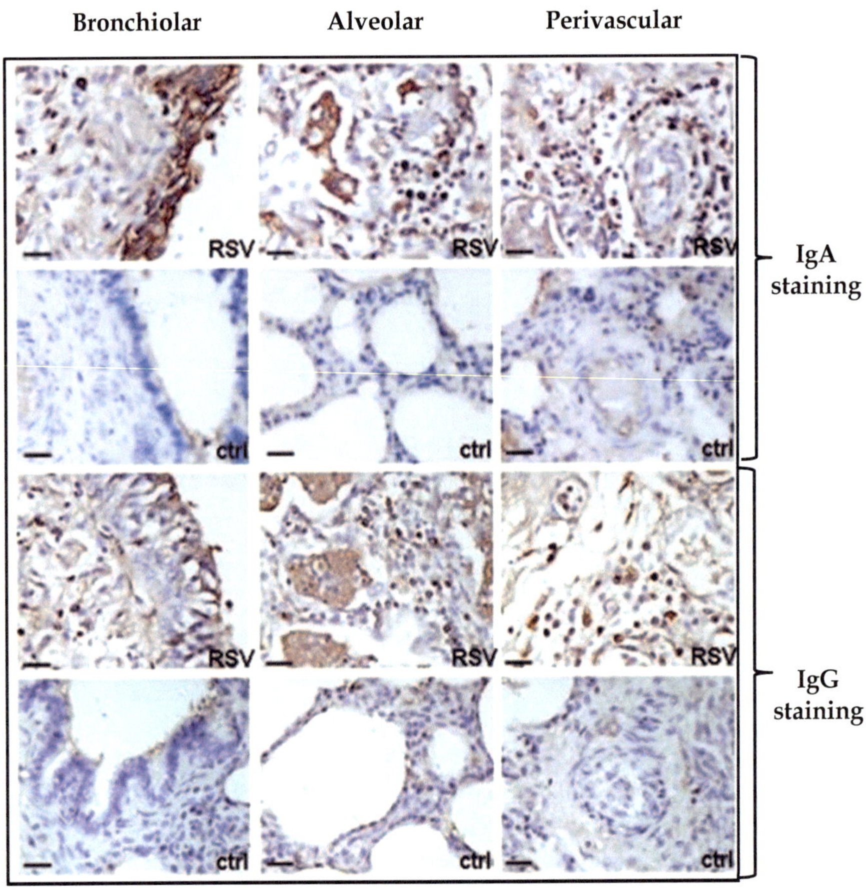

Fig. 7. Detection of immunoglobulin isotypes in samples from individuals with respiratory syncytial virus lower respiratory tract infection (RSV LRTI). IgA (upper panels) and IgG (lower panels) were detected by immunohistochemistry analysis in formalin-fixed, paraffin-embedded lung tissue obtained at autopsy from infants who died of acute RSV LRTI (RSV) or asphyxia (ctrl). Representative fields from bronchiolar (left), alveolar (middle) and perivascular (right) spaces are shown. (original magnification, x40). (Reed *et al*, Innate immune signals modulate antiviral and polyreactive antibody responses during severe respiratory syncytial virus infection, The Journal of Infectious Diseases, 2007, 199, 8, 1128-38, by permission of Oxford University Press)

Denditric cells (DC) are professional antigen presenting cells and essential for inducing adaptive immune response against pathogens. They are found in the peripheral blood or patrolling within tissues in contact with the external environment, such as the skin or the inner lining of the nose/lungs. However, little is known about the extent of their involvement during natural RSV infection and only one publication investigated their presence in fatal RSV cases (Johnson *et al*, 2007). Very few DCs were detected in the lungs and were mainly localised within bronchiolar epithelium and the peribronchiolar connective tissue. It is possible that their low number is a consequence of their migration from the lungs to the lymph nodes after detection and capture of the RSV antigens during the early inflammatory process.

2.3.3 Neutrophils and eosinophils

According to Johnson *et al* (2007), neutrophils were also a component of the inflammatory infiltrate, albeit to a lesser extent than macrophages or lymphocytes. In contrast to the diffuse distribution of mononuclear cells, neutrophils are more densely focalised between the pulmonary or bronchiolar arteries and the airway lumen. This suggests that these cells are responding to chemotractant molecules secreted by the bronchiolar epithelium only, whereas factors attracting mononuclear cells are produced by epithelial cells and cells within the lung parenchyma (Johnson *et al*, 2007). As mentioned above, neutrophils are principally found in the connective tissue of the peribronchiolar area (submuscularis), in the bronchiolar and alveolar lumens but have not been observed within the alveolar interstitium (Johnson *et al*, 2007; Welliver *et al*, 2007). They can also be detected crossing through gaps of the muscular layer and in the basal part of the bronchiolar epithelium, confirming their ability to migrate through tissues towards the airway lumen (Johnson *et al*, 2007).

Noticeably, the histopathology observations regarding the intra-luminal infiltration of macrophages, lymphocytes, neutrophils and eosinophils concur with the cell composition of nasopharyngeal (NPL) and broncho-alveolar lavages (BAL) collected from infants hospitalised with severe bronchiolitis. However, the ratios of cell types are significantly different, with neutrophils consistently being the largest cell population within nasal and pulmonary secretions (70 to 80%), followed by mononuclear cells (Brandenburg *et al*, 2000; Everard *et al*, 1994; Heidema *et al*, 2007; O'Donnell *et al*, 2002; Smith *et al*, 2001). This is further supported by the appearance of neutrophil precursors (myelocytes, metamyelocytes and banded neutrophils), normally residing in the bone marrow, in the peripheral blood of hospitalised RSV patients at a time when disease severity and viral load are declining (Lukens *et al*, 2010). It is likely that the migration of neutrophil progenitors from the bone marrow is a consequence of neutrophil exhaustion (and depletion of the banded-neutrophil pool in peripheral blood) due to a massive recruitment of these cells into the airways. In contrast, in autopsy cases neutrophils were often detected in the minority among the intra-luminal infiltrate compared to macrophages and lymphocytes (Aherne *et al*, 1970; Johnson *et al*, 2007; Welliver *et al*, 2007). The reason for this striking contrast is unclear and warrants further investigation.

Eosinophils can be detected as part of the peribronchiolar cell infiltrate but they are not a dominant component of the inflammatory process (Aherne *et al*, 1970; Johnson *et al*, 2007). For many years these cells were thought to be major players of the inflammatory response against RSV since a significant eosinophilia was one of the hallmarks described of the fatal enhanced disease associated with FI RSV vaccination (Graham *et al*, 2002). However, re-analysis of the FI-RSV autopsies challenged this dogma, as eosinophils were found to be a minor population among the pulmonary infiltrates with an uneven distribution across lung tissues, while neutrophilia was the principal characteristic of the inflammation (Graham *et al*, 2002; Prince *et al*, 2001). Therefore, it remains to be elucidated whether FI-RSV enhanced disease is representative of a natural primary RSV infection and to what extent eosinophils (and neutrophils) are involved in RSV pathology.

It is noteworthy that the histopathology of the FI-RSV autopsy cases displayed both similarities and discrepancies compared to recent histopathology studies of fatal RSV cases (Johnson *et al*, 2007; Welliver *et al*, 2007). For instance, in the former cases, Prince *et al* (2001) observed a peribronchiolar inflammation composed of 10% neutrophils, 10% macrophages and 80% lymphocytes, while the bronchial exudate contained 50% neutrophils, 30% macrophages and 20% lymphocytes. Eosinophils represented 1-2% of the inflammatory cells of the sections (Prince *et al*, 2001), whereas Graham *et al* (2002) observed many eosinophils. Also, according to the original publication describing the autopsies of the FI-RSV recipients, the alveoli contained scattered infiltrates of neutrophils and macrophages, or of neutrophils and mononuclear cells, depending on the pulmonary lobe examined (Chin *et al*, 1969). While the infiltration of macrophages and lymphocytes in the peribronchiolar and alveolar areas are consistent between reports, discrepancies regarding the amount of infiltrating eosinophils and neutrophils remain. However, comparable disease enhancement does not occur with community-acquired natural RSV infections and re-infections, and, therefore, the relevance of FI-RSV-associated pathogenesis to natural infection is unclear (Collins and Graham, 2008). It is interesting to note that the histopathological hallmarks of fatal RSV bronchiolitis or pneunmonia from normal infants were also identifiable in fatal RSV cases of immunocompromised children and adults (Ebbert *et al*, 2002; Hertz *et al*, 1989; Padman *et al*, 1985). However, the mortality and morbidity is a lot higher in the latter groups, reaching 50% of infected patients (Graham *et al*, 2002).

3. Factors associated with severe RSV infection

RSV epidemics usually occur over the winter months in temperate climates and in the rainy season in hotter climates. In the Northern hemisphere peak epidemic months are commonly November to January (Brandenburg, 2000; Garcia *et al*, 2010; Houben *et al*, 2011). Approximately 70% of children encounter their first infection before the age of one, while almost all children are infected at least once before the age of 2 years (Brandenburg, 2000; Rietweld, 2003;) and over 50% will have been infected twice (Brandenburg, 2000). About 40% of young children infected for the 1st time show signs of lower respiratory tract involvement, with some developing severe complications necessitating hospital admission (Brandenburg, 2000). Overall, 0.5 - 2.5% of infants are hospitalised with RSV infection during their first year of life, and 7 - 21% of these children require ventilation support due to respiratory failure (Brandenburg, 2000; Rietweld, 2003). RSV is the most common cause of bronchiolitis hospitalisation, with one study showing that RSV accounted for 60 - 70% of all hospitalisations with bronchiolitis (Garcia *et al*, 2010).

Deciphering the factors associated with severe RSV disease is complicated by the fact that many published studies define disease severity, and patient inclusion criteria in severe cohorts, differently. Factors such as requirement for mechanical ventilation, admission to paediatric ICU, days in hospital and oxygen saturation levels are commonly used, either alone or together. There are clearly defined groups of infants that are at high risk of severe RSV. These include infants with congenital heart disease, bronchopulmonary dysplasia, congenital or acquired immunodeficiencies or prematurity (<32 weeks gestation). However, the majority of infants hospitalised with RSV have no known high risk factors. The mechanisms leading to severe LRT disease, and possibly death, are still poorly understood. It is likely that a multitude of factors influence the course of disease during an infection. We postulate that the interrelation of various elements associated with the virus, the host and the environment will shape the outcome of RSV disease.

3.1 Viral factors

3.1.1 RSV subgroup

RSV has a single serotype with two major antigenic subgroups (A and B). Both subgroups have a worldwide geographical distribution and circulate independently, while their seasonal distribution is similar each year (Brandenburg, 2000; Collins and Graham, 2008; Rietweld, 2003). In several epidemiology studies, 3 patterns of subgroup A and B circulations within communities could be observed: a strong predominance of RSV A strains, relatively equal proportions of RSV A and B strains and, occasionally, a strong predominance of RSV B strains (Hall *et al*, 1990; Imaz *et al*, 2000; Mufson *et al*, 1988; Taylor *et al*, 1989). Numerous studies have investigated the relationship between disease severity and RSV subgroups but the data are inconclusive. In some studies infections with RSV A strains were associated with increased severity in children (Hall, *et al*, 1990; Imaz *et al*, 2000; Mufson *et al*, 1988; Taylor *et al*, 1989; Walsh *et al*, 1997), while others failed to detect any significant correlation with the subgroup (DeVincenzo *et al*, 2004; Fodha *et al*, 2007; Martinello *et al*, 2002). It is possible that the simultaneous circulation of multiple strains of each subgroup during an epidemic, the year-to-year variation in virus population, the alternated subgroup predominance and the geographical location of the study may explain discrepancies between reports (Collins and Graham, 2008; Fletcher *et al*, 1997; Hall *et al*, 1990; Martinello *et al*, 2002). Interestingly, in several studies of hospitalised children RSV A subgroup infections led to higher mean viral loads compared to RSV B (Devincenzo *et al*, 2004; Fodha *et al*, 2007; Perkins *et al*, 2005). However, in view of the discrepancies, the biological significance of strain variation in relation to disease severity remains unclear.

3.1.2 RSV strain/genetic variation

The antigenic homology between RSV subgroups is approximately 25%. The fusion protein (RSV F) is the most conserved with 90% amino acid sequence identity and 50% antigenic homology between RSV A and B subgroups. The G protein (RSV G) is the most divergent, showing only 53% amino acid relatedness and 1 to 7% antigenic homology (Brandenburg, 2000; Collins et Graham, 2008; Rietweld, 2003). Thus, phylogenetic studies have targeted the G gene to differentiate between RSV strains. For instance, Martinello *et al* (2002) investigated the association between RSV G genotypes and disease severity in children during two RSV seasons. They found that clade RSV A GA3 isolates correlated significantly with increased clinical severity scores compared to other subgroup A clades (GA2, GA4) and B isolates. Previous reports also addressed this issue, although with a different classification of RSV strains. Specifically, Hall *et al* (1990) grouped RSV A and B strains on the basis of their reaction with various monoclonal antibodies to RSV G protein. Their data suggested an association between one RSV strain (A2) and higher rates of intensive care admission. Furthermore, two studies used restriction length polymorphism (RFLP), either of N and F genes (Savon *et al*, 2006) or N and G genes (Fletcher *et al*, 1997), to define RSV strains. Both studies concluded that RSV genotypes F1N4 (RSV F and N clades) and G were associated either with longer hospital stay (Savon *et al*, 2006) or various degrees of disease severity, according to their severity criteria (Fletcher *et al*, 1997). However, in our view these observations warrant further investigation. Overall, from our current understanding it is reasonable to assume that among the multiple strains simultaneously circulating during an RSV season some could be associated with increased severity.

3.1.3 Viral load

It is evident from the few published studies available that the importance of viral load in relation to RSV disease severity remains controversial. Studies addressing this issue determined viral loads in nasal aspirates from naturally infected infants following hospitalisation or within the community (Buckingham *et al*, 2000; DeVincenzo, 2004; DeVincenzo *et al*, 2005; Fodha *et al*, 2007; Houben *et al*, 2010; Wright *et al*, 2002). With the exception of the study by Wright *et al* (2002), there is a growing consensus that mean viral titres correlate significantly with disease severity. That RSV disease might be driven mainly by the viral load is a seductive idea and would correlate with other virus-associated illnesses, such as HIV, cytomegalovirus and influenza virus (DeVincenzo, 2005).

However, analyses of mean viral titres mask the fact that some individuals in non-severe cohorts may have considerably higher virus titres in their nasal aspirates than some individuals in the severe cohorts. This is clearly exemplified by Buchkingham *et al* (2000), who presented the virus load data from individuals in the severe and non-severe disease cohorts. Their data demonstrated that some individuals in the non-severe cohort had virus loads $\geq 2 \log_{10}$ pfu/ml higher than some severe cohort counterparts. Such data argue strongly against virus load as a predictor of disease severity. On the other hand, in contrast to the severe cohort, some individuals in the non-severe cohort had virus loads $\leq 2 \log_{10}$ pfu/ml, which undoubtedly skewed mean data towards reduced values. The cumulative data suggest the possibility that a certain minimum virus replication is required to cause severe illness, but the degree of replication itself may not be the defining characteristic. Interestingly, King *et al* (1993) reported that in infants co-infected with human immunodeficiency virus type 1, prolonged clinical shedding of RSV occurred without substantial disease compared to healthy controls, thereby implying a substantial role of the host immune system in RSV pathology rather than viral cytopathic effects. In our opinion, re-analyses of the published data, in which individual virus titre data are stratified into the severe and non-severe cohorts, will greatly help our understanding of this important issue.

Convincing evidence of a correlation between virus load and disease severity was provided recently in an elegant RSV challenge study in healthy adult volunteers (DeVincenzo *et al*,

2010). While symptoms were mild and restricted to the URT, virus growth and disease severity kinetics paralleled one another, suggesting that the efficiency of virus replication was driving symptom severity. A similar temporal association of virus shedding and respiratory symptom scores and mucus weight in RSV-challenged healthy adults was described by Lee *et al.* (2004). Moreover, the secretion of specific pro-inflammatory chemokines paralleled the viral load and the severity of the disease, hence acting as potentially interesting biomarkers (IL-6, IL-8/CXCL8, RANTES/CCL5, TNF-α, MIP-1α/CCL3). This is consistent with Noah & Becker (2000), who reported that IL-8/CXCL8, RANTES/CCL5, MIP-1α/CCL3 and MCP-1/CCL2 concentrations increased in nasal lavages recovered during virus shedding from infected adult volunteers. Surprisingly, infectivity, virus growth kinetics and disease severity appeared to be independent of the initial virus inoculum titres (10^3 to $10^{5.38}$ pfu) under the experimental conditions described (DeVincenzo *et al*, 2010). This contrasted with the work by Hall *et al* (1981), in which infectivity and the onset of virus shedding was greatly influenced by the initial inoculum ($10^{5.2} >> 10^{3.2}$ $TCID_{50}$) of the adult volunteers. It is possible, however, that these discrepancies might be explained, in part at least, by the use of different RSV strains and/or the fact that volunteers were pre-screened for relatively low virus neutralising antibody titres before inclusion in the study by DeVincenzo *et al* (2010). The latter hypothesis is consistent with Lee *et al* (2004), who found a significant correlation between pre-inoculation RSV neutralisation antibody titres and infection rates, irrespective of the infecting doses tested.

As the RSV challenge studies cited above were undertaken in healthy adults, who were undoubtedly repeatedly exposed to RSV infections prior to inclusion, great care must be taken in extrapolating these data and conclusions to infants undergoing primary infection. First, in contrast to the adult challenge experiments, in which symptoms were invariably restricted to the URT, a large proportion of infants undergoing their first RSV infection have symptomatic LRT involvement. Second, such infants are, by definition, immunologically naive relative to RSV and do not possess the plethora of anti-RSV memory T and B cell/antibody responses evident in adults. Third, young infants in particular, in whom the peak of severe RSV disease occurs, are thought to be immunologically immature and are therefore likely to respond quite differently to infection compared with adults.

3.2 Host factors

3.2.1 High-risk profiles in infants

As indicated above, underlying heart and lung conditions are factors predisposing to severe RSV disease. Patients with diseases such as congenital heart disease (CHD) or bronchopulmonary dysplasia (BPD) are often associated with RSV infections of greater severity. These conditions are associated with more frequent admission to ICU, prolonged hospitalisation, increased requirement and duration for supplemental oxygen, the need for mechanical ventilation, increased severity scores and death (Brandenburg, 2000; DeVincenzo *et al*, 2005; Garcia *et al*, 2011; Kaneko *et al*, 2001; Rietweld, 2003; Thorburn K, 2009; Wang *et al*, 1995; Wright *et al*, 2002). The precise reasons for aggravated illness in these infants are unclear but pre-existing lung diseases will significantly reduce an infant's functional pulmonary reserve capacity, rendering RSV more likely to overwhelm quickly and easily the infant's defences. Prematurity (Brandenburg, 2000; Fodha *et al*, 2007; Garcia *et al*, 2011; Rietweld, 2003; Wang *et al*, 1995) and acquired or congenital immunodeficiency status (Brandenburg, 2000; Ebbert *et al*, 2002; Hertz *et al*, 1989; Padman *et al*, 1985; Rietweld, 2003) are also important predisposing factors for severity.

It is thought that the reduced transplacental acquisition of maternal antibodies in pre-term compared to full-term infants may partially explain the aggravated disease associated with RSV infection of premature infants (DeVincenzo *et al*, 2005). Indeed, in a longitudinal study, it was shown that infants with higher maternal neutralizing antibodies had a lower risk of RSV hospitalisation and that once infected they developed significantly reduced severity of disease (Glezen *et al*, 1981). Importantly, although prematurity, congenital heart and lung conditions (Wang *et al* 1995; Rietweld, 2003), and immunodeficiencies (Graham *et al*, 2002; Hall *et al*, 1986; Wang *et al* 1995) have been associated with higher mortality rates in infants, the majority of children admitted to hospital with a RSV infection do not have these high risk factors (Brandenburg, 2000; Wang *et al*, 1995).

3.2.2 Cytokine and chemokine responses

A considerable body of information supports the idea that RSV pathogenesis is, at least in part, immune mediated. In essence, an over-exuberant immune response to infection is thought to cause considerable "collateral" damage in the lungs. The drivers for much of these immune responses to infection are cytokines and chemokines. These are small secreted proteins that are induced following interaction of pathogen-associated molecular patterns with pathogen recognition receptors, such as Toll-like receptors, on host cells. They include an expanding family of proteins, whose interaction with specific cellular receptors stimulates a range of signal transduction cascades resulting in a plethora of immunological functions. Functions of cytokines and chemokines include chemoattraction and activation of immune cells, such as neutrophils, lymphocytes, monocytes/macrophages and dendritic cells, i.e., hallmarks of RSV pathogenesis. Therefore, an over-exuberant cytokine/chemokine response is likely to be associated with RSV immunopathogenesis.

In this regard, regulated upon activation, normal T cell expressed and secreted (RANTES/CCL5), macrophage inflammatory protein 1α (MIP-1α/CCL3), monocytes chemotactic protein 1 (MCP-1/CCL2), IL-1β, IL-6, IL-8/CXCL8, IL-10, IL-18, tumours necrosis factor α (TNFα) and interferon γ-induced protein 10 (IP-10/CXCL10) are among a range of cytokines/chemokines demonstrating increased expression in nasal aspirates, BALs or blood from RSV infected infants (Barmejo-Martin *et al*, 2007; Garofalo *et al*, 2001; McNamara *et al*, 2004; McNamara *et al*, 2005; Murai *et al*, 2007; Noah *et al*, 2002; Roe *et al*, 2011; Van Benten *et al*, 2003). Furthermore, the levels of some of these molecules correlated with disease severity. For example, Garofalo *et al* (2001) reported that MIP-1α/CCL3 was markedly increased in nasopharyngeal secretions from infants with severe RSV bronchiolitis compared to those with RSV-URTI only or mild bronchiolitis. Similarly, Van Benten *et al* (2003) found that increased numbers of IL-18 positive cells in nasal brushes from RSV-infected infants was specific for bronchiolitis, as similar increases were not detected in infants with only RSV-URTI.

Despite the strong evidence of correlations between cytokine and chemokine expression levels and RSV infections, it is still unclear whether these relationships are temporal or causal in relation to RSV-induced disease and disease severity. The functions of some of these molecules are consistent with a causal role, but formal proof in humans will be very difficult to achieve. In support of a causal role, an elegant study by Juntti *et al* (2009) indicated that IL-6 and IL-8 responses following LPS stimulation of cord blood samples were predictive of disease severity following later infection. In essence, cord blood from infants subsequently hospitalised with RSV had higher combined IL-6 and IL-8 responses to LPS stimulation than cord blood from RSV-infected infants treated as outpatients. However, another limitation of these studies is the fact that only RSV infection was confirmed in the infants - co-infections with other respiratory pathogens were not considered. Therefore, the possibility remains that some of the data on cytokine/chemokine expression level correlations with RSV disease severity might be compromised by co-infections at the time of sampling.

3.2.3 Genetic polymorphisms

As outlined above, the majority of infants hospitalised with RSV have no underlying high-risk profiles. Furthermore, only a small proportion of infants from any given birth cohort end up with severe RSV disease. This suggests the possibility that genetic polymorphisms may be implicated in predisposing infants to severe disease. A number of groups have attempted to address this question using genetic association studies. Not surprisingly, in view of their correlations with severe RSV disease, much of the initial work focussed on specific cytokine/chemokine genes and their receptors. A comprehensive list of these haplotypes and polymorphisms associated with severe RSV disease was recently provided by Miyairi and DeVincenzo (2008), T Tregoning and Schwarze (2010) and Zeng *et al* (2011). They include such cytokine genes as IL-4, IL-8, IL-10, IL-13 and IL-18, and receptor genes like CCR5, CD14, CX3CR1, IL4RA and TLR4. Confirmation of these associations may provide the basis for identifying, from birth, otherwise healthy infants who are at risk of severe RSV disease. It would also provide the rationale for including such infants in the high risk groups that currently benefit from the immunoprophylaxis provided by palivizumab, an anti-RSV F monoclonal antibody administered to high risk infants before and during the RSV season. However, much work remains to be done to validate these genetic associations.

3.3 Environmental factors

The environment also plays a role on the extent of RSV infection as some of these factors can impact on the exposure to the virus or lung functions. Thus, day care attendance or crowded living conditions (siblings) are recognised risk factors for RSV hospitalisation, lower respiratory tract involvement (Rietweld, 2003) and admission to ICU (DeVincenzo *et al*, 2005). This association with disease severity is likely a consequence of the high infectivity of the virus. A recent survey of RSV infection in the community attempted to define several significant predictors of RSV LRTI (Houben *et al*, 2010). As expected, they included day care and siblings but other factors such as a high parental education level, a date of birth outside RSV season (April to September) and, surprisingly, a birth weight >4 kg. However, no association was identified with maternal smoking. Thus, this study concluded that the risk of RSV-LRTI was 10 times higher for children who attended day care, had older siblings, had high parental education level, a birth weight >4 kg and were born between April and September. A comprehensive review of the literature on RSV disease risk factors by Simoes

(2003) drew similar conclusions regarding day care attendance and crowding/siblings as important environmental factors for severe RSV-LRTI. However, in contrast to Houben *et al* (2010), birth during the first half of the RSV season (September to November) was found to be a risk factor.

4. Conclusions

In this chapter we have attempted to provide a comprehensive overview of the consequences of RSV infection in humans, with particular emphasis on severe disease characteristics in otherwise healthy infants. There is a general consensus that RSV disease is a mulitfactorial phenomenon implicating virus, host and environmental elements. However, the mechanisms by which RSV causes disease in humans remain largely unknown. Ethical and clinical constraints provide challenging obstacles to elucidating these mechanisms directly in human subjects. Animal models of RSV disease have undoubted roles to play in addressing specific concepts relating to RSV pathogenesis, e.g., gene knockout studies, which cannot be undertaken in humans. However, as they are generally only capable of modelling some aspects of RSV pathogenesis in humans, extrapolating data derived from animal models to human RSV disease has been less than spectacular to date. In our opinion, ultimate success in deciphering the molecular mechanisms of RSV disease in humans is likely to come from studies directly in humans and/or in authentic *ex-vivo/in-vitro* human tissue models. A comprehensive understanding of RSV pathogenesis in humans is the first step in addressing these issues and, ultimately, to finding prophylactic and/or therapeutic solutions for this devastating viral pathogen.

5. References

Aherne W., Bird T., Court S.D., Gardner P.S. & McQuillin J., (1970). Pathological changes in virus infections of the lower respiratory tract in children. *J.Clin.Pathol.* Vol. 23, No. 1, pp. (7-18), 0021-9746; 0021-9746

Bermejo-Martin J.F., Garcia-Arevalo M.C., De Lejarazu R.O., Ardura J., Eiros J.M., Alonso A., Matias V., Pino M., Bernardo D., Arranz E. & Blanco-Quiros A. (2007) Predominance of Th2 cytokines, CXC chemokines and innate immunity mediators at the mucosal level during severe respiratory syncytial virus infection in children. Eur. Cytokine Netw. Vol. 18, No. 3, pp. (162-167), 1148-5493; 1148-5493.

Brandenburg A.H., Kleinjan A., van Het Land B., Moll H.A., Timmerman H.H., de Swart R.L., Neijens H.J., Fokkens W. & Osterhaus A.D., (2000). Type 1-like immune response is found in children with respiratory syncytial virus infection regardless of clinical severity. *J.Med.Virol.* Vol. 62, No. 2, pp. (267-277), 0146-6615; 0146-6615

Brandenburg A.H., (2000). Respiratory Syncytial Virus Infections in Infants: Determinants of Clinical Severity. (PhD), pp. (11), 90-9014084-0

Brouard J. & Dubus J.C., (2001). Clinique et physiopathologie de la bronchiolite a virus respiratoire syncytial, In:Infection virales respiratoires - tome 2 Bronchopne-umopathies virales, F. Freymuth. , pp. (19), Elsevier, 2-84299-338-1, France, Gap

Buckingham S.C., Bush A.J. & Devincenzo J.P., (2000). Nasal quantity of respiratory syncytical virus correlates with disease severity in hospitalized infants. *Pediatr.Infect.Dis.J.* Vol. 19, No. 2, pp. (113-117), 0891-3668; 0891-3668

Chin J., Magoffin R.L., Shearer L.A., Schieble J.H. & Lennette E.H., (1969). Field evaluation of a respiratory syncytial virus vaccine and a trivalent parainfluenza virus vaccine in a pediatric population. *Am.J.Epidemiol.* Vol. 89, No. 4, pp. (449-463), 0002-9262; 0002-9262

Collins P.L. & Graham B.S., (2008). Viral and host factors in human respiratory syncytial virus pathogenesis. *J.Virol.* Vol. 82, No. 5, pp. (2040-2055), 1098-5514; 0022-538X

DeVincenzo J.P., (2004). Natural infection of infants with respiratory syncytial virus subgroups A and B: a study of frequency, disease severity, and viral load. *Pediatr.Res.* Vol. 56, No. 6, pp. (914-917), 0031-3998; 0031-3998

DeVincenzo J.P., (2005). Factors predicting childhood respiratory syncytial virus severity: what they indicate about pathogenesis. *Pediatr.Infect.Dis.J.* Vol. 24, No. 11 Suppl, pp. (S177-83, discussion S182), 0891-3668; 0891-3668

DeVincenzo J.P., El Saleeby C.M. & Bush A.J., (2005). Respiratory syncytial virus load predicts disease severity in previously healthy infants. *J.Infect.Dis.* Vol. 191, No. 11, pp. (1861-1868), 0022-1899; 0022-1899

DeVincenzo J.P., Wilkinson T., Vaishnaw A., Cehelsky J., Meyers R., Nochur S., Harrison L., Meeking P., Mann A., Moane E., Oxford J., Pareek R., Moore R., Walsh E., Studholme R., Dorsett P., Alvarez R. & Lambkin-Williams R., (2010). Viral load drives disease in humans experimentally infected with respiratory syncytial virus. *Am.J.Respir.Crit.Care Med.* Vol. 182, No. 10, pp. (1305-1314), 1535-4970; 1073-449X

Downham M.A., Gardner P.S., McQuillin J. & Ferris J.A., (1975). Role of respiratory viruses in childhood mortality. *Br.Med.J.* Vol. 1, No. 5952, pp. (235-239), 0007-1447; 0007-1447

Ebbert J.O. & Limper A.H., (2005). Respiratory syncytial virus pneumonitis in immunocompromised adults: clinical features and outcome. *Respiration.* Vol. 72, No. 3, pp. (263-269), 0025-7931; 0025-7931

Everard M.L., Swarbrick A., Wrightham M., McIntyre J., Dunkley C., James P.D., Sewell H.F. & Milner A.D., (1994). Analysis of cells obtained by bronchial lavage of infants with respiratory syncytial virus infection. *Arch.Dis.Child.* Vol. 71, No. 5, pp. (428-432), 1468-2044; 0003-9888

Fisher R.G., Gruber W.C., Edwards K.M., Reed G.W., Tollefson S.J., Thompson J.M. & Wright P.F., (1997). Twenty years of outpatient respiratory syncytial virus infection: a framework for vaccine efficacy trials. *Pediatrics.* Vol. 99, No. 2, pp. (E7), 1098-4275; 0031-4005

Fletcher J.N., Smyth R.L., Thomas H.M., Ashby D. & Hart C.A., (1997). Respiratory syncytial virus genotypes and disease severity among children in hospital. *Arch.Dis.Child.* Vol. 77, No. 6, pp. (508-511), 1468-2044; 0003-9888

Fodha I., Vabret A., Ghedira L., Seboui H., Chouchane S., Dewar J., Gueddiche N., Trabelsi A., Boujaafar N. & Freymuth F., (2007). Respiratory syncytial virus infections in hospitalized infants: association between viral load, virus subgroup, and disease severity. *J.Med.Virol.* Vol. 79, No. 12, pp. (1951-1958), 0146-6615; 0146-6615

Garcia C.G., Bhore R., Soriano-Fallas A., Trost M., Chason R., Ramilo O. & Mejias A., (2010). Risk factors in children hospitalized with RSV bronchiolitis versus non-RSV bronchiolitis. *Pediatrics.* Vol. 126, No. 6, pp. (e1453-60), 1098-4275; 0031-4005

Garofalo R.P., Patti J., Hintz K.A., Hill V., Ogra P.L. and Welliver R.C. (2001). Macrophage inflammatory protein 1α (not T helper type 2 cytokines) is associated with severe forms of respiratory syncytial virus bronchiolitis. J. Infect. Dis. Vol 184, No. 4, pp. (393-399), 0022-1899; 0022-1899.

Glezen W.P., Paredes A., Allison J.E., Taber L.H. & Frank A.L., (1981). Risk of respiratory syncytial virus infection for infants from low-income families in relationship to age, sex, ethnic group, and maternal antibody level. *J.Pediatr.* Vol. 98, No. 5, pp. (708-715), 0022-3476; 0022-3476

Graham B.S., Rutigliano J.A. & Johnson T.R., (2002). Respiratory syncytial virus immunobiology and pathogenesis. *Virology.* Vol. 297, No. 1, pp. (1-7), 0042-6822; 0042-6822

Hall C.B., Douglas Jr R.G., Schnabel K.C. & Geiman J.M. (1981). Infectivity of respiratory syncytial virus by various routes of inoculation. *Infect. Immun.* Vol. 33, No. 3, pp. (779-783), 0019-9567; 0019-9567.

Hall C.B., Long C.E. & Schnabel K.C., (2001). Respiratory syncytial virus infections in previously healthy working adults. *Clin.Infect.Dis.* Vol. 33, No. 6, pp. (792-796), 1058-4838; 1058-4838

Hall C.B., Walsh E.E., Schnabel K.C., Long C.E., McConnochie K.M., Hildreth S.W. & Anderson L.J., (1990). Occurrence of groups A and B of respiratory syncytial virus over 15 years: associated epidemiologic and clinical characteristics in hospitalized and ambulatory children. *J.Infect.Dis.* Vol. 162, No. 6, pp. (1283-1290), 0022-1899; 0022-1899

Heidema J., Lukens M.V., van Maren W.W., van Dijk M.E., Otten H.G., van Vught A.J., van der Werff D.B., van Gestel S.J., Semple M.G., Smyth R.L., Kimpen J.L. & van Bleek G.M., (2007). CD8+ T cell responses in bronchoalveolar lavage fluid and peripheral blood mononuclear cells of infants with severe primary respiratory syncytial virus infections. *J.Immunol.* Vol. 179, No. 12, pp. (8410-8417), 0022-1767; 0022-1767

Henderson F.W., Hu S.C. & Collier A.M., (1978). Pathogenesis of respiratory syncytial virus infection in ferret and fetal human tracheas in organ culture. *Am.Rev.Respir.Dis.* Vol. 118, No. 1, pp. (29-37), 0003-0805; 0003-0805

Hertz M.I., Englund J.A., Snover D., Bitterman P.B. & McGlave P.B., (1989). Respiratory syncytial virus-induced acute lung injury in adult patients with bone marrow transplants: a clinical approach and review of the literature. *Medicine (Baltimore).* Vol. 68, No. 5, pp. (269-281), 0025-7974; 0025-7974

Houben M.L., Bont L., Wilbrink B., Belderbos M.E., Kimpen J.L., Visser G.H. & Rovers M.M., (2011). Clinical prediction rule for RSV bronchiolitis in healthy newborns: prognostic birth cohort study. *Pediatrics.* Vol. 127, No. 1, pp. (35-41), 1098-4275; 0031-4005

Houben M.L., Coenjaerts F.E., Rossen J.W., Belderbos M.E., Hofland R.W., Kimpen J.L. & Bont L., (2010). Disease severity and viral load are correlated in infants with primary respiratory syncytial virus infection in the community. *J.Med.Virol.* Vol. 82, No. 7, pp. (1266-1271), 1096-9071; 0146-6615

Imaz M.S., Sequeira M.D., Videla C., Veronessi I., Cociglio R., Zerbini E. & Carballal G., (2000). Clinical and epidemiologic characteristics of respiratory syncytial virus subgroups A and B infections in Santa Fe, Argentina. *J.Med.Virol.* Vol. 61, No. 1, pp. (76-80), 0146-6615; 0146-6615

Johnson J.E., Gonzales R.A., Olson S.J., Wright P.F. & Graham B.S., (2007). The histopathology of fatal untreated human respiratory syncytial virus infection. *Mod.Pathol.* Vol. 20, No. 1, pp. (108-119), 0893-3952; 0893-3952

Juntti H., Osterlund P., Kokkonen J., Dunder T., Renko M., Pokka T., Julkunen I. & Uhari M. (2009). Cytokine responses in cord blood predict the severity of later respiratory syncytial virus infection. *J. Allergy Clin. Immunol.* Vol. 124, No. 1, pp. (52-58), 1097-6825; 0091-6749.

Kaneko M., Watanabe J., Ueno E., Hida M. & Sone T., (2001). Risk factors for severe respiratory syncytial virus-associated lower respiratory tract infection in children. *Pediatr.Int.* Vol. 43, No. 5, pp. (489-492), 1328-8067

King J.C.,Jr, Burke A.R., Clemens J.D., Nair P., Farley J.J., Vink P.E., Batlas S.R., Rao M. & Johnson J.P., (1993). Respiratory syncytial virus illnesses in human immunodeficiency virus- and noninfected children. *Pediatr.Infect.Dis.J.* Vol. 12, No. 9, pp. (733-739), 0891-3668; 0891-3668

Kurlandsky L.E., French G., Webb P.M. & Porter D.D., (1988). Fatal respiratory syncytial virus pneumonitis in a previously healthy child. *Am.Rev.Respir.Dis.* Vol. 138, No. 2, pp. (468-472), 0003-0805; 0003-0805

Lee F.E., Walsh E.E., Falsey A.R., Betts R.F. & Treanor J.J., (2004). Experimental infection of humans with A2 respiratory syncytial virus. *Antiviral Res.* Vol. 63, No. 3, pp. (191-196), 0166-3542; 0166-3542

Levenson R.M. & Kantor O.S., (1987). Fatal pneumonia in an adult due to respiratory syncytial virus. *Arch.Intern.Med.* Vol. 147, No. 4, pp. (791-792), 0003-9926; 0003-9926

Lukens M.V., van de Pol A.C., Coenjaerts F.E., Jansen N.J., Kamp V.M., Kimpen J.L., Rossen J.W., Ulfman L.H., Tacke C.E., Viveen M.C., Koenderman L., Wolfs T.F. & van Bleek G.M., (2010). A systemic neutrophil response precedes robust CD8(+) T-cell activation during natural respiratory syncytial virus infection in infants. *J.Virol.* Vol. 84, No. 5, pp. (2374-2383), 1098-5514; 0022-538X

Martinello R.A., Chen M.D., Weibel C. & Kahn J.S., (2002). Correlation between respiratory syncytial virus genotype and severity of illness. *J.Infect.Dis.* Vol. 186, No. 6, pp. (839-842), 0022-1899; 0022-1899

McNamara P.S., Flanagan B.F., Hart C.A. & Smyth R.L. (2005) Production of chemokines in the lungs of infants with severe respiratory syncytial virus bronchiolitis. J. Infect. Dis. Vol. 191, No. 8, pp. (1225-1232), 0022-1899; 0022-1899.

McNamara P.S., Flanagan B.F., Selby A.M., Hart C.A. & Smyth R.L. (2004) Pro- and anti-inflammatory responses in respiratory syncytial virus bronchiolitis. *Eur. Respir. J.* Vol. 23, No. 1, pp. (106-112), 0903-1936; 0903-1936

Miyairi I. and DeVincenzo J.P. (2008). Human genetic factors and respiratory syncytial virus disease severity. Clin. Microbiol. Rev. Vol. 24, No. 4, pp. (686-703), 1098-6618; 0893-8512

Mufson M.A., Belshe R.B., Orvell C. & Norrby E., (1988). Respiratory syncytial virus epidemics: variable dominance of subgroups A and B strains among children, 1981-1986. *J.Infect.Dis.* Vol. 157, No. 1, pp. (143-148), 0022-1899; 0022-1899

Murai H., Terada A., Mizuno M., Asai M., Hirabayashi Y., Shimizu S., Morishita T., Kakita H., Hussein M.H., Ito T., Kato I., Asai K. & Togari H. (2007) IL-10 and RANTES are elevated in nasopharyngeal secretions of children with respiratory syncytial virus infection. *Allergol. Internat.* Vol. 56, No. 2, pp. (157-163), 1323-8930; 1323-8930.

Noah T.L. & Becker S. (2000). Chemokines in nasal secretions of normal adults experimentally infected with respiratory syncytial virus. *Clin. Immunol.* Vol. 97, No. 1, pp. (43-49), 1521-6616; 1521-6616.

Noah T.L., Ivins S.S., Murphy P., Kazachkova I., Moats-Staats B. & Henderson F.W. (2002) Chemokines and inflammation in the nasal passages of infants with respiratory syncytial virus bronchiolitis. *Clin. Immunol.* Vol. 104, No. 1, pp. (86-95), 1521-6616; 1521-6616.

Neilson K.A. & Yunis E.J., (1990). Demonstration of respiratory syncytial virus in an autopsy series. *Pediatr.Pathol.* Vol. 10, No. 4, pp. (491-502), 0277-0938; 0277-0938

O'Donnell D.R. & Carrington D., (2002). Peripheral blood lymphopenia and neutrophilia in children with severe respiratory syncytial virus disease. *Pediatr.Pulmonol.* Vol. 34, No. 2, pp. (128-130), 8755-6863; 1099-0496

Padman R., Bye M.R., Schidlow D.V. & Zaeri N., (1985). Severe RSV bronchiolitis in an immunocompromised child. *Clin.Pediatr.(Phila).* Vol. 24, No. 12, pp. (719-721), 0009-9228; 0009-9228

Perkins S.M., Webb D.L., Torrance S.A., El Saleeby C., Harrison L.M., Aitken J.A., Patel A. & DeVincenzo J.P., (2005). Comparison of a real-time reverse transcriptase PCR assay and a culture technique for quantitative assessment of viral load in children naturally infected with respiratory syncytial virus. *J.Clin.Microbiol.* Vol. 43, No. 5, pp. (2356-2362), 0095-1137; 0095-1137

Reed J.L., Welliver T.P., Sims G.P., McKinney L., Velozo L., Avendano L., Hintz K., Luma J., Coyle A.J. & Welliver RC S., (2009). Innate immune signals modulate antiviral and polyreactive antibody responses during severe respiratory syncytial virus infection. *J.Infect.Dis.* Vol. 199, No. 8, pp. (1128-1138), 0022-1899; 0022-1899

Rietveld E., (2003). Respiratory Syncytial Virus Infections in Young Children Risk Assessment and Prevention. (PhD), pp. (183), 90-9017574-1

Roe M.F., Bloxham D.M., Cowburn A.S. & O'Donnell D.R. (2011) Changes in helper lymphocyte chemokine receptor expression and elevation of IP-10 during acute respiratory syncytial virus infection in infants. *Exp. Allergy Immunol.* Vol. 22, No. 2, pp. (229-234), 1399-3038; 0905-6157

Savon C., Goyenechea A., Valdes O., Aguilar J., Gonzalez G., Palerm L., Gonzalez G. & Perez Brena P., (2006). Respiratory syncytial virus group A and B genotypes and disease severity among Cuban children. *Arch.Med.Res.* Vol. 37, No. 4, pp. (543-547), 0188-4409; 0188-4409

Simoes E.A. (2003). Environmental and demographic risk factors for respiratory syncytial virus lower respiratory tract disease. *J. Pediatr.* Vol. 143, No. 5 Suppl. pp. (S118-S126), 0022-3476; 0022-3476

Smith P.K., Wang S.Z., Dowling K.D. & Forsyth K.D., (2001). Leucocyte populations in respiratory syncytial virus-induced bronchiolitis. *J.Paediatr.Child Health.* Vol. 37, No. 2, pp. (146-151), 1034-4810; 1034-4810

Spann K.M., Tran K.C., Chi B., Rabin R.L. & Collins P.L., (2004). Suppression of the induction of alpha, beta, and lambda interferons by the NS1 and NS2 proteins of human respiratory syncytial virus in human epithelial cells and macrophages [corrected. *J.Virol.* Vol. 78, No. 8, pp. (4363-4369), 0022-538X; 0022-538X

Taylor C.E., Morrow S., Scott M., Young B. & Toms G.L., (1989). Comparative virulence of respiratory syncytial virus subgroups A and B. *Lancet.* Vol. 1, No. 8641, pp. (777-778), 0140-6736; 0140-6736

Thorburn K., (2009). Pre-existing disease is associated with a significantly higher risk of death in severe respiratory syncytial virus infection. *Arch.Dis.Child.* Vol. 94, No. 2, pp. (99-103), 1468-2044; 0003-9888

Tregoning J.S. & Schwarze J., (2010). Respiratory viral infections in infants: causes, clinical symptoms, virology, and immunology. *Clin.Microbiol.Rev.* Vol. 23, No. 1, pp. (74-98), 1098-6618; 0893-8512

Van Benten I.J., van Drunen C.M., Koopman L.P., KleinJan A., van Middelkoop B.C., de Waal L., Osterhaus A.D., Neijens H.J. & Fokkens W.J. (2003). RSV-induced bronchiolitis but not upper respiratory tract infection is accompanied by an increased nasal IL-18 response. J. Med. Virol. Vol. 71, No. 2, pp. (290-297), 0146-6615; 0146-6615

Van Benten I.J., van Drunen C.M., Koopman L.P., van Middelkoop B.C., Hop W.C., Osterhaus A.D., Neijens H.J. & Fokkens W.J., (2005). Age- and infection-related maturation of the nasal immune response in 0-2-year-old children. *Allergy.* Vol. 60, No. 2, pp. (226-232), 0105-4538; 0105-4538

Walsh E.E., McConnochie K.M., Long C.E. & Hall C.B. (1997). Severity of respiratory syncytial virus infection is related to virus strain. *J. Infect. Dis.* Vol. 175, No. 4, pp. (814-820), 0022-1899; 0022-1899

Wang E.E., Law B.J. & Stephens D., (1995). Pediatric Investigators Collaborative Network on Infections in Canada (PICNIC) prospective study of risk factors and outcomes in patients hospitalized with respiratory syncytial viral lower respiratory tract infection. *J.Pediatr.* Vol. 126, No. 2, pp. (212-219), 0022-3476; 0022-3476

Welliver T.P., Reed J.L. & Welliver RC S., (2008). Respiratory syncytial virus and influenza virus infections: observations from tissues of fatal infant cases. *Pediatr.Infect.Dis.J.* Vol. 27, No. 10 Suppl, pp. (S92-6), 0891-3668; 0891-3668

Welliver T.P., Garofalo R.P., Hosakote Y., Hintz K.H., Avendano L., Sanchez K., Velozo L., Jafri H., Chavez-Bueno S., Ogra P.L., McKinney L. & Reed J.L., (2007). Severe human lower respiratory tract illness caused by respiratory syncytial virus and influenza virus is characterized by the absence of pulmonary cytotoxic lymphocyte responses. Vol. 195, No. 8, pp. (1126-1136), 0022-1899; 0022-1899

Wright P.F., Gruber W.C., Peters M., Reed G., Zhu Y., Robinson F., Coleman-Dockery S. & Graham B.S., (2002). Illness severity, viral shedding, and antibody responses in infants hospitalized with bronchiolitis caused by respiratory syncytial virus. *J.Infect.Dis.* Vol. 185, No. 8, pp. (1011-1018), 0022-1899; 0022-1899

Zeng R., Li C., Li N., Wei L. & Cui Y., (2011). The role of cytokines and chemokines in severe respiratory syncytial virus infection and subsequent asthma. *Cytokine.* Vol. 53, No. 1, pp. (1-7), 1096-0023; 1043-4666

Zhang L., Peeples M.E., Boucher R.C., Collins P.L. & Pickles R.J., (2002). Respiratory syncytial virus infection of human airway epithelial cells is polarized, specific to ciliated cells, and without obvious cytopathology. *J.Virol.* Vol. 76, No. 11, pp. (5654-5666), 0022-538X; 0022-538X

Zhao D.C., Yan T., Li L., You S. & Zhang C., (2007). Respiratory syncytial virus inhibits interferon-alpha-inducible signaling in macrophage-like U937 cells. *J.Infect.* Vol. 54, No. 4, pp. (393-398), 1532-2742; 0163-4453.

6

Detection of Bacteriophage in Droplets

Phillipa Perrott and Megan Hargreaves
Queensland University of Technology
Australia

1. Introduction

The economic costs associated with illnesses like influenza and the common cold are in the order of billions of dollars, arising from medical treatment, lost income and decreased productivity of ill workers. Acute respiratory diseases can be more severe for the young, elderly or immuno-compromised, causing complications and death in many cases.

Transmission of respiratory diseases, including of respiratory syncytial virus (RSV), can be via small droplets that are able to remain suspended in the air and subsequently be inhaled by a susceptible host (Centers for Disease Control, 2010). However, little information is available on the specifics of transmission via aerosol droplets. A greater understanding of the fate of viruses in droplets, and the effect of physical factors that govern aerosol spread, is needed to control the spread of viral infections. The research undertaken in this study addresses some questions surrounding aspects of virus transmission via the aerosol route, in order to contribute to a more comprehensive understanding of this issue.

1.1 Transmission of viral infections

Respiratory infections can be spread by direct contact with an infected person, or by indirect contact with an intermediate contaminated object (fomite) (Goldmann, 2000). However, the mode of transmission of which the least information is available, is airborne transmission. This occurs when droplets, also known as bioaerosols, evaporate and become droplet nuclei,which are small residue droplets with diameters of less than 5 µm, that can remain suspended in the air for long periods of time (Fiegel et al., 2006). Droplet nuclei are thus associated with long distance transmission.

Virus survival and spatial distribution of droplets are dependent on a number of factors, including droplet size and atmospheric conditions. Our knowledge of the mechanisms by which viruses are released into the air by humans or animals is somewhat limited, as is the nature of the association between the virus and its carrier particles. Furthermore, understanding of the mechanisms responsible for transport and spread of the agents in common types of indoor environments such as residential apartments, buildings, hotels and hospitals is also very limited.

While studies have been conducted to characterise the distribution of such virus-containing droplets, results have varied widely. Most of these studies have used models to simulate natural aerosolisation, and until recently, no studies had examined the natural cough droplet distribution of infected human subjects. A greater understanding of the fate of viruses in droplets, and the effect of physical factors that govern aerosol spread, is needed to control the spread of viral infections.

Respiratory syncytial virus (RSV) is a medically important virus, and is one of the two major causes of lower respiratory tract (LRT) infections in infants and young children. Recently, it has also been recognised as important pathogens in adults, although the symptoms are less distinct and often the viral cause is not initially correctly identified (Hall, 2001). Additionally, there are no effective means of controlling the spread of this virus.

There are two subtypes of RSV, serotypes A and B (Liolios et al., 2001). RSV is responsible for approximately 90,000 hospitalisations and 4,500 deaths in children aged six months and younger of the same age group, each year in the US alone. Stockton and colleagues stated that although the incidence of RSV in infants is known and widely documented, its contribution to morbidity and mortality in adults is unknown, and possibly under-diagnosed (Stockton et al., 1998).

Of the recognised mechanisms by which respiratory viruses can spread, some consider bioaerosols to be the principal mode of transmission (Couch et al., 1986). Others believe that direct and indirect contact is more to blame for spread of the disease. This issue remains contentious, with support on both sides, and evidence varying widely. However, it is generally agreed by most experts that airborne transmission of viruses is an issue requiring further investigation. As methods for droplet measurement and virus detection continue to become more sophisticated, more data is becoming available.

1.2 Bioaerosols

Bioaerosols have been defined as a collection of aerosolised biological particles (Cox and Wathes, 1995), which can vary depending on source, dispersal mechanisms and environmental conditions (Pillai, 2002). Bioaerosols themselves can be pathogenic, or can act as a vehicle for the dissemination of pathogens (Pillai and Ricke, 2002), such as fungi, bacteria or viruses. It is thought that many infections, particularly respiratory infections, can be transmitted between persons via airborne droplets from an infected person to an uninfected person. These droplets, or infectious aerosols, contain pathogens, which upon contact or inhalation may cause disease in a susceptible person. Therefore, bioaerosols contribute substantially to the transmission of many infectious diseases. Researchers, however, are unable to reach a consensus as to the significance of the airborne route in the transmission of respiratory diseases, due to a shortage of evidence for either argument. This can be attributed to past inadequate technologies, which were unable to fully recognise all facets of bioaerosol distribution. However, even with the aid of the more sophisticated technology that has become available over the last couple of decades, agreement between experts has still not been attained.

Infectious bioaerosols can be generated from a number of sources, including sewage treatment plants (Carducci et al., 1999), toilets (Barker and Jones, 2005), and infected people. In this study, we are only interested in the latter, as they are undeniably implicated in the spread of respiratory infections like RSV. Droplets evaporate very quickly once they are released (in the order of milliseconds), and their size decreases to approximately half the original size of the droplet (Nicas et al., 2005). Weber states that "there is no unique and generally agreed upon classification of airborne droplets, for example, concerning the aerodynamic diameter which defines the cut-off size between droplet nuclei and large droplets" (Weber and Stilianakis, 2008) (page 362). Droplet nuclei are generally considered to be smaller than 10 µm in aerodynamic diameter, although some studies cite 5 µm as the cut off.

It has been shown that viruses are more effectively spread by aerosol than bacteria or fungi (Carducci et al., 1999). Barker and Jones (2005)reported that in a controlled study on aerosols generated from toilets, twice as many viruses survived as bacteria. Viral diseases thought to be transmitted by infectious aerosol range from relatively mild conditions such as the common cold to more severe diseases, including severe acute respiratory syndrome (SARS), smallpox and influenza (Tseng and Li, 2005, Wang et al., 2005).

1.2.1 Bioaerosol production

The emission of respiratory droplets by people can occur via breathing, talking, coughing or sneezing (Edwards et al., 2004). Droplets are created when currents of air pass over the mucous linings in the respiratory tract, creating disturbances in the surface of the mucous. This can lead to the creation of droplets which break away from the bulk of the liquid (Fiegel et al., 2006). The production of droplets and aerosols is a complex process in the body, with many factors influencing the properties of the resulting particles.

Droplets expelled from the respiratory tract differ in size depending on the exact point of creation. This is due to the physiology of the respiratory tract: as the diameter of the respiratory tract varies, air pressure and speed change accordingly (Morawska, 2006). For example, the trachea has a larger diameter than bronchioles, so the air pressure and speed is lower, and the resulting droplets theoretically should be larger in size and fewer in number. Talking and breathing activities generally tend to create droplets which are larger and fewer in numbers. Droplets from these activities are typically created in the mouth. Activities such as coughing produce droplets which are much smaller, and in greater numbers, usually from the lower sections of the respiratory tract. Droplets produced from coughing and sneezing have been reported to range in size from 1 to 100 µm by one study (Kowalski and Bahnfleth, 1998) and from 1 to 20 µm by another study (Knight, 1973). Papineni and Rosenthal (1997) reported that the quantity of droplets produced was highest in coughing compared to other respiratory activities.

The properties of mucous and respiratory fluids will most probably introduce a further influential element in the creation of the resulting droplets. Edwards (1991) noted that high surface tension of mucous, which is found in infected individuals, favours the formation of relatively larger droplets; similarly, lower viscosity favours the formation of smaller droplets (Burkdolder and Berg, 1974). Differing compositions of respiratory fluids will require varying flow velocities in the respiratory tract to produce droplets, due to changed adhesion forces of the respiratory fluids (Papineni and Rosenthal, 1997). In an infected individual, these fluids will usually be more viscous, and therefore it can be inferred that droplets produced by such an individual will be different from that of a healthy individual. Therefore, droplets will vary in size, in the number of droplets produced, according to the type of respiratory activity and the health status of the individual.

The creation of the droplet does not only affect the droplet physically, in terms of its fate in the environment, but ultimately it dictates whether or not the droplet will contain an infectious particle. In this regard, we must consider the general pathologies of respiratory infections. The precise location of the infection in the respiratory tract is certainly the most important factor here. Some viruses, for instance rhinoviruses and other viruses causing the common cold, preferentially localise infection in the upper respiratory tract. Other viruses favour the lower respiratory tract. Parainfluenza viruses and respiratory syncytial viruses both replicate in the nasopharyngeal epithelium, and after a few days spread to the lower respiratory tract (Hall, 2001).

1.2.2 Bioaerosol transport

An area of specific interest of the three stages of aerosol transmission is transport of droplets. Bioaerosol transport in the air has been widely documented in field or model studies. However, fewer studies have examined the aerial transport and fate of droplets emitted by humans during breathing, coughing, sneezing or talking (Nicas et al., 2005). Even fewer studies have examined the detection of respiratory viruses in infected individuals; before 2007 there were no known studies that had achieved this.

Morawska (2006) stated that the most important factor affecting particle fate is particle size. Additionally, particle size has a significant effect on the biological properties of a droplet. The initial size and concentration of the droplets alters dramatically upon release into the atmosphere, mostly due to evaporation. Droplets of pure liquid evaporate completely; thus, the degree by which the droplet evaporates is largely dependent on the water content and composition of the droplet. Interestingly, a recent study found that the dynamic evaporation of respiratory aerosols was very similar in speed to pure water droplets of a similar size; however this study only investigated dynamic evaporation in the order of seconds, and the findings do not preclude further drying of droplets over minutes or hours (Morawska et al., 2008). Furthermore, it investigated droplets expelled by healthy individuals. If during respiratory infection, droplets have a higher mucous content (and thus less water content), the particle size may not decrease in size upon release, compared to a droplet with less mucous content (and more water content).

Once the droplets have been released into the air, they are subjected to a number of forces that determine their distance and time of travel; these include Brownian motion, gravity, electrical forces, thermal gradients, electromagnetic radiation, turbulent diffusion, inertial forces and relative humidity (Pillai and Ricke, 2002). Brownian motion, which refers to the collision of the droplets with other molecules in the air, increases with rising temperature and decreasing size; particles larger than 1 μm are generally more affected by gravity than Brownian motion (Pillai and Ricke, 2002) and may settle rapidly out of the air (Papineni and Rosenthal, 1997, Foarde et al., 1999). Other factors affecting droplet fate are the size, shape and quantity of the droplets.

Information regarding droplets expelled by healthy individuals is relatively abundant. It has been reported that the size of droplets released by humans can range from 0.5 μm to 200 μm (Erdal and Esmen, 1995). Morawska and colleagues (2008) identified three distinct modes of aerosols during common expiratory respiratory activities: breath mode aerosol with a count median diameter (CMD) of <1 μm; a vocal cord vibration aerosol with a CMD near 3 μm; and a saliva aerosol mode near 10 μm. The number and concentration of particles is highly variable from person to person. Edwards and colleagues (2004) studied the release of droplets by 11 subjects and were able to separate them into two groups based on the number of particles they exhaled. Whilst 'high-producers' expelled an average of 500 particles per litre per six hours, 'low-producers' expelled an average of less than 500 particles per litre per six hours. However, it must be noted that the subjects in the preceding studies were healthy volunteers, and that the droplets produced from healthy individuals are likely to be dynamically distinct from the droplets produced by infected people.

Information on droplets expelled by infected individuals is vital to the understanding of transmission of infection, however, this issue has not been appropriately pursued. Additionally, publications describing particle size are not always clear as to whether droplet measurements refer to the initial droplet size (size before evaporation) or the dry droplet size (after evaporation) (Morawska et al., 2009). This difference is important, as evaporation plays a very important part in droplet fate. It is imperative to know the final size and composition of the droplets in question, so that their fate can be accurately predicted.

The majority of reports published on bioaerosol transport have agreed on the most influential factors that affect virus transport in the air. The most commonly investigated environmental condition that has been documented is relative humidity (RH). It has been reported that some respiratory illnesses are less frequent in high RH (Wang et al., 2005); however this is not the case for all viruses, as one study found that rhinoviruses had a higher recovery rate at high RH. Lipid-enveloped viruses tend to have a greater stability at lower RH, usually below 40 % (Benbough, 1971, Pillai and Ricke, 2002).

A review by Fiegel and co-workers (2006) concluded that both inhaled and exhaled bioaerosols could act as vectors for deep-lung and environmental transport of airborne disease. They also concluded that it is likely that a small percentage of the population would be responsible for dissemination of the majority of exhaled bioaerosols.

Tang and co-workers (2006) conducted a review into aerosol transmission of infectious diseases within healthcare premises. From the data they gathered, the authors found evidence that infectious organisms are able to be transmitted over both short and long distances, and that some organisms associated only with short-range transmission can also cause outbreaks over greater distances via transmission of evaporated droplets. This review concluded that personal protective equipment is needed to prevent person-to-person short-range transmission of infectious diseases.

1.2.3 Bioaerosol reception

The reception of droplets and subsequent risk of infection relies on the deposition of droplets in the respiratory tract, which in turn depends on a number of factors. The size of the droplet will determine the depth to which the droplet is able to penetrate the airways. A study conducted by Hatch (1961) found that the retention of particles in the respiratory tract is close to 100 % for particles with a diameter of about 5μm; retention drops to about 20 % for particles of about 0.25 -0.5 μm and then increases again to reach 60 % for sub-microscopic particles (smaller than 0.1 μm). The majority of droplets that are 20 μm in diameter deposit in the nasal passages, with a small fraction depositing in the pharynx and larger bronchi (Knight, 1980). Foarde (1999) stated that nearly all 2 μm particles are deposited in the respiratory tract, whilst Daigle and colleagues (2003) found that deposition of particles increased as their size decreased.

The smaller the particles, the more likely they are to impact on the lower respiratory tract. Proctor (1966) stated that although few deposition studies have been conducted, it is likely that particles smaller than 5 μm will penetrate to the lower respiratory tract. It has been reported that the main mechanism for deposition of particles with a diameter less than 0.5 μm is diffusion (Daigle et al., 2003), which can occur in the alveoli of the lungs (Wilson et al., 2002). Diffusion by smaller particles is more harmful because they can diffuse rapidly through the alveolar membrane into the blood (Hogan et al., 2005).

Hinds (1982) described the fate of aerosol particles deposited in the respiratory tract as follows: the upper respiratory tract has a mucous lining that is propelled, along with the deposited particles, up toward the pharynx and swallowed; whereas the lower respiratory tract, including the alveolar regions, has no mucous lining, and clearance of particles is much slower and less efficient (Hinds, 1982).

Once a bioaerosol has deposited in the respiratory tract, whether or not a disease state will eventuate is determined by the following: whether or not the virus in question is still intact and able to infect a cell; the location of deposition in the respiratory tract, and whether or not the virus can bind to the cells; and the immunological status of the individual.

The spread of particles, and in particular bioaerosols, in indoor environments is a complex process, involving many factors. To understand more comprehensively the potential spread of disease in these situations, a more thorough understanding is required of both virus persistence in droplets and the physical factors which significantly affect it.

1.3 Methods to study bioaerosol transport

Bacteriophages have played a key role in various types of research. A particularly important application of bacteriophages is their use as models or surrogates. In these systems, they are used in place of other viruses to give an indication of how the virus in question may respond to particular conditions. Bacteriophages are viruses that infect bacteria, and are thus are not harmful to humans. This use of bacteriophage is important because they do not pose serious health risks and are relatively easy to propagate in the laboratory; therefore there are reduced risks and costs associated with the experiments. They are also readily available and have relatively simple detection assays (Van Cuyk et al., 2004). Many bacteriophages exist, and are classified based on their morphology. Like other viruses, the genome can consist of either single- or double-stranded DNA or single- or double-stranded RNA (Nelson, 2004).

Surrogate bacteriophages are selected based on a simple set of general criteria. In an aerosol study, it is important to choose a bacteriophage that has similar aerosol characteristics to the specific viruses (in terms of aerodynamics and survival). MS2 is a commonly used bacteriophage in surrogate studies, including some studies investigating virus transmission in the air. Foarde and co-workers (1999) chose to use MS2 as a surrogate for various viruses including influenza, as it had similar shape and aerosol characteristics as human viruses, despite the fact that it is slightly smaller and non-enveloped. In another study, MS2 was used along with another *E. coli* phage, T3, to determine the best method for studying airborne viruses (Hogan et al., 2005). It was chosen as a surrogate as it had suitable size and shape, similar to that of commonly tested airborne viruses. Barker and Jones (2005) used MS2 to examine aerosol contamination caused by toilets. Furthermore, it has been used to compare the efficiencies of common air samplers (Tseng and Li, 2005).

An increasing number of studies have investigated the detection and/or survival of viruses in droplets; however extensive study of the persistence of respiratory viruses in aerosols has not been undertaken, nor has it been performed on the MS2 which is often used as a surrogate. Of particular interest is the quantification of virus survival when limiting factors are applied. As so few studies have been conducted regarding the actual aerosol characteristics of MS2 or common respiratory viruses, it is logical to begin with simulated studies so that they can provide a basis of comparison and assist in our knowledge and application of these methods to studies involving infected individuals. Moreover, it is important to simulate these studies as closely as possible to real-life so that fewer external factors need to be taken into account.

1.4 Studies of aerosolised virus

From previous simulated droplet experiments, it is known that virus survival and spatial distribution of droplets are dependent on a number of governing factors including aerodynamic droplet size and atmospheric conditions. Extensive studies examining the effect of temperature and relative humidity have also been conducted. Given that these factors have been described in the literature quite satisfactorily, they were not examined in this study. Instead, other limiting physical factors were investigated.

Prior to 1995, virtually all studies that examined viral transport in aerosols used culture methods, by employing a suitable host cell layer to examine for infected regions or plaques. The number of plaques was taken to indicate the number of intact virus particles, hence the unit of PFU (plaque-forming-units) per unit volume was used. PFU has traditionally been used for such studies. However, it is now thought that only a fraction of viruses present may be capable of forming a plaque in a host layer after the aerosolisation process, due to physical damage to the virion, and thus the traditional methods very probably underestimate the actual number of infectious viruses remaining in the aerosols.

In addition, there is no accurate information available as to how many intact virus particles are required for the infection of a host cell. Instinctively, the answer would be that just one virus particle per host cell was required, but this has not yet been proven conclusively. The general lack of research in this area can be attributed to a lack of suitable virus detection methods.

The rapid development of PCR techniques has allowed more suitable application of this technique to the problem of detecting viruses in aerosols over the past decade. The shift towards the molecular detection method polymerase chain reaction, or PCR, in recent aerosol research, has presented a timely opportunity to design a method which allows collection, detection, and quantification of viruses in an air sample. This has allowed us to detect not only the "culturable" or intact virions in the aerosols, but all intact virus RNA. In developing such a method, it was important to note the likelihood of low viral concentrations in respiratory aerosols.

2. Study of MS2 bacteriophage and respiratory viruses in aerosols

The objective of our research was to develop a PCR assay to detect viruses in aerosols, and to characterise the fate of bacteriophage MS2 in aerosols produced from four different aerosol types, whilst varying physical factors.

2.1 Development of PCR assays to study viruses in aerosols

Respiratory viruses can be spread by infectious aerosols, generated from infected persons. However, detection of viruses in aerosols is not sensitive enough to confirm the characteristics of virus aerosols. The aim of this study was to develop assays for respiratory syncytial virus (RSV) and MS2 bacteriophage, which are sufficiently sensitive to be used in aerosol studies. To achieve this, a two-step, nested real-time PCR assay was developed. Outer primer pairs were designed to nest each existing real-time PCR assay. The sensitivities of the nested real-time PCR assays were compared to those of existing real-time PCR assays. Both nested real-time PCR assays were applied in an aerosol study to compare their abilities to detect bacteriophage in air samples. Assays were also described for influenza A (H1N1 and H3N3), influenza B, and parainfluenza virus 1, and are described in Perrott et. al (2009).

2.1.1 Methods

Primer sets for the nested real-time PCR assays were designed based on previously described TaqMan® assays for each virus (see table 1). Using Primer Express®, an outer primer pair was designed to nest each TaqMan® primer/probe set. The outer primer pairs were used in the first round of amplification, which included a reverse transcription step (RT-PCR), followed by a second round of amplification using the TaqMan® primers and probe.

The first step of the assay was a conventional PCR and was performed using SuperScript™ III One-Step RT-PCR with Platinum® Taq DNA polymerase mastermix (Invitrogen, Vic., Australia). For the second step (TaqMan® assay), Universal mix (Applied Biosystems) was prepared by adding primers and probe to the reaction mix. The assays were performed on an Applied Biosystems ABI 7500 System, and results are reported in cycle threshold (Ct) values.

Organism	Reference	Primer set	Primer name	Sequence (5′ -3′)
Human Respiratory Syncytial Virus	This study	Outer	RSV-F1	TATTTGCATCGCCTTACAGTC
			RSV-R1	CTAAGGCCAAAGCTTATACAG
		Inner	RSVF	AGTAGACCATGTGAATTCCCTGC
			RSVR	GTCGATATCTTCATCACCATACTTT TCTGTTA
		Probe	RSV probe	TCAATACCAGCTTATAGAAC
MS2	This study	Outer	MS2-F5O	TGA ACA AGC AAC CGT TAC CCC
			MS2-R5O	TAT CAG GCT CCT TAC AGG CAG C
	O'Connell et al., 2006	Inner	MS2F5	GCT CTG AGA GCG GCT CTA TTG
			MS2R5	CGT TAT AGC GGA CCG CGT
		Probe	MS2-5 probe	CCGAGACCAATGTGCGCCGTG

Table 1. All primers and probes used in this study are shown in this table. This includes the outer (or nesting) primer pairs as well as the existing TaqMan® primers and probes.

2.1.2 Results and discussion

The real-time PCR assay for RSV detected the virus with a titre of 10^4 $TCID_{50}$ at 25.64 Ct, with an endpoint of 10 $TCID_{50}$, detected at 36.06 Ct (see figure 1). The nested real-time PCR assay detected the 10^4 $TCID_{50}$ titre of virus at 15.97 Ct, nearly 10 cycles earlier than the real-time PCR assay. Moreover, the nested real-time PCR assay had an endpoint of 1 $TCID_{50}$, amplifying at 31.22 Ct. The PCR products had to be diluted 1:1000, due to an excess of product resulting from the first round PCR, which exhausted the reagents and prevented the reaction from proceeding after about 8 cycles. An excellent distribution for a 10-fold dilution series for this virus was displayed by this assay, with distribution intervals between 2.85 cycles and 4.98 cycles. The virus was detected at an average of 8.93 cycles earlier by the nested real-time PCR assay than the real-time PCR assay, after the PCR products were diluted 1:1000.

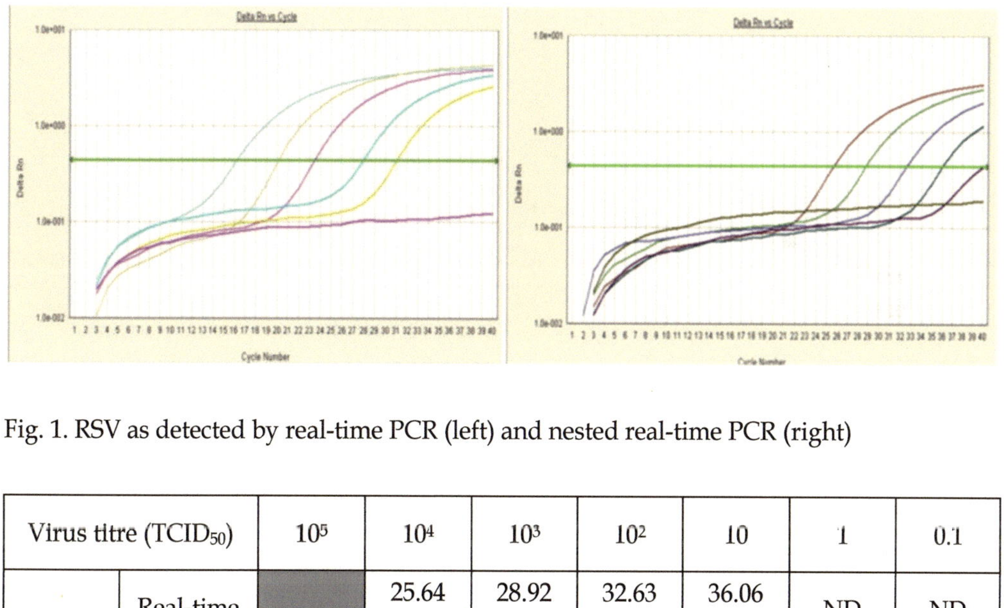

Fig. 1. RSV as detected by real-time PCR (left) and nested real-time PCR (right)

Virus titre ($TCID_{50}$)		10^5	10^4	10^3	10^2	10	1	0.1
RSV	Real-time		25.64 Ct	28.92 Ct	32.63 Ct	36.06 Ct	ND	ND
	Nested		15.97 Ct	19.79 Ct	23.39 Ct	28.37 Ct	31.22 Ct	ND
Virus titre (PFU)			10^4	10^3	10^2	10	1	0.1
MS2	Real-time		23.11 Ct	26.33 Ct	30.63 Ct	33.50 Ct	ND	ND
	Nested		7.42 Ct	9.27 Ct	12.39 Ct	16.02 Ct	19.18 Ct	19.31 Ct

Table 2. This table shows the results of the real-time and nested real-time PCR assays for detection of RSV and MS2 at several concentrations. The results displayed are cycle threshold values.

For MS2, the real-time PCR assay, as described by O'Connell et al (2006), had an endpoint of 10 PFU, detected at 33.50 Ct. In contrast, the nested real-time PCR assay was able to detect as low as 0.1 PFU at 19.31 cycles. Furthermore, the nested assay was also able to detect MS2 at much earlier cycles in comparison with the non-nested assay. Whilst the highest dilution (10^4 PFU) was detected by the real-time PCR assay at 23.11 Ct, it was detected by the nested real-time PCR assay at 7.42 Cts. The nested real-time PCR assay for MS2 improved the detection of the virus dilutions by an average of 17.11 cycles in comparison to the real-time PCR assay. The distribution of the series, using the nested real-time PCR assay, was good and intervals were from 1.85 cycles to 3.63 cycles.

Both the real-time PCR assay for MS2 and the nested real-time PCR assay for MS2 were used to detect MS2 bacteriophages from samples collected by gravitational settling, in order to determine which assay was more sensitive. Whilst the real-time PCR assay was only able to detect the virus from one air sample, the nested real-time PCR assay amplified MS2 from 14 out of the 16 samples, as seen in figure 2. All amplified samples were detected from 8.65 to 37.73 Cts.

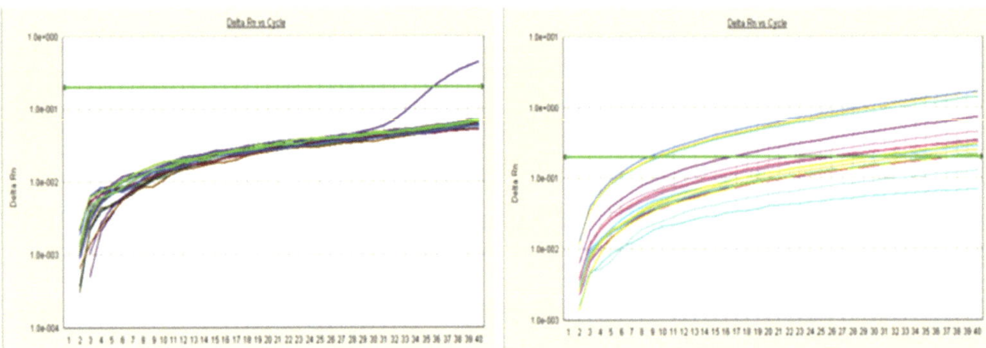

Fig. 2. The application of the real-time assay (left) and the nested real-time assay (right) to air samples

Further to the development of the nested real-time PCR, it was necessary to develop a standard curve to quantify the collected viruses. It was decided that a synthetic RNA standard was the most appropriate option; this circumvented the problem of extraneous DNA and RNA in viral RNA extracted from the viruses, which can give a falsely increased amount of RNA. The synthetic RNA was constructed from DNA oligonucleotides and underwent several clean up steps to ensure the quality of the RNA was appropriate for PCR.

Quantification of MS2 bacteriophage in aerosol samples using this method is described in the following section.

2.2 Bacteriophage in aerosols

The objective of this study was to apply the PCR method to detect the presence of the viral RNA in aerosols, and to compare its sensitivity and accuracy for estimation of viruses through detection of RNA, with that of the traditional plaque assay.

2.2.1 Methods

A Perspex chamber of approximately 150 L was used for all air testing experiments. Aerosols were created and delivered into the chamber with the Collison six-jet nebuliser (BGI Inc, Waltham, US), operated at a flow rate of six litres per minute (L/min), the air flow required to produce aerosols with a size of around 2 µm. Aerosol collection was performed using a six stage Andersen impactor. A collection plate with an *E. coli* overlay was placed into each of the six stages and each experiment was performed in triplicate. Plaques were counted the following day, and the positive-hole correction method was applied. Average (mean) counts were then calculated for each experiment.

We explored the following factors: concentration of virus in the nebulising suspension (10^5 to 10^3 PFU/mL); elapsed time between aerosolisation and sampling (0, 2, 5, 10 and 20 minutes); and the type of droplets ('wet droplets' were delivered directly into the chamber from the Collison, and 'dry droplets' which were mixed with sterile air at about 12 L/min, in order to dry the droplets before they were delivered into the chamber). Aerosolisation was performed for 30 seconds for each experiment.

Two types of nebulising suspension were used: traditionally-used phosphate buffered saline (PBS) and an artificial mucous (0.4 %), as described by King et. al (1985). Theoretically, the artificial mucous simulates an infected persons respiratory secretions more accurately than a water-like, non-viscous fluid. Thus, four droplet types were tested.

2.2.2 Results and discussion

2.2.2.1 Effect of droplet type

The UV-APS showed that the majority of droplets produced by the six-jet Collison nebuliser, when operating at six L/min, ranged in aerodynamic diameter from less than 0.523µm to 2.1 µm. The four types of droplets created by the Collison (wet and dry droplets from the artificial mucous suspension and the PBS suspension) differed slightly in size (see table 3). The droplets with the largest diameter were the wet droplets generated from PBS, with a mode of 0.980 µm. In comparison, the mode of the dry droplets from the same suspension was 0.965 µm. The artificial mucous droplets were smaller again: wet droplets from this suspension had a mode 0.910 µm; dry droplets had a mean diameter of 0.835 µm.

Sample	Median (µm)	Aerodynamic mean (µm)	Geometric mean (µm)	Mode (µm)	Concentration of droplets/cm³
PBS wet	1.100	1.226	1.166	0.980	15,000
PBS dry	1.023	1.087	1.057	0.965	2303
AM wet	0.915	0.976	0.935	0.910	1842
AM dry	0.850	0.884	0.860	0.835	412

Table 3. Size distributions and droplet concentration of the four types of droplets used in this study, as measured using the UV-APS

The number of droplets was considerably different. There was a much higher concentration of droplets created from the PBS suspension, especially when wet droplets were aerosolised from the PBS suspension. A concentration of 15,000 droplets per cm³ was measured using the UV-APS, whereas when wet droplets were aerosolised from the artificial mucous suspension, a concentration of only 1842 droplets per cm^3 was recorded. When dry droplets were aerosolised from the PBS suspension, the average number of droplets per cm^3 was 2303; from the artificial mucous suspension, an average of 412 droplets per cm^3 was recorded.

2.2.2.2 Effect of elapsed time on MS2 as detected by the plaque assay and the PCR assay

When MS2 was aerosolised in PBS wet droplets, the recovery rates of MS2 RNA copies were higher than those of the infectious particles. When wet droplets were collected immediately after aerosolisation (elapsed time = 0 minutes), 0.171 % of the infectious viruses were recovered from the original challenge by the plaque assay. However, the nested real-time PCR assay detected 1.03 % of the RNA copies, an average of 1,324,558 (± 780,684) RNA copies, from the original challenge. After a time elapse of two minutes, infectious MS2 levels as detected by the plaque assay, dropped to 0.001 %. However, the recovery rate of RNA copies dropped to only 0.42 % when detected by the nested real-time PCR assay, with an average of 547,496 (± 381,113) RNA copies detected. After five minutes elapsed time, the plaque assay showed that levels of infectious viruses dropped to 0.004 %, and then to 0.0002 % after 10 minutes elapsed between aerosolisation and collection. No infectious viruses were detected at the 20 minutes elapsed time point. The nested real-time PCR assay, on the other hand, detected 636,653 (± 274,203) RNA copies after five minutes elapsed, equating to 0.49 % of the original challenge. The virus level then decreased to 0.28 % at ten minutes with 365,052 (± 174,191) RNA copies detected; and at the last time point of 20 minutes elapsed time, the virus recovery rate rose slightly with 267,856 (± 490,294) RNA copies detected (0.38 %).

When MS2 was aerosolised from artificial mucous droplets, the nested real-time PCR assay was able to detect more relative RNA copies than infectious particles when collected after 20 minutes elapsed time. Using the plaque assay, 3.474 % of the infectious particles generated from the artificial mucous suspension were recovered initially (data not shown here, see Section 5.3.1); this dropped to zero viruses detected at the 20 minutes time point. However, the nested real-time PCR assay detected 1.70 % of the original RNA copies immediately after release, which then dropped to 0.84 % after a 20 minute elapse time.

When aerosolised in PBS dry droplets, the recovery, rate as measured by RNA copies, was comparable to the MS2 infectivity recovery rates. Upon immediate collection, 0.087% of the original challenge remained infectious; whilst 0.04% of the RNA copies were recovered from the original challenge, with 48,010 (± 6,859) RNA copies detected by the nested real-time PCR assay. The level of infectious viruses then dropped after a two minutes elapse to 0.037%; meanwhile, an average of 9,677 (± 4437) RNA copies were detected, this indicated a recovery rate of 0.017% of the RNA copies from the original challenge. Infectivity remained at a similar level after five minutes elapsed: 0.032% of infectious MS2 was recovered as opposed to 0.007% of the RNA copies, which equated to an average of 9,643 (± 7,281) RNA copies. After ten minutes elapsed however, the level of infectious viruses dropped to 0.001%. The nested real-time PCR assay showed that the rate remained at 0.006% of the original RNA copies. Finally, after 20 minutes elapsed, 0.011% of the original viruses remained infectious, whilst the rate of recovery of the RNA copies was 0.004%, with 4,567 (± 1,751) RNA copies detected.

When aerosolised in artificial mucous dry droplets, only 0.0003 % of the RNA copies were detected by the PCR. This is probably due to an experimental error. After a 20 minute elapsed time, 0.012 % of the RNA copies were recovered. This is in comparison to the plaque assay which measured a relative recovery rate of 1.688 % infectious particles upon immediate collection. No infectious MS2 was detected after 20 minutes had elapsed.

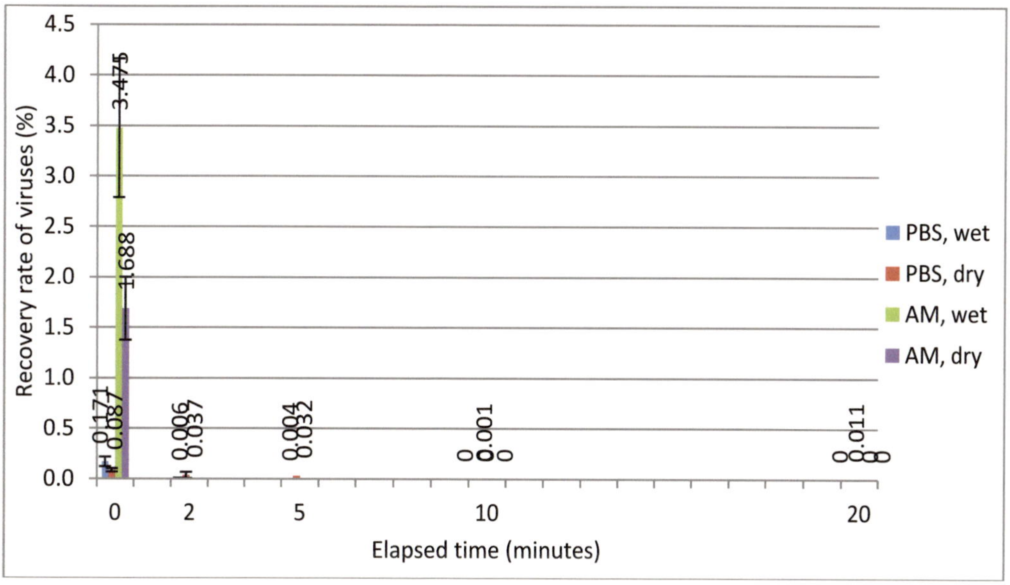

Fig. 3. The relative recovery of MS2 from the four different droplet types. Recoveries have been normalised to an initial challenge of 10^5 PFU, collected after different elapsed times of zero minutes, two minutes, five minutes and ten minutes

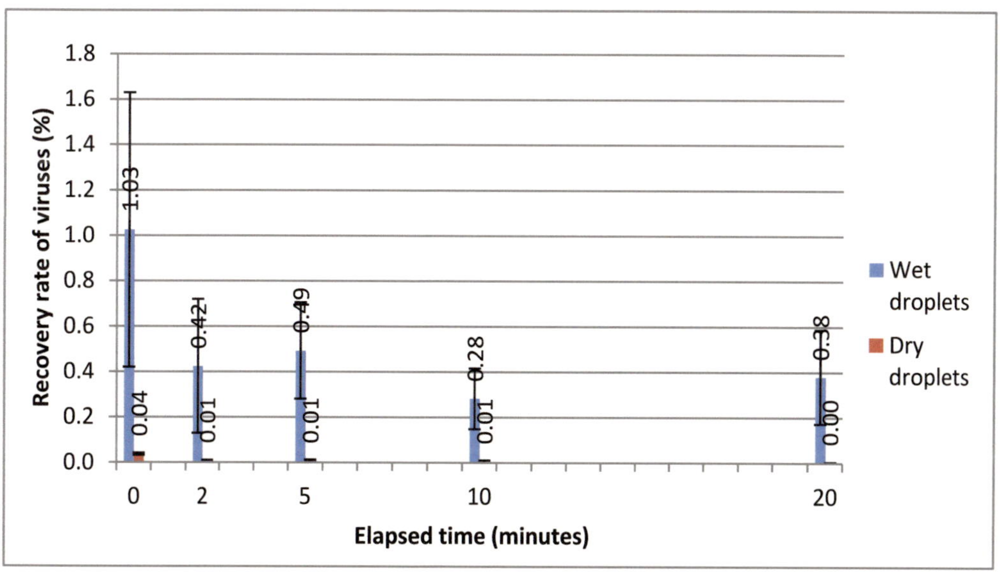

Fig. 4. Recovery of MS2 RNA copies from droplets generated from a PBS nebulising suspension and collected after varying elapsed times, detected by the nested real-time PCR assay

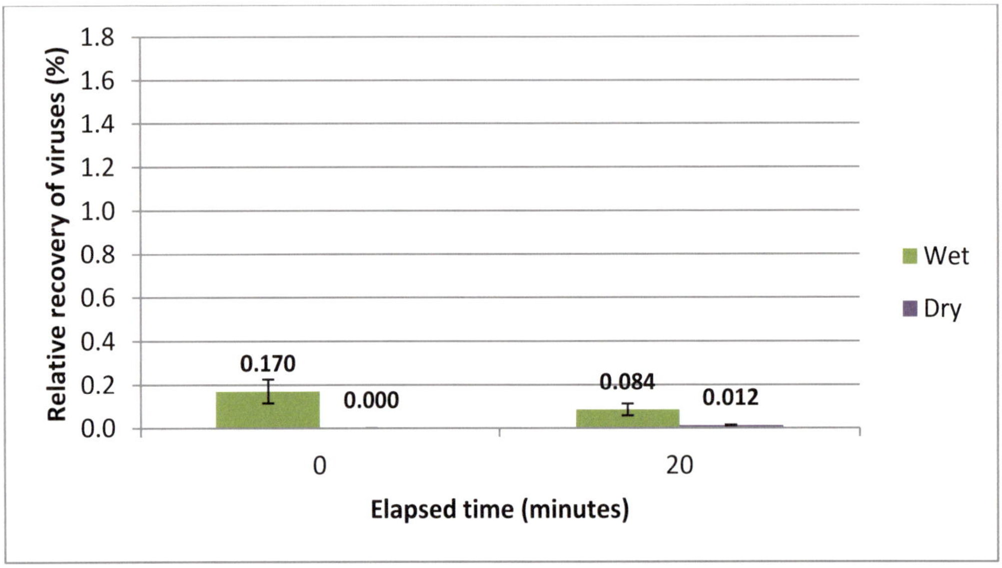

Fig. 5. Recovery of MS2 RNA copies from droplets generated from an artificial mucous suspension after varying elapsed times, as detected by the nested real-time PCR assay

A possible explanation for the almost immediate decay in MS2 infectivity, when held in the artificial mucous suspension, is that the suspension actually had a degrading effect on virus infectivity over time, as observed in an experiment examining this at different temperatures and times. It showed that when MS2 was held on ice, the numbers of infective MS2 dramatically decreased: after 20 minutes, 58.58 % of the viruses were no longer able to form plaques, whereas when they were held in broth (used to propagate MS2 bacteriophage) and the PBS, the levels dropped by only 8.07 % and 23.08 % respectively. Given that the nebulising suspensions, within the Collison nebuliser, were kept on ice during the experiments and between replicates, this could certainly explain why the decay of MS2 infectivity was so pronounced.

Utrup and Frey found that 25 minutes following the initial aerosolisation, the levels of detectable MS2 had dropped by 28 % relative to the sample taken five minutes after aerosolisation (Utrup and Frey, 2004). This is a higher recovery than ours, however their methods and equipment differed, so realistically the results cannot be directly compared.

2.2.2.3 Effect of virus concentration in the nebulising suspension

For the PBS droplets, the results from the nested real-time PCR assay were similar to the plaque assay results, however, in all circumstances, the nested real-time PCR assay detected more viruses (relative to the original amount aerosolised) than the plaque assay (see figure 6 and 7). From a challenge of 10^5 PFU (equivalent to 1.3 x 10^8 RNA copies), an average of 1,324,558 (± 780,684) RNA copies were recovered (1.03 %) from wet droplets. A challenge of 10^4 PFU (1.3 x 10^7 RNA copies) yielded an average recovery of 7013.23 (± 2685) copies, equating to 0.05 %; and an average of 518.13 (± 518.13) copies were recovered from the 10^3 PFU (1.3 x 10^6 RNA copies) challenge (0.04 %). When dry droplets were aerosolised from the PBS suspension, the average recoveries, as measured by the nested real-time PCR assay, were also higher than the recoveries given by the plaque assay. An average of

48,010 (± 6,859) RNA copies was recovered from the 10^5 PFU challenge (0.037 %). Virus recovery increased slightly to 0.042 % when aerosolised from the 10^4 PFU challenge, with 5408 (± 3193) RNA copies detected by the nested real-time PCR assay. No RNA was detected from the 10^3 PFU challenge.

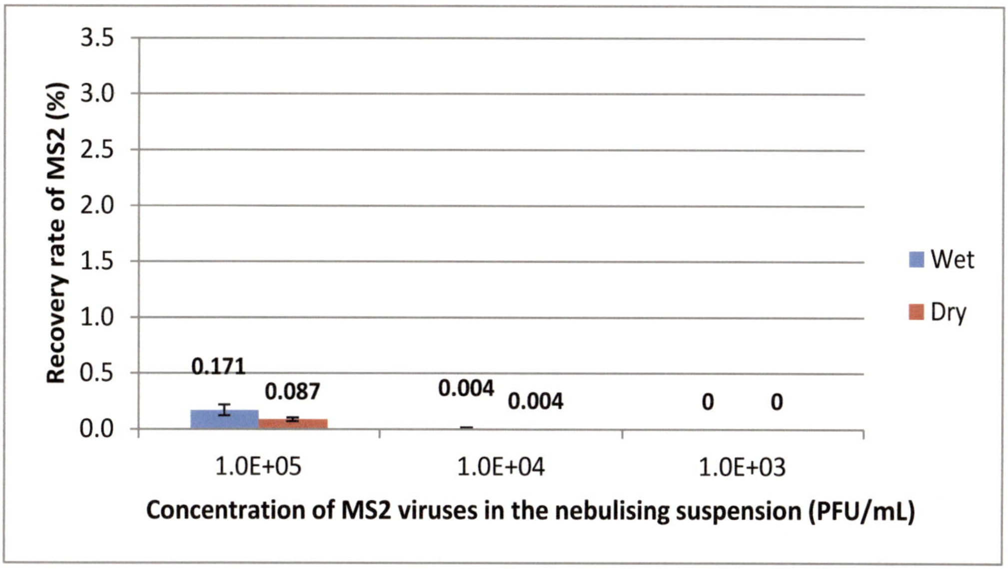

Fig. 6. Recovery of infectious MS2 from droplets generated from a PBS nebulising suspension of varying MS2 concentrations, as detected by the plaque assay

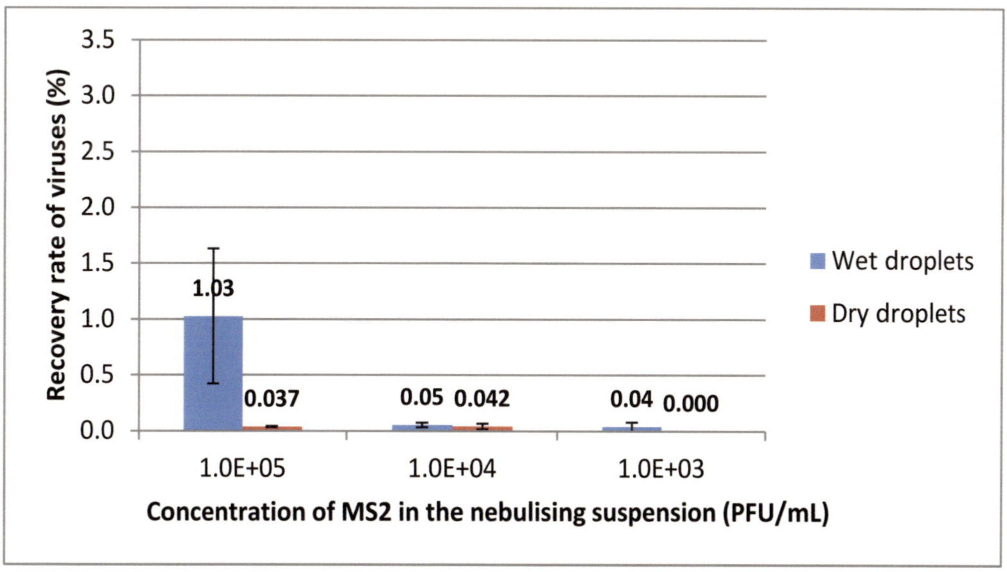

Fig. 7. Recovery of MS2 RNA copies from aerosols generated from PBS nebulising suspensions of varying MS2 concentrations, as detected by the nested real-time PCR assay

Similar to the plaque assay results, no explainable trend was apparent when the nested real-time PCR assay was used to detect MS2 in droplets from nebulising suspensions of varying concentrations (see figures 6-3 and 6-4). In the standard experiment for wet droplets, an average of 219,496 (± 71,923) RNA copies, or 0.17 % of the viruses from the original challenge introduced into the chamber was detected. This recovery dropped to 0.012 % from a nebulising suspension of 10^4 PFU/mL, with 1546 (± 1053) RNA copies detected; the recovery level then increased to 0.060%, or 775 (± 204) RNA copies, from the suspension containing 10^3 PFU/mL of MS2.

When aerosolised in dry droplets, the average rate of recovery increased with decreasing virus concentration in the nebulising suspension. This is not to say that the total numbers of RNA copies increased; rather the amount recovered relative to what was introduced into the chamber. The standard experiment yielded very low results (most likely as a result of experimental error) with a recovery rate of 0.0003 %, equivalent to 368 (± 306) RNA copies. The proportion of viruses recovered from the original suspensions of 10^4 PFU/mL increased to 0.068 % with the detection of 8765 (± 3118) RNA copies; this rate increased again for viruses aerosolised from the suspension of 10^3 PFU/mL, with 1222 (± 631) RNA copies detected, a relative recovery of 0.095 %. For the 10^5 PFU/mL challenge, more infectious MS2 was recovered than RNA copies in the dry droplets (in relative terms of recovery). However, for the challenges with lower PFU, relatively more RNA copies were recovered from the original challenge than infectious MS2.

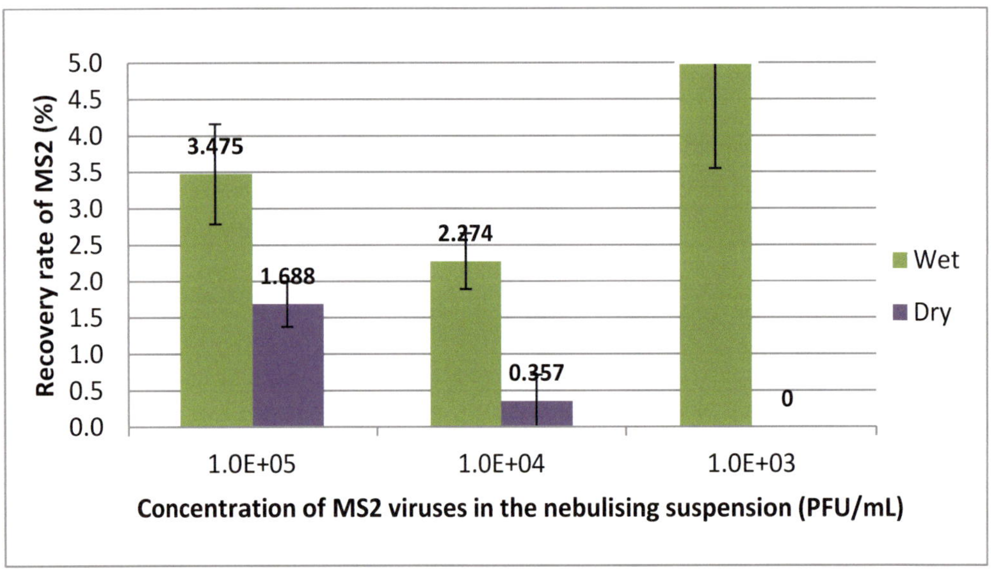

Fig. 8. Recovery of infectious MS2 from aerosols generated from artificial mucous nebulising suspensions of varying virus concentration, as detected by the plaque assay

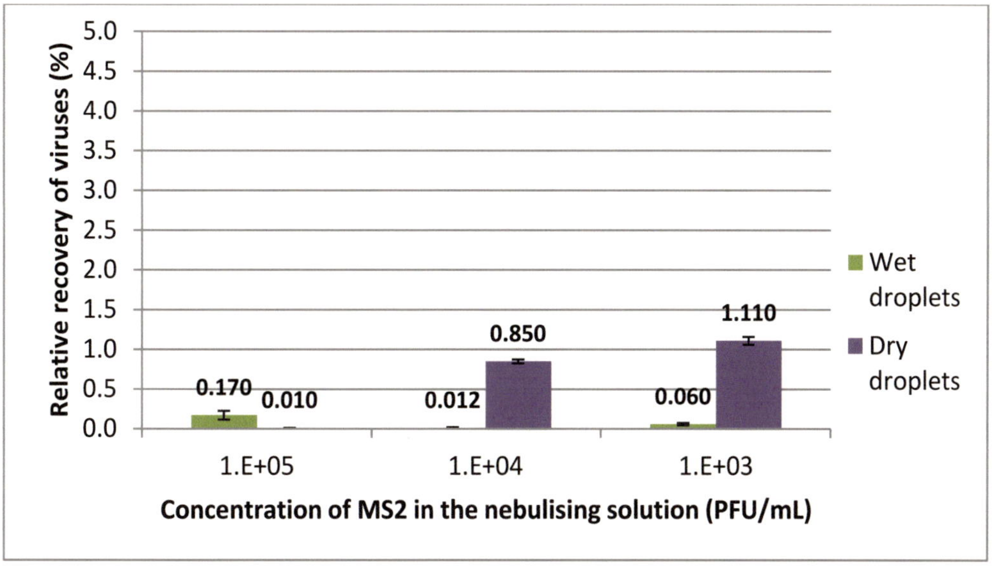

Fig. 9. Recovery of MS2 RNA copies from droplets generated from an artificial mucous suspension of varying MS2 concentration, as detected by the nested real-time PCR assay

3. Conclusions

We characterised four different droplet types and found that each droplet type had a significantly different effect on the persistence of viruses in the droplets. Most importantly, we demonstrated that the artificial mucous had a protective effect on virus infectivity, under certain conditions. We also showed that MS2 could be recovered from PBS droplets, with relative recovery rates of up to 0.17 % as detected by the plaque assay, and up to 1.03 % as detected by the nested real-time PCR assay. When aerosolised from artificial mucous droplets, MS2 was recovered with relative recovery rates of up to 3.474 % as detected by the plaque assay, and up to 1.110 % as detected by the PCR assay.

We showed that when held in a PBS nebulising suspension, infectious MS2 bacteriophage could be detected by the plaque assay up to ten minutes following aerosolisation in wet droplets, and up to, and possibly beyond, 20 minutes after aerosolisation in dry droplets. When MS2 was aerosolised from the artificial mucus suspension, it was not detected in the air by the plaque assay at ten minutes or 20 minutes following aerosolisation (from wet or dry droplets). However, we believe this is due to the result of a combination of effects including: the decay over time of MS2 virus infectivity when held in artificial mucous suspension on ice; the damage inflicted by impaction onto the agar; and the reduced viral load in the droplets.

When the concentration of MS2 was varied in the PBS nebulising suspension, the lower limit of detection of infectious viruses, using the plaque assay, was 10^4 PFU/mL for both wet and dry droplets. When the concentration was varied in the artificial mucus suspension, the plaque assay detection limit was a nebulising suspension virus concentration of 10^4 PFU/mL for the dry droplets and 10^3 PFU/mL for the wet droplets.

The differences between the PBS nebulising suspension and the artificial mucous suspension were interesting: it was clear that the artificial mucous suspension had a protective effect on the MS2 infectivity on immediate release. Based on the standard experiment, more than 20 times the amount of viruses remained infectious (intact) when aerosolised from the artificial mucous suspension in comparison to droplets produced from the PBS suspension. It may follow that the physical properties of human mucous will have a protective effect on the viruses.

The nested real-time PCR assay generally favoured the detection of MS2 in droplets. However, considering that there are a lot more viral copies of RNA present in a given sample than viruses which can form a plaque (an estimated 1292 copies to one PFU), this is not surprising. It is of course very likely that we will find more RNA copies than infectious viruses in a sample. Overall, the nested real-time PCR assay results were fairly comparable to the plaque assay in terms of trends against the variables tested.

4. Significance

This study sought to address the issue of to what extent viruses could survive given optimal conditions. It did not take into account all of the numerous factors which might influence aerial transmission including, but not limited to: bioaerosol production (location of virus in the respiratory tract; production of suitable droplets which viruses can be carried within, etc); transport (environmental factors such as temperature, relative humidity, UV desiccation etc); and reception of aerosols (deposition of droplets, location of deposition, ability of viruses to bind to, infect and replicate in cells). In other words, aside from the factors we have investigated here, the virus needs to also overcome the aerosolisation process, the transport process, remain infectious and find a suitable host in which to initiate disease.

In addition to contributing to knowledge in the field of respiratory virus transmission, this study has developed several methods for studying both bacteriophage and respiratory viruses in air samples. Methods developed include: sensitive, quantitative nested real-time PCR assays for RSV as well as MS2 bacteriophage; aerosol collection methods for collecting bacteriophage using host-overlay agar plates; and an aerosol collection method for pathogenic viruses, suitable for applying PCR analysis.

Sensitive, quantitative, nested, real-time PCR assays were developed as part of this study, and successfully applied to aerosol studies using MS2 bacteriophage and influenza virus. The assays were used in combination with synthetic RNA controls for preparation of standard curves against which the unknown samples were quantified. The PCR method we have developed here is not a perfect solution to the problems encountered in detecting viruses in droplets; however it is a strong step in the right direction. As evidenced by the large error and standard deviation values, it is clear that there are still problems with accurately quantifying viruses in air samples. However, we have developed an assay which is very sensitive and can detect viruses in droplets where plaque assays cannot. The information in this study, as well as the method development, can be applied to the study of respiratory viruses in droplets.

We examined small droplets with a range of diameters spanning 0.65 - 2.1 µm, which is consistent with the range of respiratory droplets as reported by several studies (Knight, 1973, Erdal and Esmen, 1995, Kowalski and Bahnfleth, 1998, Morawska et al., 2008). It is the transmission and recovery of intact viruses within these droplets, which become droplet nuclei, that pertains to the aerosol spread of respiratory viruses. We have shown that these droplets can potentially be vehicles of virus transmission, notwithstanding the other factors which affect airborne infection (as mentioned above). Furthermore, droplets that equilibrate to a size smaller in diameter than 0.65 µm were not considered here, as they were not within the size range of the Andersen sampler. This does not mean that the viruses are not intact, but that our limit of detection cannot provide for such a small particle.

We have also conducted aerosol research with influenza virus, which provided surprisingly robust and stable results (data not shown), considering prior assumptions that it is a labile virus. The recovery of influenza was neither higher nor lower than that of the MS2 bacteriophage, overall. Rather, it was much more consistent with respect to the levels of virus remaining in the droplets. Whether or not this is due to the nature of virus stability is a question that cannot be answered absolutely by this study. It is possible that the differences in the efficacies of the nested real-time PCR assays may have contributed to this finding. In any case, it is possible that this may be the case for similar studies with RSV.

In future studies, the elapsed times could be extended to up to hours, to see how long the relative amounts of RNA copies remain stable, and to see at approximately what endpoint they can still be detected. Again, the comparable levels of viruses aerosolised in wet droplets were much higher than the corresponding experiments where dry droplets were aerosolised.

5. Acknowledgements

Thanks to the Australian Research Council for providing funding for this study and thanks to Lidia Morawska and the International Laboratory for Air Quality and Health (ILAQH) who provided equipment and expertise. Thanks also to Queensland Health Forensic and Scientific Services, who provided the laboratory space and equipment, and to Public Health Virology who also were integral in the completion of this research.

6. References

Barker, J. & Jones, M. V. (2005). The potential spread of infection caused by aerosol contamination of surfaces after flushing a domestic toilet. *J Appl Microbiol,* Vol. 99, No. 2, pp 339-347,1364-5072 (Print).

Benbough, J. E. (1971). Some factors affecting the survival of airborne viruses. *J Gen Virol,* Vol. 10, No. 3, pp 209-220

Burkdolder, H. C. & Berg, J. C. (1974). *AIChE J.,* Vol. 20, No. 872-880

Carducci, A., Gemelli, C., Cantiani, L., Casini, B. & Rovini, E. (1999). Assessment of microbial parameters as indicators of viral contamination of aerosol from urban sewage treatment plants. *Lett Appl Microbiol,* Vol. 28, No. 3, pp 207-210,0266-8254 (Print).

Centers for Disease Control. 2010. *Respiratory Syncytial Virus - Transmission and Prevention* [Online]. Atlanta. Available: http://www.cdc.gov/rsv/about/transmission.html [Accessed 13 July 2011].

Couch, R. B., Kasel, J. A., Glezen, W. P., Cate, T. R., Six, H. R., Taber, L. H., Frank, A. L., Greenberg, S. B., Zahradnik, J. M. & Keitel, W. A. (1986). Influenza: its control in persons and populations. *J Infect Dis,* Vol. 153, No. 3, pp 431-440,0022-1899 (Print).

Cox, C. S. & Wathes, C. M. 1995. Bioaerosols in the environment. *Bioaerosols handbook.* Boca Raton: CRC Press.

Daigle, C. C., Chalupa, D. C., Gibb, F. R., Morrow, P. E., Oberdorster, G., Utell, M. J. & Frampton, M. W. (2003). Ultrafine particle deposition in humans during rest and exercise. *Inhal Toxicol,* Vol. 15, No. 6, pp 539-552,0895-8378 (Print).

Edwards, D. A., Brenner, H. & Wasan, D. T. 1991. *Processes and Rheology.* Boston: Butterworth-Heinemann.

Edwards, D. A., Man, J. C., Brand, P., Katstra, J. P., Sommerer, K., Stone, H. A., Nardell, E. & Scheuch, G. (2004). Inhaling to mitigate exhaled bioaerosols. *Proc Natl Acad Sci U S A,* Vol. 101, No. 50, pp 17383-17388,0027-8424 (Print).

Erdal, S. & Esmen, N. A. (1995). Human head model as an aerosol sampler: Calculation of aspiration efficiencies for coarse particles using an idealized human head model facing the wind. *J Aerosol Sci,* Vol. 26, No. 2, pp 253-272

Fiegel, J., Clarke, R. & Edwards, D. A. (2006). Airborne infectious disease and the suppression of pulmonary bioaerosols. *Drug Discov Today,* Vol. 11, No. 1-2, pp 51-57

Foarde, K. K., Hanley, J. T., Ensor, D. S. & Roessler, P. (1999). Development of a method for measuring single-pass bioaerosol removal efficiencies of a room cleaner. *Aerosol Sci Tech,* Vol. 30, No. 223-234

Goldmann, D. A. (2000). Transmission of viral respiratory infections in the home. *Pediatr Infect Dis J,* Vol. 19, No. 10, pp S97-S102,0891-3668.

Hall, C. B. (2001). Respiratory syncytial virus and parainfluenza virus. *N Engl J Med,* Vol. 344, No. 25, pp 1917-28,0028-4793 (Print) 0028-4793 (Linking).

Hatch, T. F. (1961). Distribution and deposition of inhaled particles in respiratory tract. *Bacteriol Rev,* Vol. 25, No. 237-240,0005-3678 (Print).

Hinds, W. C. 1982. *Aerosol Technology: Properties, Behaviour and Measurement of Airborne Particles,* New York, John Wiley & Sons.

Hogan, C. J., Jr., Kettleson, E. M., Lee, M. H., Ramaswami, B., Angenent, L. T. & Biswas, P. (2005). Sampling methodologies and dosage assessment techniques for submicrometre and ultrafine virus aerosol particles. *J Appl Microbiol,* Vol. 99, No. 6, pp 1422-34,1364-5072 (Print).

King, M., Brock, G. & Lundell, C. (1985). Clearance of mucus by simulated cough. *J Appl Physiol,* Vol. 58, No. 6, pp 1776-1782

Knight, V. 1973. *Viral and Mycoplasmal Infections of the Respiratory Tract,* Philadelphia, Lea & Febiger.

Knight, V. (1980). Viruses as agents of airborne contagion. *Ann N Y Acad Sci,* Vol. 353, No. 147-56

Kowalski, W. J. & Bahnfleth, W. (1998). Airborne respiratory diseases and mechanical systems for control of microbes. *Heating, Piping, and Air Conditioning,* Vol. 70, No. 7, pp 34,0017940X.

Liolios, L., Jenney, A., Spelman, D., Kotsimbos, T., Catton, M. & Wesselingh, S. (2001). Comparison of a multiplex reverse transcription-PCR-enzyme hybridization assay with conventional viral culture and immunofluorescence techniques for the detection of seven viral respiratory pathogens. *J Clin Microbiol,* Vol. 39, No. 8, pp 2779-2783,0095-1137 (Print).

Morawska, L. (2006). Droplet fate in indoor environments, or can we prevent the spread of infection? *Indoor Air,* Vol. 16, No. 5, pp 335-47,0905-6947 (Print) 0905-6947 (Linking).

Morawska, L., Johnson, G., Ristovski, Z., Hargreaves, M., Mengersen, K. L., Corbett, S., Chao, C., Li, Y. & Katoshevski, D. (2009). Size distribution and sites of origin of droplets expelled during expiratory activities. *J Aerosol Sci,* Vol. 40, No. 3, pp 256-269

Morawska, L., Johnson, G. R., Ristovski, Z., Hargreaves, M., Mengersen, K. L., Chao, C., Wan, M. P., Li, Y., Xie, X. & Katoshevski, D. 2008. Droplets expelled during human expiratory activities and their origin. *11th International Conference on Indoor Air Quality and Climate.*

Nelson, D. (2004). Phage taxonomy: we agree to disagree. *J Bacteriol,* Vol. 186, No. 21, pp 7029-31,0021-9193 (Print).

Nicas, M., Nazaroff, W. W. & Hubbard, A. (2005). Toward understanding the risk of secondary airborne infection: emission of respirable pathogens. *J Occup Environ Hyg,* Vol. 2, No. 3, pp 143-54,1545-9624 (Print).

Papineni, R. S. & Rosenthal, F. S. (1997). The size distribution of droplets in the exhaled breath of healthy human subjects. *J Aerosol Med,* Vol. 10, No. 2, pp 105-16,0894-2684 (Print).

Perrott, P., Smith, G., Ristovski, Z., Harding, R. & Hargreaves, M. (2009). A nested real-time PCR assay has an increased sensitivity suitable for detection of viruses in aerosol studies. *J Appl Microbiol,* Vol. 106, No. 5, pp 1438-47

Pillai, S. D. 2002. Bioaerosols and public health. *In:* INSAM, H., RIDDECH, N. & KLAMMER, S. (eds.) *Microbiology of composting.* Berlin: Springer-Verlag GmbH & Co.

Pillai, S. D. & Ricke, S. C. (2002). Bioaerosols from municipal and animal wastes: background and contemporary issues. *Can J Microbiol,* Vol. 48, No. 8, pp 681-96

Proctor, D. F. (1966). Airborne disease and the upper respiratory tract. *Bacteriol Rev,* Vol. 30, No. 3, pp 498-513

Stockton, J., Ellis, J. S., Saville, M., Clewley, J. P. & Zambon, M. C. (1998). Multiplex PCR for typing and subtyping influenza and respiratory syncytial viruses. *J Clin Microbiol,* Vol. 36, No. 10, pp 2990-2995,0095-1137 (Print).

Tang, J. W., Li, Y., Eames, I., Chan, P. K. S. & Ridgway, G. L. (2006). Factors involved in the aerosol transmission of infection and control of ventilation in healthcare premises. *J Hosp Infect,* Vol. 64, No. 2, pp 100-114

Tseng, C. C. & Li, C. S. (2005). Collection efficiencies of aerosol samplers for virus-containing aerosols. *J Aerosol Sci,* Vol. 36, No. 5-6, pp 593-607

Utrup, L. J. & Frey, A. H. (2004). Fate of bioterrorism-relevant viruses and bacteria, including spores, aerosolized into an indoor air environment. *Exp Biol Med (Maywood),* Vol. 229, No. 4, pp 345-350,1535-3702 (Print).

Van Cuyk, S., Siegrist, R. L., Lowe, K. & Harvey, R. W. (2004). Evaluating microbial purification during soil treatment of wastewater with multicomponent tracer and surrogate tests. *J Environ Qual,* Vol. 33, No. 1, pp 316-329,0047-2425 (Print).

Wang, B., Zhang, A., Sun, J. L., Liu, H., Hu, J. & Xu, L. X. (2005). Study of SARS transmission via liquid droplets in air. *J Biomech Eng,* Vol. 127, No. 1, pp 32-38,0148-0731 (Print).

Weber, T. P. & Stilianakis, N. I. (2008). Inactivation of influenza A viruses in the environment and modes of transmission: a critical review. *J Infect,* Vol. 57, No. 5, pp 361-373

Wilson, S. C., Morrow-Tesch, J., Straus, D. C., Cooley, J. D., Wong, W. C., Mitlohner, F. M. & McGlone, J. J. (2002). Airborne microbial flora in a cattle feedlot. *Appl Environ Microbiol,* Vol. 68, No. 7, pp 3238-3242

Part 2

Epidemiologic and Diagnostic Aspects of RSV Infection

7

Life-Threatening RSV Infections in Children

Martin C.J. Kneyber
Department of Paediatric Intensive Care, Beatrix Children's Hospital
University Medical Center Groningen, University of Groningen, Groningen
The Netherlands

1. Introduction

During the middle of the 20th century, Chanock and co-workers recovered an cytopathogenic agent from lung secretions of young infants with lower respiratory tract disease (LRTD). This agent was found out to be similar to an agent that was identified in an outbreak of infection in chimpanzees resembling the common cold (Chanock et al, 1957; Morris J.A. et al, 1956). Because of its characteristic cytopathologic findings in tissue culture where it forms syncytia of epithelial cells, the virus was named *respiratory syncytial virus* (Chanock et al, 1957). From serological studies it was observed that almost all children have been infected by RSV by the age of two years (Glezen et al, 1986). Since then, RSV has been identified as the most important causative agent of viral LRTD (Hall, 2001). Approximately 100.000 infants are annually admitted with RSV induced bronchiolitis in the United States, and the number of hospitalizations is increasing (Shay et al, 1999). Because of this, RSV associated disease imposes a major burden on health care resources (Leader et al, 2003). Furthermore, RSV is increasingly being recognized as an important pathogen causing severe LRTD in elderly and immunocompromised patients (Falsey et al, 2005).

This chapter reflects on the current knowledge about RSV in critically ill children admitted to the pediatric intensive care unit (PICU) and its possible therapeutic options.

2. Epidemiology of RSV

RSV (genus *pneumoviridae,* family of *paramyxoviridae*) is a single stranded enveloped RNA virus. The RSV genome codes for ten major proteins (Hacking et al, 2002). Of these proteins, the F (fusion) and the G (attachment) glycoprotein are the major surface antigenic determinants. Two antigenic strains of RSV, group A and group B, can be identified. Both groups co-circulate together but also independently from each other during annual epidemics (Hall et al, 1990). The clinical spectrum of RSV associated disease extends from mild upper respiratory tract infection to severe lower respiratory tract infection including bronchiolitis and pneumonia (Hall, 2001). Re-infections occur frequently, although they tend to be mild (Henderson et al, 1979).

Severe RSV infection necessitating mechanical ventilation (MV) occurs in 2 - 16% of previously healthy infants (Leclerc et al, 2001). This percentage may increase up to 30 - 35% among high-risk patients such as children with congenital heart disease (CHD), chronic lung disease (CLD), compromised immune function, postnatal age less than 6 weeks and premure birth (i.e. less than 37 weeks gestational age) (Wang et al, 1996). The mean duration of conventional MV may be as long as 10 days, but in a proportion of ventilated patients alternatives mode such high-frequency oscillatory ventilation (HFOV) or extra-corporeal membrane oxygenation (ECMO) are necessitated when severe impaired oxygenation or ventilation persists (Guerguerian et al, 2004; Leclerc et al, 2001). Usually mortality rates are less than 1% for previously healthy infants, although these percentages may increase up to 10% among high-risk infants (Shay et al, 2001).

3. Clinical manifestations of RSV in the PICU

RSV LRTD is usually referred to as "bronchiolitis" because of the clinical presence of audible airflow limitation on expiration in a significant proportion of infected infants and the classic hyperinflation on chest radiograph. In infants admitted to the PICU an increase in total respiratory system resistance compatible with obstructive disease has also been demonstrated (Gauthier et al, 1998; Hammer et al, 1995; Hammer et al, 1997; Mallory Jr et al, 1989). Nevertheless, RSV LRTD is in fact a heterogeneous disease, implicating that it is incorrect to label all RSV LRTD as bronchiolitis (Isaacs, 1998). This is of importance because of the proposed differences in ventilatory strategies needed to treat obstructive or restrictive disease (Frankel et al, 1999). Furthermore, identification of the clinical phenotype aids in targeting a specific population of infants for a therapeutic modality.

In critically ill children RSV LRTD can also be characterized as a restrictive disease (Frankel et al, 1999). Hammer and co-workers evaluated 37 mechanically ventilated infants with RSV and were able to categorize them as having obstructive or restrictive disease based upon the findings from pulmonary function testing (PFT) (Hammer et al, 1997). Ten infants had decreased respiratory system compliance (Crs) compatible with restrictive disease in conjunction with four-quadrant alveolar consolidation on chest radiograph compared to healthy controls. The remaining 27 had increased respiratory system resistance (Rrs), compatible with obstructive disease. Infants with restrictive disease required prolonged ventilation compared to infants with obstructive disease. However, infants with underlying diseases such as prematurity and/or chronic lung disease were not excluded in their analysis. Especially among infants with restrictive disease there were three infants with CLD. By including these infants, it cannot be ruled out they had pre-existing lung abnormalities that might contribute to altered respiratory system mechanics. For instance, prematurely born infants with CLD have higher Rrs that predisposed them to suffer from symptomatic RSV LRTD compared to controls (Broughton et al, 2006). Hence, the issue of clinical phenotype is still subject of scientific debate.

Unfortunately, in most PICU's PFT is not done routinely. Alternatively, ventilatory indices characterizing the efficacy of gas exchange might be used. These include the oxygenation index (OI) and the alveolar-arterial oxygen gradient (Aa-DO_2). Tasker and co-workers found an Aa-DO_2 > 400 mmHg during the first 24 hours of mechanical ventilation and mean airway pressure (MAP) > 10 cm H_2O associated with radiographic appearances suggestive of RSV restrictive disease (Tasker et al, 2000). All infants were previously healthy, and had upon PICU admission four-quadrant alveolar consolidation on their chest radiograph. However, their definition of severe RSV LRTD was based upon a chest radiograph scoring system developed for prematurely born infants with infant respiratory distress syndrome (IRDS) and has not been validated for patients with RSV to our knowledge (Maconochie et al, 1991). Furthermore, their findings have not been validated yet. We have retrospectively studied parameters for gas exchange in 53 mechanically ventilated infants with RSV LRTD admitted between 1995 and 2005, and were unable to detect significant differences in oxygenation index (OI) or alveolar-arterial oxygen gradient (Aa-DO_2) between infants with radiological classified restrictive disease and obstructive disease (manuscript in preparation). We further observed a comparable duration of MV between infants with obstructive and restrictive disease. Our findings strengthen our assumption that RSV LRTD is a heterogeneous disease that cannot be strictly dichotomized into a restrictive and obstructive disease.

RSV is also a neurotrophic virus. Our group has found that it causes apnoea (defined by a cessation of respiration or a bradycardia with accompanying cyanosis for a period of 20 seconds or longer) in approximately one out of every five patients presenting with RSV (Kneyber et al, 1998). In fact, apnoea may be the presenting symptom without any other symptoms of respiratory tract infection. The odds for MV were 6.5-fold increased among infants who present with RSV - associated apnoea. The exact mechanism underlying RSV-associated apnoea is unknown, although it has been observed that the apnoea is of central origin (Rayyan et al, 2004).

Cardiovascular compromise during RSV infection has been reported by various authors. Severe RSV infection may mimic shock (Njoku et al, 1993). Nearly half of all infants admitted to the PICU were found to have elevated cardiac enzyme levels (Checchia et al, 2000; Eisenhut et al, 2004). Cardiovascular support either by fluid boluses or inotropic drug use is not seldomly necessitated in ventilated infants (Checchia et al, 2000; Eisenhut et al, 2004; Kim et al, 1997). Life-threatening disturbances of the cardiac rhythm have also been described in critically ill patients with RSV (Playfor et al, 2005; Thomas et al, 1997).

There is much controversy whether or not severe RSV infection is associated with increased occurrence of the syndrome of inappropriate antidiuretic hormone secretion (SIADH). One group of investigators have reported that 33% infants admitted to the PICU developed hyponatraemia (serum sodium < 136 mmol/L) (Hanna et al, 2003). Four of them had a hyponatraemic seizure upon PICU admission. Van Steensel-Moll and co-workers observed increased ADH levels in mechanically ventilated children compared with non-ventilated children (Steensel-Moll et al, 1990). However, these were not significantly correlated with serum sodium levels.

4. Bacterial co-infections

Many if not all infants admitted to the PICU with RSV LRTD have antibiotics prescribed. Clinicians often assume that a concurrent bacterial pulmonary infection is probably (partially) accountable for the development of respiratory failure due to RSV. Nevertheless, the occurrence of severe infections is low. Randolph *et al* retrospectively studied the number of positive cultures from blood, urine, cerebrospinal fluid and endotracheal aspirates upon PICU admission among 63 mechanically ventilated previously healthy infants (Randolph et al, 2004). All of these infants were treated with antibiotics. They observed a low percentage (< 2%) of concurrent bacterial blood stream infection. In addition, 24 (38.1%) had positive cultures from endotracheal aspirates that could be linked to either possible or probable bacterial pneumonia. These observations were supported by the findings of Bloomfield *et al*

(Bloomfield et al, 2004). They observed bacteraemia in 6 children out of 208 PICU admissions. Four infants were mechanically ventilated. All of them were prematurely born or had congenital heart disease. Our group has also studied retrospectively the occurrence of concurrent bacterial infection in 65 mechanically ventilated infants during 1996 - 2001 (Kneyber et al, 2005a). In 38 of these infants microbiological investigations were performed. All had antibiotics upon PICU admission. We found only one positive culture from blood and 37.5% positive cultures from endotracheal aspirates compatible with bacterial pneumonia. Infants with concurrent bacterial infection had similar CRP concentrations and white blood cell counts compared to infants with negative cultures. In addition, the presence of bacterial pulmonary infection upon PICU admission was undetectable by the OI as this was equal among infants with and without positive cultures. There were two additional remarkable finding from our study. First, concurrent bacterial infection occurred almost exclusively in previously healthy, term born infants. Second, infants with positive concurrent bacterial infection required prolonged ventilatory support (14.3 ± 2.4 versus 10.6 ± 1.0 days).

All retrospectively made observations were confirmed by a study from Thorburn *et al* (Thorburn et al, 2006). Their group prospectively collected endotracheal aspirates in 165 mechanically ventilated infants during three consecutive RSV seasons. They observed that 21.8% had concurrent bacterial pneumonia upon PICU admission. Strikingly, these infants also required prolonged ventilatory support compared to infants without bacterial pneumonia. Only 36% of these infants had antibiotics on PICU admission. The majority of bacterial pneumonias occurred in infants with pre-existing morbidity.

It may thus be concluded that at least in (significant) proportion of infants hospitalised to the PICU with severe RSV LRTD a bacterial pneumonia (partially) contributes to the development of respiratory failure. Whereas others report such findings among children with pre-existing morbidity, we were unable to confirm this. At present therefore, it seems rational to refrain from the routine use of antibiotics in children admitted to the PICU. Immediate investigation of the endotracheal aspirate may identify those children in whom antibiotics are justified, although this hypothesis calls for further study such as a randomized controlled trial.

5. Pathophysiology

The pathophysiological mechanisms underlying RSV-induced respiratory failure with subsequent necessitation of MV are not fully elucidated. Various pathways can be proposed that most likely interact with each other, including viral load and strain, pre-exististing structural abnormalities and the host immune response. Pre-existing structural abnormalities of the respiratory system may predispose prematurely born children and children with CLD or CHD to a severe disease course. Prematurely born but otherwise healthy infants have an underdeveloped respiratory system that is easily compromised by the direct toxic effects of an infectious agent, such as epithelial necrosis due to invading virus (Welliver, 2003). Young children with CLD have structural abnormal airways that collapse easily as well as structural pulmonary abnormalities predisposing them to severe disease necessitating MV (Welliver, 2003).

Viral strain is not accountable for disease severity. We observed that the need for PICU admission and MV is equally distributed among infants with RSV group A and B (Kneyber et al, 1996). In contrast, the effect of viral load on disease severity is less clear. Conflicting data have been reported on differences in viral load between ventilated and non-ventilated infants. DeVincenzo *et al* were unable to find significant differences in viral load obtained from nasal washes between previously healthy ventilated (n = 22) and non-ventilated infants (n = 119) (5.185 versus 4.963 log pfu/mL) (DeVincenzo et al, 2005). Others, however, observed significantly higher nasal viral load among ventilated (n = 15) versus non-ventilated previously healthy infants (n = 24) (5.06 ± 0.34 vs. 3.91 ± 0.35 log pfu/mL, p = .022) (Buckingham et al, 2000). Only one group of investigators has exclusively focused on differences in viral load among ventilated infants. Van Woensel *et al* found a higher viral load in tracheal aspirates of infants (n = 14) who met criteria for "severe RSV LRTD" (PaO_2/FiO_2 ratio ≤ 200 mmHg and a mean airway pressure (MAP) > 10 cmH_2O (72.0 ± 28.0 RNA copies) compared to infants (n = 8) with "mild" disease (21.1 ± 9.2 RNA copies, p = .20) (van Woensel et al, 2003a). At present, there are no reports on differences in viral load among various categories of mechanically ventilated high-risk infants. Further studies are awaited.

Various authors have postulated that the immune response against RSV plays an important role in determining disease severity, especially when there is no pre-existing disease (Bont et al, 2002). It is subject of debate whether or not the immune response against RSV is protective or disease-enhancing. Results from animal studies have led to the assumption that an overshoot of the T-cell response towards a T - helper 2 profile may be responsible for severe disease (Cannon et al, 1988). This skwewing towards a T - helper 2 response has not been universally confirmed to occur in children with RSV LRTD (Bont et al, 2002).

A good humoral immune response is necessary to prevent severe RSV LRTD. Low titers of neutralising antibodies have been found to be associated with severe RSV LRTD (Glezen et al, 1981; Karron et al, 1999). Yet, this may specifically apply for infants born prematurely as in general they lack sufficient titers of protective immunoglobulin G neutralising antibodies because placental transport of IgG occurs late in gestation, near the end of the third trimester. Early post-natal life is associated with a physiological immune deficiency defined by hyporesponsiveness of mononuclear phagocytes to stimuli and a diminished T - cell response (Marchant et al, 2005; Marodi, 2006). This low level of immune response could very young previously healthy infants render susceptible for severe disease.

Next to this, a good cellular immune response is also necessary to prevent severe RSV LRTD. Low numbers of T - cells are found in peripheral blood samples of ventilated infants compared to non-ventilated infants, although this also may suggest recruitment of activated T - cells to the lungs (de Weerd et al, 1998). More importantly, low levels of IFN-γ (a T - helper 1 cell cytokine) were found in nasopharyngeal aspirates of mechanically ventilated children compared to non-ventilated children (Bont et al, 2001). In addition, monocyte-derived interleukin (IL) 12 was observed to be inversely related to the duration of MV. IL-12 promotes the differentiation of naïve CD4 -positive T cells into T-helper 1 cells (Ramshaw et al, 1997). Finally, mononuclear cells of ventilated infants exhibited diminished ex-vivo lymphoproliferative responses and the capacity to produce IFN-γ and IL-4 compared to non-ventilated infants.

It may thus be concluded that severe RSV LRTD in healthy term and pre-term born infants originates from an immature immune system so that they cannot neutralise the virus sufficiently. For children with pre-existing abnormalities of the respiratory system it is probably the combination of both. In addition, it cannot be ruled out that genetic polymorphisms also play an important role in the host susceptibility for severe RSV LRTD. Future research should be directed towards understanding the pathophysiological mechanisms underlying severe RSV LRTD and are eagerly awaited.

6. Treatment of severe RSV LRTD

Therapeutic management of mechanically ventilated infants with severe RSV LRTD can either be curative or supportive. Curative treatment includes the virostatic drug ribavirin or corticosteroids, whereas bronchodilators and exogenous surfactant are supportive.

Three reports reporting the efficacy of ribavirin were reviewed systematically in a Cochrane review (Randolph et al, 2000). Results from a total number of 104 mechanically ventilated infants were pooled. The use of ribavirin was associated with a significant decrease in the duration of MV (mean difference 1.2 days (95% confidence interval -.2 to -3.4, p = 0.03). Normal saline was used as placebo in two studies, whereas sterile water was used in the third study. However, the beneficial effect of ribavirin was discarded when the one study using sterile water instead for normal saline for control was excluded from analysis. This could be explained by the serious side-effect of sterile water, being induction of bronchospasmn. Thus, there is not rationale for the use of ribavirin. Furthermore, is not easy to administer and is associated with teratogenic side-effects.

Others have explored the efficiacy of corticosteroids (Buckingham et al, 2002; van Woensel et al, 1997; van Woensel et al, 2003b; van Woensel et al, 2011). Unfortunately, the results of these studies cannot be easily compared because of the different dosing and duration of treatment. Van Woensel *et al* initially performed a post-hoc analysis of 14 mechanically ventilated infants in their original trial of prednisolone 1 mg/kg for seven days versus placebo in hospitalised children with RSV (van Woensel et al, 1997). They observed a non-significant difference in mean duration of MV (4.7 ± 2.91 versus 6.3 ± 4.23 days). Subsequently, they designed a randomised clinical trial in mechanically ventilated infants comparing dexamethason 0.15 mg/kg/day every 6 hours for 48 hours with placebo in 85 patients (van Woensel et al, 2003b). No significant difference in mean duration of MV between the two treatment arms was found. Yet, post-hoc analysis suggested that corticosteroids might be beneficial among ventilated infants who met criteria for mild disease as derived by Tasker *et al* (Tasker et al, 2000). Similar results were obtained in a study including 41 mechanically ventilated infants (Buckingham et al, 2002). Recently, Van Woensel *et al* have completed a third RCT (the so-called STAR-trial) based upon the post-hoc analysis from their second RCT (van Woensel et al, 2011). Eighty-nine patients were stratified according to oxygenation abnormalities: $PaO_2/FiO_2 < 200$ and MAP > 10 cmH_2O (N = 45) vs $PaO_2/FiO_2 > 200$ and MAP < 10 cmH_2O (N = 44) and randomized to either dexamethason 0.15 mg/kg/day every 6 hours for 48 hours with placebo. The study showed that the duration of MV was not significantly reduced in both stratification arms by dexamethason. Hence, the use of corticosteroids cannot be supported.

The efficacy of bronchodilators for ventilated infants with RSV LRTD has been explored in three different studies (Derish et al, 1998; Hammer et al, 1995; Mallory, Jr. et al, 1989). Mallory and co-workers observed a ≥ 30% improvement of peak expiratory flow at 25% (MEF_{25}) of functional residual capacity (FRC) in 13 out of 14 mechanically ventilated children with RSV LRTD (Mallory, Jr. et al, 1989). Pulmonary function was assessed by deflation flow-volume curve analysis. Hammer *et al* performed a more elegant study by excluding infants with restrictive disease (Hammer et al, 1995a). However, only 10 out of 20 infants with obstructive RSV LRTD responded to nebulised albuterol (defined by a ≥ 2-fold improvement of intra-individual coefficient of variation for MEF_{25} en Rrs. Derish *et al* included 25 infants and observed a significant increase in PEF at FRC and decrease in Rrs in some patients (Derish et al, 1998). Of note, all three studies incorporated infants with pre-existing morbidity, and none were designed to detect an effect on the duration of MV and/or PICU stay. The routine use of bronchodilators, therefore, seems unjustified. Recently, Levin and co-workers confirmed the absence of beneficial effect of bronchodilators (i.e. norepinephrine, levalbuterol, and racemic albuterol) (Levin et al, 2008).

Low levels of surfactant phospholipids and proteins as well as a diminished function of surfactant (lowering surface tension at the alveolar-capillary level) has been described (Kneyber et al, 2005b). Hence, the the use of exogenous surfactant seems highly rational. Its effect on disease course has been explored in three RCTs (Luchetti et al, 1998; Luchetti et al, 2002; Tibby et al, 2000). The group of Luchetti *et al* performed two studies investigating porcine surfactant versus no placebo (Luchetti et al, 1998; Luchetti et al, 2002). In their first study 20 children with bronchiolitis of whom 20% were RSV positive were randomized to receive either 50 mg/kg porcine surfactant once, or nothing (Luchetti et al, 1998). In their second, and methodologically more sound, study 40 children with RSV LRTD were randomized (Luchetti et al, 2002). Not only oxygenation improved in both studies, but the mean duration of MV was also significantly different between the surfactant and the placebo group (4.4 ± .4 vs 8.9 ± 1.0 days in the first study and 4.6 ± .8 vs 5.8 ± .7 days in the second study). These findings were confirmed by a study by Tibby *et al*, randomizing 19 infants to receive either 100 mg/kg bovine surfactant twice or air placebo (Tibby et al, 2000). Furthermore, a trend towards a reduced duration of MV was observed (126 hours vs 170 hours in the control group). Taken together, the findings of these three studies strongly call for a RCT with duration of MV as primary endpoint.

MV remains the mainstay of supportive therapy for infants with RSV - induced respiratory failure. Interestingly, there are no randomized controlled trials (RCT) on for instance various ventilatory strategies (volume controlled versus pressure controlled) or the level of positive end-expiratory pressure (PEEP) (Leclerc et al, 2001). MV with heliox has been scantily studied among infants with RSV LRTD. From a pathophysiological point of view MV with heliox seems rational. Heliox has a density that is one-seventh that of air, resulting in a decreased resistance to gas flow (Gupta et al, 2005). There is one trial investigating the effect of MV with heliox in various concentrations in ten infants with RSV LRTD (Gross et al, 2000). No beneficial effect could be demonstrated. As the study has methodological flaws, and no attempt was made to discriminate clinical phenotype of RSV LRTD, the role of MV with heliox requires further study. Our group has undertaken a pilot-study in 13 ventilated infants with RSV LRTD. Heliox 60/40 (i.e. 60% helium and 40% oxygen in the inspired gas) significantly reduced the Rrs compared with conventional gas mixture although CO_2 exchange was not improved (Kneyber et al, 2009). Our findings warrant follow-up in a large RCT.

Until now, the mainstay of therapy for mechanically ventilated infants with RSV LRTD has been symptomatic. Judging the outcomes of the various RCTs, it is highly unlikely that this will change in the near future. The only promising therapeutic modality seems exogenous surfactant, although this has no direct curative effect.

7. Prevention

Vaccination against RSV will not readily be available, but passive immunisation can be applied (Kneyber et al, 2004). Passive immunization can be achieved through palivizumab, which is a monoclonal antibody directed against the F - glycoprotein. Presently, its use is advised for (a) infants not older than 12 months without CLD born after a gestation of 28 weeks, (b) infants not older than six months without CLD born after a gestation of 29 to 32 weeks, and (c) infants born after a gestation of 32 to 35 weeks with at least two of the following risk factors: attending child care, having school-aged siblings, being exposed to environmental air pollutants, having congenital abnormalities of the airways, or being diagnosed with severe neuromuscular disease. Palivizumab is also advised for children younger than two years of age with CLD or a hemodynamically significant CHD (Meissner et al, 2003).

The effect of routine passive immunization on the number of PICU admissions as well as duration of MV is not clear. In the IMpact study an overall reduction of 55% in hospitalizations was found among palivizumab recipients (N = 1002 vs 500 controls). However, the number of PICU admissions (1.3% vs 3%) or number of mechanically ventilated children (0.2% vs .7%) was not significantly affected (The IMpact-RSV Study Group, 1998). Children with congenital heart disease were separately studied (639 palivizumab recipients vs 648 controls) (Feltes et al, 2003). Again, the overall reduction of 45% in hospitalizations was not observed for the number of PICU admissions (2% vs 3.7%) or mechanically ventilated children (1.3% vs 2.2%). Two post-licensure studies after the introduction of palivizumab have been reported. Pedraz and co-workers studied the efficacy of palivizumab in four consecutive RSV seasons (non-prophylaxed children (N = 1583) admitted between 1998 - 2000, and prophylaxed (N = 1919) children admitted between 2000 - 2002) in Spain (Pedraz et al, 2003). The number of children admitted to the PICU (13% vs 20%) or requiring MV (8% vs 11%) were comparable. Similar observations were made in a national survey performed in Israel during two consecutive RSV seasons (2000 - 2002), including 296 children (Prais et al, 2005). It thus seems that monthly prophylaxis with palivizumab does not have an effect on the occurrence of severe RSV LRTD necessitating PICU admission and/or MV. This suggests that not only virological and/or immunological factors are (partially) responsible for the development of severe RSV LRTD.

8. Long term effects

Long-term follow-up studies of children hospitalised with RSV LRTD have irrespective of age consistently shown impaired pulmonary function compared with children who had no apparent infecting agent, mainly characterized by an obstructive pattern (i.e. increased airway resistance) (Cassimos et al, 2008; Dezateux et al, 1997; Singleton et al, 2003; Stein et al, 1999). This increase in airway resistance coincides with episodes of recurrent wheezing resembling childhood asthma in up to 50% of children, and not results in a high use of asthma medications but also in a substantial decrease in parental-reported health-related quality of life of the child (Bont et al, 2000; Bont et al, 2004; Kneyber et al, 2000; Stein et al, 2004). Importantly, in general there is no data available on pulmonary function after being mechanically ventilated for RSV LRTD (Ermers et al, 2009). Mechanical ventilation is life-saving for patients with RSV induced respiratory failure. Yet, numerous experimental studies have shown that mechanical ventilation induces a pulmonary inflammation that aggravates lung injury leading to irreversible damage. This has been labelled "double-hit principle" (Tremblay et al, 1998; Tremblay et al, 2006). More specifically, lung inflammation and programmed cell death were enhanced by mechanical ventilation in a mouse model of RSV LRTD (Bem et al, 2009).

9. Conclusion

RSV is an important cause of serious morbidity annually occurring in paediatric critical care units. At present, the mainstay of therapy for mechanically ventilated infants is still symptomatic. The routine use of ribavirin or corticosteroids cannot be recommended. However, there are new and promising (supportive) treatment modalities emerging such as the use of exogenous surfactant or mechanical ventilation with heliox. Future research should also be directed towards a better understanding of the pathophysiological mechanisms underlying severe RSV LRTD to gain insight why infants need to ventilated and what the effects of mechanical ventilation in combination with RSV itself are on long term outcome. Only then it will be possible to develop new curative treatments and to identify patients who might benefit from such a treatment. In the mean time, we continue our endless care and devotion to these infants.

10. References

Bem RA, van Woensel JB, Bos AP, Koski A, Farnand AW, Domachowske JB, Rosenberg HF, Martin TR & Matute-Bello G. (2009) Mechanical ventilation enhances lung inflammation and caspase activity in a model of mouse pneumovirus infection. *Am.J.Physiol Lung Cell Mol.Physiol.* Vol. 296, issue 1, pp. L46-L56,

Bloomfield P, Dalton D, Karleka A, Kesson A, Duncan G & Isaacs D. (2004) Bacteraemia and antibiotic use in respiratory syncytial virus infections. *Arch Dis Child.* Vol. 89, issue 4, pp. 363-367,

Bont L, Aalderen WM & Kimpen JL. (2000) Long-term consequences of respiratory syncytial virus (RSV) bronchiolitis. *Paediatr.Respir.Rev.* Vol. 1, issue 3, pp. 221-227,

Bont L, Heijnen CJ, Kavelaars A, van Aalderen WM, Brus F, Draaisma JM, Pekelharing-Berghuis M, Diemen-Steenvoorde RA & Kimpen JL. (2001) Local interferon-gamma levels during respiratory syncytial virus lower respiratory tract infection are associated with disease severity. *J Infect.Dis.* Vol. 184, issue 3, pp. 355-358,

Bont L & Kimpen JL. (2002) Immunological mechanisms of severe respiratory syncytial virus bronchiolitis. *Intensive Care Med.* Vol. 28, issue 5, pp. 616-621,

Bont L, Steijn M, van Aalderen WM & Kimpen JL. (2004) Impact of wheezing after respiratory syncytial virus infection on health-related quality of life. *Pediatr.Infect.Dis.J.* Vol. 23, issue 5, pp. 414-417,

Broughton S, Bhat R, Roberts A, Zuckerman M, Rafferty G & Greenough A. (2006) Diminished lung function, RSV infection, and respiratory morbidity in prematurely born infants. *Arch Dis Child.* Vol. 91, issue 1, pp. 26-30,

Buckingham SC, Bush AJ & DeVincenzo JP. (2000) Nasal quantity of respiratory syncytical virus correlates with disease severity in hospitalized infants. *Pediatr Infect Dis J*. Vol. 19, issue 2, pp. 113-117,

Buckingham SC, Jafri HS, Bush AJ, Carubelli CM, Sheeran P, Hardy RD, Ottolini MG, Ramilo O & DeVincenzo JP. (2002) A randomized, double-blind, placebo-controlled trial of dexamethasone in severe respiratory syncytial virus (RSV) infection: effects on RSV quantity and clinical outcome. *J Infect.Dis*. Vol. 185, issue 9, pp. 1222-1228,

Cannon MJ, Openshaw PJ & Askonas BA. (1988) Cytotoxic T cells clear virus but augment lung pathology in mice infected with respiratory syncytial virus. *J Exp.Med*. Vol. 168, issue 3, pp. 1163-1168,

Cassimos DC, Tsalkidis A, Tripsianis GA, Stogiannidou A, Anthracopoulos M, Ktenidou-Kartali S, Aivazis V, Gardikis S & Chatzimichael A. (2008) Asthma, lung function and sensitization in school children with a history of bronchiolitis. *Pediatr.Int*. Vol. 50, issue 1, pp. 51-56,

Chanock R, Roizman B & Myers R. (1957) Recovery from infants with respiratory illness of a virus related to chimpanzee coryza agent (CCA). I. Isolation, properties and characterization. *Am J Hyg*. Vol. 66, issue 3, pp. 281-290,

Checchia PA, Appel HJ, Kahn S, Smith FA, Shulman ST, Pahl E & Baden HP. (2000) Myocardial injury in children with respiratory syncytial virus infection. *Pediatr.Crit Care Med*. Vol. 1, issue 2, pp. 146-150,

de Weerd W, Twilhaar WN & Kimpen JL. (1998) T cell subset analysis in peripheral blood of children with RSV bronchiolitis. *Scand.J Infect.Dis*. Vol. 30, issue 1, pp. 77-80,

Derish M, Hodge G, Dunn C & Ariagno R. (1998) Aerosolized albuterol improves airway reactivity in infants with acute respiratory failure from respiratory syncytial virus. *Pediatr Pulmonol*. Vol. 26, issue 1, pp. 12-20,

DeVincenzo JP, El Saleeby CM & Bush AJ. (2005) Respiratory syncytial virus load predicts disease severity in previously healthy infants. *J Infect Dis*. Vol. 191, issue 11, pp. 1861-1868,

Dezateux C, Fletcher ME, Dundas I & Stocks J. (1997) Infant respiratory function after RSV-proven bronchiolitis. *Am.J.Respir.Crit Care Med*. Vol. 155, issue 4, pp. 1349-1355,

Eisenhut M, Sidaras D, Johnson R, Newland P & Thorburn K. (2004) Cardiac Troponin T levels and myocardial involvement in children with severe respiratory syncytial virus lung disease. *Acta Paediatr*. Vol. 93, issue 7, pp. 887-890,

Ermers MJ, Rovers MM, van Woensel JB, Kimpen JL & Bont LJ. (2009) The effect of high dose inhaled corticosteroids on wheeze in infants after respiratory syncytial virus infection: randomised double blind placebo controlled trial. *BMJ*. Vol. 338, issue b897-

Falsey AR, Hennessey PA, Formica MA, Cox C & Walsh EE. (2005) Respiratory Syncytial Virus Infection in Elderly and High-Risk Adults. *The New England Journal of Medicine*. Vol. 352, issue 17, pp. 1749-1759,

Feltes TF, Cabalka AK, Meissner HC, Piazza FM, Carlin DA, Top FH, Jr., Connor EM & Sondheimer HM. (2003) Palivizumab prophylaxis reduces hospitalization due to respiratory syncytial virus in young children with hemodynamically significant congenital heart disease. *J Pediatr*. Vol. 143, issue 4, pp. 532-540,

Frankel LR & Derish MT. (1999) Respiratory syncytial virus induced respiratory failure in the pediatric patient. *New Horiz*. Vol. 7, issue 335-346,

Gauthier R, Beyaert C, Feillet F, Peslin R, Monin P & Marchal F. (1998) Respiratory oscillation mechanics in infants with broncholitis during mechanical ventilation. *Pediatr Pulmonol.* Vol. 25, issue 18-31,

Glezen WP, Paredes A, Allison JE, Taber LH & Frank AL. (1981) Risk of respiratory syncytial virus infection for infants from low-income families in relationship to age, sex, ethnic group, and maternal antibody level. *J Pediatr.* Vol. 98, issue 5, pp. 708-715,

Glezen WP, Taber LH, Frank AL & Kasel JA. (1986) Risk of primary infection and reinfection with respiratory syncytial virus. *Am J Dis Child.* Vol. 140, issue 6, pp. 543-546,

Gross MF, Spear RM & Peterson BM. (2000) Helium-oxygen mixture does not improve gas exchange in mechanically ventilated children with bronchiolitis. *Crit Care.* Vol. 4, issue 3, pp. 188-192,

Guerguerian AM, Farrell C, Gauthier M & Lacroix J. (2004) Bronchiolitis: what's next? *Pediatr Crit Care Med.* Vol. 5, issue 5, pp. 498-500,

Gupta VK & Cheifetz IM. (2005) Heliox administration in the pediatric intensive care unit: an evidence-based review. *Pediatr Crit Care Med.* Vol. 6, issue 2, pp. 204-211,

Hacking D & Hull J. (2002) Respiratory syncytial virus--viral biology and the host response. *J Infect.* Vol. 45, issue 1, pp. 18-24,

Hall CB. (2001) Respiratory syncytial virus and parainfluenza virus. *N.Engl J Med.* Vol. 344, issue 25, pp. 1917-1928,

Hall CB, Walsh EE, Schnabel KC, Long CE, McConnochie KM, Hildreth SW & Anderson LJ. (1990) Occurrence of groups A and B of respiratory syncytial virus over 15 years: associated epidemiologic and clinical characteristics in hospitalized and ambulatory children. *J Infect.Dis.* Vol. 162, issue 6, pp. 1283-1290,

Hammer J, Numa A & Newth CJ. (1995) Albuterol responsiveness in infants with respiratory failure caused by respiratory syncytial virus infection. *J Pediatr.* Vol. 147, issue 1295-1298,

Hammer J, Numa A & Newth CJ. (1997) Acute respiratory distress syndrome caused by respiratory syncytial virus. *Pediatr Pulmonol.* Vol. 23, issue 176-183,

Hanna S, Tibby SM, Durward A & Murdoch IA. (2003) Incidence of hyponatraemia and hyponatraemic seizures in severe respiratory syncytial virus bronchiolitis. *Acta Paediatr.* Vol. 92, issue 4, pp. 430-434,

Henderson FW, Collier AM, Clyde WA, Jr. & Denny FW. (1979) Respiratory-syncytial-virus infections, reinfections and immunity. A prospective, longitudinal study in young children. *N.Engl.J Med.* Vol. 300, issue 10, pp. 530-534,

Isaacs D. (1998) Is bronchiolitis an obsolete term? *Curr Opin Pediatr.* Vol. 10, issue 1-3,

Karron RA, Singleton RJ, Bulkow L, Parkinson A, Kruse D, DeSmet I, Indorf C, Petersen KM, Leombruno D, Hurlburt D, Santosham M & Harrison LH. (1999) Severe respiratory syncytial virus disease in Alaska native children. RSV Alaska Study Group. *J Infect Dis.* Vol. 180, issue 1, pp. 41-49,

Kim KK & Frankel LR. (1997) The need for inotropic support in a subgroup of infants with severe life-threatening respiratory syncytial viral infection. *J.Investig.Med.* Vol. 45, issue 8, pp. 469-473,

Kneyber MC, Blusse vO-A, van VM, Uiterwaal CS, Kimpen JL & van Vught AJ. (2005a) Concurrent bacterial infection and prolonged mechanical ventilation in infants with respiratory syncytial virus lower respiratory tract disease. *Intensive Care Med.* Vol. 31, issue 5, pp. 680-685,

Kneyber MC, Brandenburg AH, de Groot R, Joosten KF, Rothbarth PH, Ott A & Moll HA. (1998) Risk factors for respiratory syncytial virus associated apnoea. *Eur.J Pediatr.* Vol. 157, issue 4, pp. 331-335,

Kneyber MC, Brandenburg AH, Rothbarth PH, de Groot R, Ott A & Steensel-Moll HA. (1996) Relationship between clinical severity of respiratory syncytial virus infection and subtype. *Arch.Dis.Child.* Vol. 75, issue 2, pp. 137-140,

Kneyber MC & Kimpen JL. (2004) Advances in respiratory syncytial virus vaccine development. *Curr.Opin.Investig.Drugs.* Vol. 5, issue 2, pp. 163-170,

Kneyber MC, Plotz FB & Kimpen JL. (2005b) Bench-to-bedside review: Paediatric viral lower respiratory tract disease necessitating mechanical ventilation--should we use exogenous surfactant? *Crit Care.* Vol. 9, issue 6, pp. 550-555,

Kneyber MC, van Heerde M, Twisk JW, Plotz FB & Markhors DG. (2009) Heliox reduces respiratory system resistance in respiratory syncytial virus induced respiratory failure. *Crit Care.* Vol. 13, issue 3, pp. R71-

Kneyber MCJ, Steyerberg EW, de Groot R & Moll HA. (2000) Long-term effects of respiratory syncytial virus (RSV) bronchiolitis in infants and young children: a quantitative review. *Acta Paediatr.* Vol. 89, issue 6, pp. 654-660,

Leader S & Kohlhase K. (2003) Recent trends in severe respiratory syncytial virus (RSV) among US infants, 1997 to 2000. *J Pediatr.* Vol. 143, issue 5, Supplement 1, pp. 127-132,

Leclerc F, Scalfaro P, Noizet O, Thumerelle C, Dorkenoo A & Fourier C. (2001) Mechanical ventilatory support in infants with respiratory syncytial virus infection. *Pediatr.Crit Care Med.* Vol. 2, issue 3, pp. 197-204,

Levin DL, Garg A, Hall LJ, Slogic S, Jarvis JD & Leiter JC. (2008) A prospective randomized controlled blinded study of three bronchodilators in infants with respiratory syncytial virus bronchiolitis on mechanical ventilation. *Pediatr.Crit Care Med.* Vol. 9, issue 6, pp. 598-604,

Luchetti M, Casiraghi G, Valsecchi R, Galassini E & Marraro G. (1998) Porcine-derived surfactant treatment of severe bronchiolitis. *Acta Anaesthesiol Scand.* Vol. 42, issue 805-810,

Luchetti M, Ferrero F, Gallini C, Natale A, Pigna A, Tortorolo L & Marraro G. (2002) Multicenter, randomised, controlled study of porcine surfactant in severe respiratory syncytial virus-induced respiratory failure. *Pediatr.Crit Care Med.* Vol. 3, issue 261-268,

Maconochie I, Greenough A, Yuksel B, Page A & Karani J. (1991) A chest radiograph scoring system to predict chronic oxygen dependency in low birth weight infants. *Early Human Develop.* Vol. 26, issue 37-43,

Mallory Jr GB, Motoyama EK, Koumbourlis AC, Mutich RL & Nakayama DK. (1989) Bronchial reactivity in infants with acute respiratory failure with viral bronchiolitis. *Pediatr Pulmonol.* Vol. 6, issue 253-259,

Marchant A & Goldman M. (2005) T cell-mediated immune responses in human newborns: ready to learn? *Clin.Exp Immunol.* Vol. 141, issue 1, pp. 10-18,

Marodi L. (2006) Innate cellular immune responses in newborns. *Clin.Immunol.* Vol. 118, issue 2-3, pp. 137-144,

Meissner HC & Long SS. (2003) Revised indications for the use of palivizumab and respiratory syncytial virus immune globulin intravenous for the prevention of respiratory syncytial virus infections. *Pediatrics*. Vol. 112, issue 6 Pt 1, pp. 1447-1452,

Morris J.A., Blount R.E. & Savage RE. (1956) Recovery of cytopathogenic agent from chimpanzees with coryza. *Proc.Soc.Exp Biol Med*. Vol. 92, issue 3, pp. 544-549,

Njoku DB & Kliegman RM. (1993) Atypical extrapulmonary presentations of severe respiratory syncytial virus infection requiring intensive care. *Clin.Pediatr.(Phila)*. Vol. 32, issue 8, pp. 455-460,

Pedraz C, Carbonell-Estrany X, Figueras-Aloy J & Quero J. (2003) Effect of palivizumab prophylaxis in decreasing respiratory syncytial virus hospitalizations in premature infants. *Pediatr Infect Dis J*. Vol. 22, issue 9, pp. 823-827,

Playfor SD & Khader A. (2005) Arrhythmias associated with respiratory syncytial virus infection. *Paediatr.Anaesth*. Vol. 15, issue 11, pp. 1016-1018,

Prais D, Danino D, Schonfeld T & Amir J. (2005) Impact of palivizumab on admission to the ICU for respiratory syncytial virus bronchiolitis: a national survey. *Chest*. Vol. 128, issue 4, pp. 2765-2771,

Ramshaw IA, Ramsay AJ, Karupiah G, Rolph MS, Mahalingam S & Ruby JC. (1997) Cytokines and immunity to viral infections. *Immunol.Rev*. Vol. 159, issue 119-135,

Randolph AG, Reder L & Englund JA. (2004) Risk of bacterial infection in previously healthy respiratory syncytial virus-infected young children admitted to the intensive care unit. *Pediatr Infect Dis J*. Vol. 23, issue 11, pp. 990-994,

Randolph AG & Wang EE. (2000) Ribavirin for respiratory syncytial virus infection of the lower respiratory tract. *Cochrane.Database.Syst.Rev*. Vol. 2, pp. CD000181-

Rayyan M, Naulaers G, Daniels H, Allegaert K, Debeer A & Devlieger H. (2004) Characteristics of respiratory syncytial virus-related apnoea in three infants. *Acta Paediatr*. Vol. 93, issue 6, pp. 847-849,

Shay DK, Holman RC, Newman RD, Liu LL, Stout JW & Anderson LJ. (1999) Bronchiolitis-associated hospitalizations among US children, 1980-1996. *JAMA*. Vol. 282, issue 15, pp. 1440-1446,

Shay DK, Holman RC, Roosevelt GE, Clarke MJ & Anderson LJ. (2001) Bronchiolitis-associated mortality and estimates of respiratory syncytial virus-associated deaths among US children, 1979-1997. *J Infect.Dis*. Vol. 183, issue 1, pp. 16-22,

Singleton RJ, Redding GJ, Lewis TC, Martinez P, Bulkow L, Morray B, Peters H, Gove J, Jones C, Stamey D, Talkington DF, DeMain J, Bernert JT & Butler JC. (2003) Sequelae of severe respiratory syncytial virus infection in infancy and early childhood among Alaska Native children. *Pediatrics*. Vol. 112, issue 2, pp. 285-290,

Steensel-Moll HA, Hazelzet JA, van der Voort E, Neijens HJ & Hackeng WH. (1990) Excessive secretion of antidiuretic hormone in infections with respiratory syncytial virus. *Arch.Dis.Child*. Vol. 65, issue 11, pp. 1237-1239,

Stein RT & Martinez FD. (2004) Asthma phenotypes in childhood: lessons from an epidemiological approach. *Paediatr.Respir.Rev*. Vol. 5, issue 2, pp. 155-161,

Stein RT, Sherrill D, Morgan WJ, Holberg CJ, Halonen M, Taussig LM, Wright AL & Martinez FD. (1999) Respiratory syncytial virus in early life and risk of wheeze and allergy by age 13 years. *Lancet*. Vol. 354, issue 9178, pp. 541-545,

Tasker RC, Gordon I & Kiff K. (2000) Time course of severe respiratory syncytial infection in mechanically ventilated infants. *Acta Paediatr*. Vol. 2000, issue 938-941,

The IMpact-RSV Study Group. (1998) Palivizumab, a humanized respiratory syncytial virus monoclonal antibody, reduces hospitalization from respiratory syncytial virus infection in high-risk infants. *Pediatrics*. Vol. 102, issue 3 Pt 1, pp. 531-537,

Thomas JA, Raroque S, Scott WA, Toro-Figueroa LO & Levin DL. (1997) Successful treatment of severe dysrhythmias in infants with respiratory syncytial virus infections: two cases and a literature review. *Crit Care Med*. Vol. 25, issue 5, pp. 880-886,

Thorburn K, Harigopal S, Reddy V, Taylor N & van Saene HK. (2006) High incidence of pulmonary bacterial co-infection in children with severe respiratory syncytial virus (RSV) bronchiolitis. *Thorax*. Vol. 61, issue 7, pp. 611-615,

Tibby SM, Hatherill M, Wright SM, Wilson P, Postle AD & Murdoch IA. (2000) Exogenous surfactant supplementation in infants with respiratory syncytial virus bronchiolitis. *Am.J.Respir.Crit Care Med*. Vol. 162, issue 4 Pt 1, pp. 1251-1256,

Tremblay LN & Slutsky AS. (1998) Ventilator-induced injury: from barotrauma to biotrauma. *Proc.Assoc.Am.Physicians*. Vol. 110, issue 6, pp. 482-488,

Tremblay LN & Slutsky AS. (2006) Ventilator-induced lung injury: from the bench to the bedside. *Intensive Care Med*. Vol. 32, issue 1, pp. 24-33,

van Woensel JB, Lutter R, Biezeveld MH, Dekker T, Nijhuis M, van Aalderen WM & Kuijpers TW. (2003a) Effect of dexamethasone on tracheal viral load and interleukin-8 tracheal concentration in children with respiratory syncytial virus infection. *Pediatr Infect Dis J*. Vol. 22, issue 8, pp. 721-726,

van Woensel JB, van Aalderen WM, de WW, Jansen NJ, van Gestel JP, Markhorst DG, van Vught AJ, Bos AP & Kimpen JL. (2003b) Dexamethasone for treatment of patients mechanically ventilated for lower respiratory tract infection caused by respiratory syncytial virus. *Thorax*. Vol. 58, issue 5, pp. 383-387,

van Woensel JB & Vyas H. (2011) Dexamethasone in children mechanically ventilated for lower respiratory tract infection caused by respiratory syncytial virus: A randomized controlled trial. *Crit Care Med*. Vol. 39, issue 7, pp. 1779-1783,

van Woensel JB, Wolfs TF, van Aalderen WM, Brand PL & Kimpen JL. (1997) Randomised double blind placebo controlled trial of prednisolone in children admitted to hospital with respiratory syncytial virus bronchiolitis. *Thorax*. Vol. 52, issue 7, pp. 634-637,

Wang EE, Law BJ, Boucher FD, Stephens D, Robinson JL, Dobson S, Langley JM, McDonald J, MacDonald NE & Mitchell I. (1996) Pediatric Investigators Collaborative Network on Infections in Canada (PICNIC) study of admission and management variation in patients hospitalized with respiratory syncytial viral lower respiratory tract infection. *J Pediatr*. Vol. 129, issue 3, pp. 390-395,

Welliver RC. (2003) Review of epidemiology and clinical risk factors for severe respiratory syncytial virus (RSV) infection. *J Pediatr*. Vol. 143, issue 5 Suppl, pp. S112-S117,

8

Epidemiology and Diagnosis of Human Respiratory Syncytial Virus Infections

Javed Akhter and Sameera Al Johani
Department of Pathology and Laboratory Medicine/King Abdulaziz Medical City
Saudi Arabia

1. Introduction

Respiratory syncytial virus (RSV) is a common winter time respiratory virus that affects persons of all ages. RSV was first isolated in children with pulmonary disease in 1957. Initially referred to as the 'chimp coryza virus', the nature of the virus to form syncytia (fusion of cells to form larger cells without any internal cell boundaries) in tissue culture subsequently resulted in the virus being named the respiratory syncytial virus. Formation of syncytia permits the virus to spread by evading host antibodies (Weir & Fisman , 2004)

Human RSV is a negative sense enveloped RNA virus and is a member of the family Paramyxoviridae, classified within the genus Pneumovirus. RSV has two subtypes A and B that are distinguished largely by differences in the viral attachment (G) protein or the nuclear (N) protein (Sato et al., 2005). During epidemics, either subtype may predominate, or both subtypes may circulate concurrently. RSV is unstable in the environment, readily inactivated by soap and water. The virus is spread through close contact with infected carriers or contaminated surfaces. Infection occurs when infected materials come in contact with the mucous membranes of the eyes, nose or mouth. It is possible that inhaled fomites are a source of infection. It can remain infectious on surfaces or fomites for 4-7 hours and can also survive on unwashed hands.

RSV is the main cause of bronchiolitis worldwide and can cause up to 70 or 80 percent of lower respiratory infections (LRIs) during high season. The lower respiratory tract includes continuation of the airways from the trachea and bronchi to the bronchioles and the alveoli (Henrickson, 2004). The common LRIs in children are pneumonia and bronchiolitis and the most common causes of viral LRIs are RSVs (Steweart et al., 2009). They tend to be highly seasonal, unlike parainfluenza viruses, the next most common cause of viral LRIs.

Environmental conditions such as temperature, relative humidity and UV-B radiation have been described in relation to RSV epidemics (Welliver, 2009). A study performed in Spain (Lapena et al., 2005) indicated that low temperature and low absolute humidity were positively associated with the number of RSV cases and low absolute humidity was independently related to RSV infection. Worldwide, RSV peaks at two temperature intervals: between 2-6°C in temperate regions and 24-30°C in tropical regions. RSV activity is greatest at 45-65% relative humidity and UV-B radiance inversely related to the number of RSV cases. The relation between RSV activity and low minimum temperature indicates that this factor enhances virus transmission. It has been described in earlier studies that transmission of RSV is inversely related to temperature in cooler climates and this may be a result of increased stability of the virus in the secretions during the colder climate. Inactivation of RSV in air has been described (Rechsteiner & Winkler, 1969); stable aerosols of RSV were prepared and kept at different relative humidity. Virus recoveries were highest at high relative humidity and the stability of the aerosol was maximal at 60% relative humidity. This indicates that humidity indeed plays an important role and may affect transmission of the virus.

1.1 Children

RSV is the largest single cause of childhood hospitalization due to lower respiratory tract disease. Infections manifest themselves as mild upper respiratory tract infections or lower respiratory tract infections: bronchitis, bronchiolitis, and pneumonia. 10% of those infected require specialised paediatric care. High risk groups for severe RSV infection include premature infants, children with congenital heart disease, cystic fibrosis and other chronic lung disease (Stensballe, 2002). This may be due to the fact that immunity has not become fully established, narrow airways, incomplete development of the lungs and relatively short bronchial tree. It also affects the elderly and immuno-compromised patients. It has been estimated that RSV causes about 500,000 deaths in children each year globally (Shay et al., 1999). Although, mortality due to RSV is very low in Western Europe, the number of child deaths due to acute respiratory infections worldwide is considerable with 70% of deaths occurring in Africa and Southeast Asia (Nair et al., 2011).

• Cause of worldwide epidemics, which can occur annually or biennially
• Most children are infected by 3 years of age
• Responsible for about 70% of cases of bronchiolitis in children
• Re-infections occur throughout life and the same serotype can re-infect children and adults
• Associated with recurrent wheeze for many years after bronchiolitis
• Low birth weight is associated with acute respiratory infections in developing countries
• Cord blood vitamin D deficiency has been associated with Respiratory Syncytial Virus Bronchiolitis

Table 1. Characteristics of RSV infection

1.2 Adults

The elderly show increased susceptibility to respiratory infections and other related complications. In community dwelling, the elderly suffer fom 1.2 to 1.6 acute respiratory infections per year accounting for 25 - 50% of respiratory illness (Nicholson et al., 1997). RSV is a significant and unrecognized cause of seasonal respiratory tract infections (RTIs) in adults, accounting for as much as 25% of excess wintertime mortality usually attributed to influenza. Nearly 80% of RSV associated underlying respiratory and circulatory deaths occur among the elderly (Ramirez, 2008). RSV is estimated to account for about 180,000 hospital admissions each year exceeding. RSV is also recognized as an important cause of viral pneumonia in adults. Clustering of RSV infected patients on wards has suggested nosocomial spread by health care workers. Preventive measures such as handwashing are important, especially in hospitals and nursing homes where there may be many immunocompromised patients. During RSV season, it is advisable to minimize contact between high-risk patients and children.

2. Epidemiology of RSV Infections

RSV is highly contagious, it is thought that of half the infants that acquire RSV infection during the first year of life, approximately 40% of these infections result in lower respiratory infections. Virtually all children will have been infected by RSV by the first 3 years of life. RSV is associated with more deaths than influenza in children aged 1-12 months. Excess deaths due to RSV and influenza virus infection have also been reported for the elderly population.

2.1 Developed countries

Epidemics of the virus occur annually and tend to start in November or December and last 4 to 5 months. In any one year, about 90,000 children will be hospitalized due to RSV and 4,500 will die. RSV epidemic patterns differ by geographic locations. In the Northern hemisphere and particularly, within the United States, RSV mostly circulates between November and March (Dawson-Caswell and Muncie 2011). However, the severity of the season, peak of activity and time of onset can vary. Communities in the Southern United States experience the earliest onset of RSV activity. Midwestern States experience the latest. The national average duration is about 15 weeks and can range from 13 to 20 weeks (MMWR, 2010). The epidemic pattern of RSV is quite different in regions of Europe (biennial epidemics in alternating cycles of approximately 9 and 15 months) than in the Western hemisphere (annual epidemics). In Australia, about 100,000 infants are infected by RSV every winter. In temperate regions of Australia, the occurrence of annual winter epidemics has been well demonstrated (Mullins et al., 2003). The incidence peaks in July, with 55-77% of all cases occurring between July and September. Most of the cases of RSV infections in Australia occur in children under the age of 4 years. Mechanisms underlying the pathogenesis induced by RSV are mostly unknown. RSV induced bronchiolitis in infancy may predispose to asthma later in life (Ghildyal et al., 2003). In Germany, Finland, Switzerland, Sweden and Croatia, there is a two year RSV cycle repeating every 23 to 25 months. Unlike Europe, Great Britain experiences a monophasic, annual RSV epidemic cycle. In some parts of the USA, RSV cycles are also monophasic and annual (Milinaric-Galinovic et al., 2008)..

2.2 Developing countries

In developing countries, respiratory diseases represent a challenge to public health because of their severity, frequency, trends, and economic impact. Data from developing countries are even more limited in the ability to provide a clear estimate of disease burden. Published in 1998, a review of the literature on RSV in tropical and developing countries identified from ten longitudinal community-based studies that RSV was the etiological agent in 2% (in India) to 73% (in Brazil) of lower respiratory infection episodes (Weber et al. 1998). Three studies (from Brazil, Uruguay, and Colombia) reported RSV as being the etiological agent in more than 50% of the community-based acute lower respiratory tract infection episodes. The authors identified the limitations associated with different methods used by the different studies to detect RSV. In general, studies that used immunofluorescence methods had higher rates of RSV detection, and the majority of the community-based longitudinal studies that had low RSV detection rates used culture alone. The same review examined the more abundant hospital-based studies in tropical and developing countries and found that RSV was detected in between 6 and 96% of cases of hospitalised lower respiratory tract infections. On average, RSV accounted for 65% of samples that were positive for a virus (range 27-96%); and 17% of acute respiratory tract infections in children admitted to hospital.

There is relatively scant information for the role of RSV in causing LRI among children in developing countries. Hence the WHO introduced standardized protocols for new studies to be undertaken in these regions. This was first performed in, Mozambique, Indonesia, Nigeria and South Africa (Robertson et al., 2004). The total incidence of LRIs occurring among children aged < 1 year was lowest in Indonesia and highest in Mozambique where 50% of children presented with an LRI and 13% were hospitalized. Among infants, RSV infections identified were 36% in Nigeria, 23% in Indonesia and 6% in Mozambique. For severe RSV attributable LRIs, the proportion was high in Indonesia but low in Mozambique. The rates of severe illness in children < 1 year in Indonesia, Mozambique and South Africa (15-16/1000 child years) are very similar to rates of hospitalization from industrialized countries eg. England (20/1000 child years), Germany (12/1000 child years), Norway (10/1000 child years), USA (20/1000 child years) and Austria (6/1000 child years). Differences in RSV rates in developing countries also depends on many social factors such fewer health centres, large families with many children facilitates more spread of infections. In some countries such as South Africa and Mozambique, the peak for RSV correlates with the presence or absence of rainfall.

2.3 RSV Infections in the Middle East

Little is known about the epidemiology of RSV infections in the Middle East and other desert climate regions of the world. The Middle East has large areas covered by desert. In summer, it is hot and can be very humid, whereas in winter, temperature can drop significantly. These weather variations can exacerbate respiratory infections (ARI) and chronic lung diseases in susceptible individuals especially asthmatics (Waness et al., 2011). Acute respiratory infections play a major role in hospitalizations in the Middle East. The number of children admitted with RSV diseases from developing countries in 2005 was more than double that estimated in 1986, and the incidence of RSV-acute lower respiratory tract (ALRI) was twice that of industrialized countries (Nair et al., 2010)

A review of RSV infections in the Middle East region (Table 2) shows that the occurrence of RSV infections is in the Winter season peaking around January as in other parts of the world, with the same age groups affected. This is in contrast to some developing countries eg. Indonesia, where the incidence of RSV LRI in the first 6 months of life is relatively low. Most cases of disease occur in older children (Simoes et al., 2011). A more precise understanding of the timing of annual RSV epidemics should assist providers in maximizing the benefit of preventive therapies.

The current data on the load and importance of viral respiratory infection and hospitalization is scarce. Recipients of bone marrow transplant have been reported to have mortality rates over 50% with RSV pneumonia. Molecular epidemiologic studies have demonstrated that RSV nosocomial outbreaks often result from multiple introductions of distinct strains from the community. In Saudi Arabia a review of RSV hospitalizations showed that the majority of cases are due to bronchopneumonia, prematurity and lung, heart disorders (Al-Muhsen, 2010). In Jordan, RSV positive children require higher rates of oxygen use and longer hospital stay, which is a financial burden for poor countries (Khuri-Bulos et al., 2010). A study in Kuwait (Hijazi et al., 1997) found that RSV was the commonest agent identified in 52% cases of bronchiolitis, 29% of pneumonia and 51% of croup. Another study in Al Ain has shown that the clinical pattern of RSV infections includes bronchiolitis in 58% of cases, bronchopneumonia in 19% of cases and pneumonia 11%. RSV was strongly associated with cool temperatures and relative humidity between 50-60% (Uduman et al., 1996). The cycle of RSV infections is also less defined in the Middle East. In Saudi Arabia, the pattern appears to show regular rates of infection with a slower peak approximately at 3 years (Fig 1). Such trends need to be monitored and extended to other Middle Eastern countries.

Children younger than 60 days and those with severe symptoms may require hospitalization. Neither antibiotics nor corticosteroids are helpful for bronchiolitis. A bronchodilator trial is appropriate for children with wheezing, but should not be continued unless there is a prompt favorable response (Jafri, 2003). Frequent hand washing and contact isolation may prevent the spread of RSV infections. Children younger than two years at high risk of severe illness, including those born before 35 weeks of gestation and those with chronic lung or cardiac problems, may be candidates for palivizumab prophylaxis for RSV infection during the peak infection season (Lieberthal et al., 2006).

Recent studies have shown that Vitamin D deficiency in healthy neonates is associated with increased risk of RSV LRTI in the first year of life (Belderbos, et al., 2011). Vitamin D supplementation during pregnancy may be a useful strategy to prevent RSV LRTI during infancy. This could be particularly significant in Saudi Arabia and other developing countries where there is a high level of vitamin D deficiency among the population.

Hajj pilgrimage is a yearly event in which >2 million Muslims from around the world gather in Mecca, Saudi Arabia. Such high density of crowding presents a risk for local outbreaks and for worldwide spread of infectious agents. ARI is the leading cause of admission to Saudi hospitals during the Hajj (Ahmed et al., 2006). The close contact among pilgrims during periods of intense congestion, their shared sleeping accommodations (mainly in tents) and the dense air pollution all combine to increase the risk of airborne respiratory disease transmission. A viral etiology of upper respiratory tract infection (URTI) is most commonly implicated at the Hajj, but bacterial super infection often follows. More than 200 viruses can cause URTI at the Hajj. The main etiologies are RSV, parainfluenza, influenza and adenovirus (Rashid et al, 2008).

Country	Seasonality of RSV (Start)	Seasonality of RSV (End)	Prevalence of RSV in Lower Respiratory Tract Infection	Study Size (patient number)	Age Group affected	Authors
Saudi Arabia (Riyadh)	November	February	83%	883	<5 years	Akhter et al., 2008
Saudi Arabia (Qassim Region)	December	February	45.4%	282	< 1 year	Meqdam M et al 2006
Saudi Arabia (Abha Region)	November	February	40%	115	< 2 years	Al Shehri et al 2005
Saudi Arabia (Riyadh)	November	February	28.5%	256	< 5 years	Al Hajjar et al 1993-1996
Kuwait	October	March	36.8 %	1,014	< 1 year	Khadada M. et al 2010
Lebanon	December	May	26.7%	120	< 6 years	Hamze A et al 2007-2008
Jordan	December	March	12.5%	200	< 2 years	Al Toum R et al 2006
Turkey	January	March	29.5%	332	< 2 years	Kanra et al 2005
UAE	November	february	28.6%	252	< 3 years	Uduman SA et al 1993 - 1995
Qatar	November	February	59.9%	257	< 1 year	Wahab et al 1996-1998
Egypt	December	February	16.4%	91	< 5 years	Fattouh et al 2011

Table 2. Seasonality of RSV Infections Observed in the Middle East

Number of Patients	Predisposing factors	Age Range	Location	Treatment	Author
94	Premature, pulmonary pathology, neurological and cardio-vascular abnormalities	<1 year	Riyadh	Oxygen supplementation, bronchodilators, antibiotics	Al Muhsen, 2010
8	Pre term, ARDS	28 weeks	Riyadh	Mechanical ventilation, support	Kilani, 2002
412	Bronchopneumonia. broncihiolitis	< 5 years	Riyadh		Bakir et al, 1998
69		< 1 year	Riyadh	Supportive, antibiotics	Jamjoom et al, 1993
51	Prematurity, chronic lung diseases, atopic dermatitis, pure formula feeding, passive smoking	< 2 years	Abha	Supportive, Oxygen	Al Shehri, 2005
128	bronchopneumonia bronchiolits Coughing tachpnea	< 1 year	Qassim	antibiotics	Meqdam, 2006

Table 3. Characterisitics of RSV Infections in hospitalized Patients in Saudi Arabia

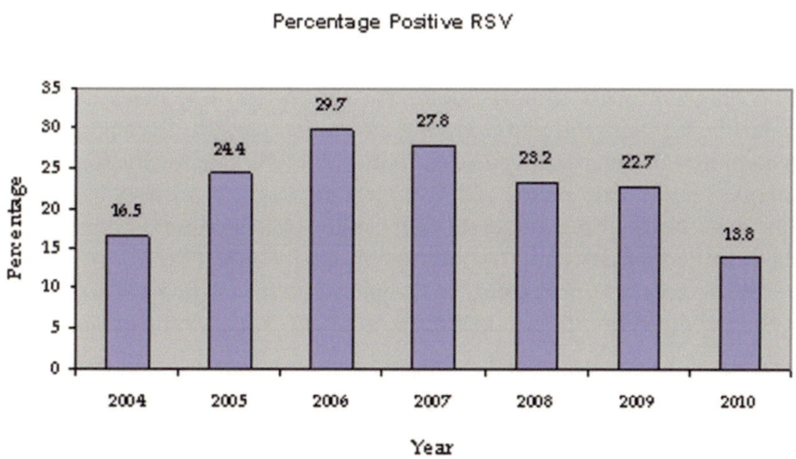

Fig. 1. Prevalence of RSV Infections between 2004 - 2010 at a tertiary Care Center in Saudi Arabia (Akhter, et al., 2008)

3. Laboratory diagnosis

Early diagnosis of RSV infection enables timely interventions to be introduced to control the spread of disease. Given the similarity in clinical presentation to influenza and human metapneumovirus, laboratory confirmation provides a definitive diagnosis of RSV infection. Clinical features of RSV infections overlap with other respiratory viruses so laboratory diagnosis is essential to establish diagnosis. Prior to the introduction of molecular diagnostics, respiratory viruses were primarily identified by virus isolation in tissue culture or antibody/antigen detection by serological methods: Specimens should be collected in the acute stage of the illness, kept moist, and refrigerated immediately.

3.1 Imaging studies

Chest radiography is frequently obtained in children with severe RSV infection. Chest radiography typically reveals hyperinflated lung fields with a diffuse increase in interstitial markings. In 20-25% of cases, focal areas of atelectasis and/or pulmonary infiltrate are also noted. Generally, these findings are neither specific to RSV infection nor predictive of the course or outcome, except for the observation that infants who have the additional findings of atelectasis and/or pneumonia may have a more severe course with their illness.

3.2 Clinical specimens

Nasopharyngeal aspirates (NPAs), swabs and washes are acceptable for culture, direct antigen detection and Nucleic acid testing (NAT) where this is available. Other acceptable specimens are endotracheal aspirates, bronchoalveolar lavage fluid and lung biopsy tissue. Swabs should be cotton, rayon or dacron-tipped, plastic-coated or aluminium shafted swabs. They should be placed into viral transport media and transported at 4°C or frozen at -70°C. Unacceptable specimens include Calcium alginate swabs or swabs in gel media, wooden swabs and dry swabs

3.3 Tissue culture methods

A cost-effective and relatively rapid approach to detecting RSV in humans is to use cell cultures in conjunction with immunofluorescence antibody (IFA) methods. Traditional cell cultures, while being sensitive, required long incubation periods. Recent advances have led to the development of enhanced cell lines that require shorter incubation periods but are also cocultivated (or contain mixed cell lines) to detect several viruses in the same culture vial (Lanley et al. 2007). The benefits of such cell line mixes in terms of providing a rapid and sensitive method for detecting respiratory viruses including RSV have been established, however, RSV detection is optimised by supplementing cell line cultures with the non-culture method of direct immunofluorescence Assay (DFA) (Leland and Ginocchia. 2007).

Viral culture is the gold standard by which other tests are compared. Specificity is not usually an issue; however, sensitivity in adults can be problematic. Adults generally shed lower titres and for a shorter period of time than children. Also, the virus is thermolabile and does not survive lengthy transit times. Culture is only 20 - 45% sensitive when compared with serology using acute and convalescent sera. The benefits of tissue culture are its broad sensitivity for a range of viruses, the necessity for infectious virus particles and its relatively low cost. Human heteroploid cells, such as HEP-2 and HeLa generally provide the best tissue culture for RSV isolation. RSV produces a characteristic CPE consisting of syncytia formation and appears in 4 to 5 days.

Mixed cell line cultures were used for the first time at a tertiary care center in Saudi Arabia to accelerate virus isolation (Akhter et al). Rapid testing algorithms allowed all respiratory syncytial virus (RSV) isolates to be detected in one day, influenza isolates to be detected in 2 days, parainfluenza isolates within 3 days, and adenovirus in 2-5 days. 92% of RSV infections occurred in children one year and under. RSV infections occurred between November and February, with a peak in January. Influenza and adenovirus outbreaks occurred in November and December. Parainfluenza occurred in 2 waves, first in November and December followed by another peak in April. RSV appears to occur in a two year cycle similar to Europe (Fig 1)

3.4 Shell vial assay

Laboratory diagnosis of RV infections has become easier and more rapid with the use of centrifugation-enhanced shell vials (SV) as the culture method. Centrifugation of the clinical specimen onto cell monolayers followed by immunofluorescence detection and identification of viral antigens in SV cultures allows a much earlier diagnosis of infection. In this technique a small bottle (vial) with a removable round glass cover slip is used to grow the cells as a monolayer on the cover slip. Nowadays mixed cell types can be put in a single monolayer providing a variety of cell types for the virus to infect in a single vial. Once these monolayers are ready to be inoculated, the growth medium is removed from the vial and the clinical sample placed directly on the monolayer. The vial is then centrifuged, the clinical sample is removed and fresh growth medium is then added to the vial. It is possible, using this technique, to identify the presence of a virus before CPE occurs by using fluorescent monoclonal antibodies to detect early and pre-early proteins. The disadvantage of this method is it is not possible to do "blind passages". Some viruses may require longer incubation to adapt to the particular cell lines. Once used, the monolayer can not be re-incubated or re-inoculated as the fixed cells and viruses are not viable (Gleaves et al., 1984).

3.5 Antigen detection

Several ELISA kits are available for the detection of RSV antigens on a solid phase. ELISA techniques offer the advantages of objective interpretation, speed, and the possibility of screening a large number of specimens. Disadvantages include a generally poorer sensitivity and a "grey zone" of equivocal results, which requires confirmation by a time-consuming blocking ELISA procedure (Casiano et al., 2003). Both direct and indirect IF utilizing either polyclonal or monoclonal antibodies are available which possess a high degree of sensitivity and specificity. The general sensitivity of IF is 80 - 90% and for monoclonal antibody 95 - 100% (Aldous et al., 2004). IF techniques are fast and easy to perform but the interpretation of results is subjective and the specimen must contain adequate nasopharyngeal cells. Detection of RSV antigens in respiratory secretions by IFA or EIA is widely used in children and removes the need to recover infectious virus but requires a significant viral load to generate a positive result. Hence, these methods are not suitable for adults as studies have shown positive rates of only 23% by IFA and 10% by EIA.

3.6 Serology

Serologic diagnosis requires paired serum specimens in most instances and is intrinsically slower than direct methods. A variety of serologic techniques are used to measure antibodies, including neutralization, hemagglutination inhibition, complement fixation, and enzyme-linked immunosorbent assay (ELISA). Measurement of complement-fixation antibodies is generally less sensitive than the other methods and does not provide a serotype-specific diagnosis. Immunocompromised hosts often fail to develop diagnostic increases in antibody titers. RSV infections reoccur throughout life diagnosis can be demonstrated by a greater ≥ 4 fold increase in RSV specific IgG. When baseline sera are available, this method is ≥ 90% sensitive for diagnosis of RSV infection in the elderly. However utility of serology is limited to its retrospective nature (Falsey et al., 2003).

3.7 Molecular methods

The principal amplification technique used for RNA viruses is reverse-transcriptase polymerase-chain reaction (RT-PCR). Detection of RNA viruses requires an additional first step in which RNA is reverse transcribed to complementary DNA before PCR amplification. Theoretically, this technique is capable of detecting a single virus within 24 hours. Detection of the amplified sequence may be done at the reaction endpoint, or by continuous monitoring (real-time PCR). Real-time PCR has the advantage of allowing the virus to be quantified (Whiley et al., 2002).

Multiplex PCR methods have been developed that allow the detection of more than one nucleic acid sequence, and therefore more than one virus type, in the same assay. These are based on the principle that products of real time cyclers can be detected simultaneously at different wavelengths of fluoresence. Other nucleic acid amplification methods have also been developed, notably nucleic acid sequence base amplification (NASBA). This technique is also known as isothermal amplification, as it does not require the repeated temperature cycling used in conventional PCR methods (Beck & Henrickson, 2010).

The advantages of PCR and related methods are considerable. The main benefit is time saving allowing hours to a result rather than several days as for a cell culture assay. PCR also requires less operator skill and training to carry out and can be automated to process large numbers of samples. It is also extremely sensitive, although it can be vulnerable to contamination and cannot distinguish infective viruses. Most PCR methods require some costly equipment and are not suitable for use outside the laboratory. Non-quantitative PCR results may also be difficult to interpret, since low numbers of virus that do not signify an infection may be detected, but this problem is largely overcome by real-time PCR. Molecuar methods can also detect several orders of magnitude less than tissue culture methods (Borg et al., 2003).

3.8 Microarrays

DNA microarrays used as 'genomic sensors' have great potential in clinical diagnostics. Microarray analysis has the capability to offer multiplex detection, Multiple microarray platforms exist, including printed double-stranded DNA and oligonucleotide arrays, in situ-synthesized arrays, high-density bead arrays, electronic microarrays, and suspension bead arrays (Wong et al., 2007). In general terms, probes are synthesized and immobilized as discrete features, or spots. Each feature contains millions of identical probes. The target is fluorescently labeled and then hybridized to the probe microarray. A successful hybridization event between the labeled target and the immobilized probe will result in an increase of fluorescence intensity over a background level, which can be measured using a fluorescent scanner. Biases inherent in random PCR-amplification, cross-hybridization effects, and inadequate microarray analysis, however, limit detection sensitivity and specificity (Miller & Tang, 2009).

3.9 Emerging technologies

There are several emerging molecular assays that have potential applications in the diagnosis and monitoring of respiratory viral infections (Takahashi et al., 2008). These techniques include direct nucleic acid detection by quantum dots, loop-mediated isothermal amplification; multiplex ligation-dependent probe amplification, amplification using arbitrary primers, target-enriched multiplexing amplification, pyrosequencing, padlock probes, solid and suspension microarrays, and mass spectrometry (Wu & Tang, 2009). Several of these systems already are commercially available to provide multiplex amplification and high-throughput detection and identification of a panel of respiratory viral pathogens. Further validation and implementation of such emerging molecular assays in routine clinical virology services will enhance the rapid diagnosis of respiratory viral infections and improve patient care.

Method of Detection	Advantage	Disadvantage
Virus Culture	Characteristic syncytial CPE allows identification Broad sensitivity	Time-consuming Need confirmatory identification method Requires expertise to maintain cell lines
Antigen Detection (IFA and EIA)	Commercial kits widely available Rapid ID Suitable for screening large numbers	Can give false results Does not allow for genotyping
PCR	Rapid addition of new viruses Detection of unidentified respiratory viruses Suitable for early detection and monitoring of viruses	Highly sensitive but sometimes false products Containment of amplicons to prevent contamination
Real Time PCR	Rapid product confirmation High Sensitivity and Specificity Automated	Limited number of virus detection in one-tube False signal High cost
Microarrays	Rapid Can screen multiple pathogens	Low sensitivity False signal

Table 4. Methods Used For Laboratory Diagnosis of RSV

4. Conclusion

Lower respiratory tract infections caused by RSV occur epidemically, and the appearance of epidemics seems to vary with latitude, altitude and climate. Onset weeks and durations of RSV seasons also vary substantially by year and location. Local RSV data are needed to accurately define the onset and offset of RSV seasons and to refine timing of passive immune prophylaxis therapy recommendations. Further studies on RSV particularly in developing countries should address these questions in more detail. RSV is an important pathogen of young children in tropical and developing countries and a frequent cause of hospital admission. Prevention of RSV disease relies on rapid diagnosis, infection control and hygiene measures, as well as providing immunoprophylaxis in select infants. The prophylaxis, however, is costly, and so targeting the recipient population and timing of administration is important for optimal effectiveness and judicious use of limited health care resources

The relative proportions of different genotypes vary from year to year with steady replacement of the dominant genotype each year, suggesting that herd immunity may play a role in the abundance of a particular genotype in a particular epidemic. A small study in Hungary (Pankovics et al., 2009) using molecular detection and genetic analysis showed that based upon the F region 96% viruses genetically belonged to type A and 4% were classified as type B human RSV. Based upon the G region, out of the type A viruses 72.7% belonged to group GA5 and 27.3% to group GA2. Viral nucleotide sequence was identical in several cases. A Japanese study (Shobugawa et al., 2009) investigated a total of 488 human RSV samples from 1,103 screened cases in a pediatric clinic in Niigata. According to the phylogenetic analysis, among the PCR-positive samples, 338 HRSV-A strains clustered into the previously reported genotypes GA5 and GA7 and two novel genotypes, NA1 and NA2, which were genetically close to GA2 strains. Another study In India (Agrawal et al., 2009) showed that 95% were group B strains and 5% group A. Similarly, an outbreak in Turkey indicated that subgroup B was highly dominant (Guney et al., 2004). In Thailand, equal infectivity and severity of both RSV subgroups has been shown (Boonyasuppayakom et al., 2007). Such knowledge has yet to be ascertained for the Middle Eastern countries. There is a dustinct need to carry out molecular typing of RSV in Saudi Arabia and other surrounding countries to further elucidate the pattern of infections, the prevalent strains circulating in the region and possible approaches for treatment. The importance of RSV infections has resulted in surveillance monitoring being conducted in Europe and other developed countries. Such coordinated strategies are important to consider in developing countries where the impact of RSV infections is greater.

5. References

Ahmed QA, Arabi YM, Memish ZA Health risks at the Hajj. Lancet 2006;367:1008–15.

Agrawal AS, Sarkar M, Ghosh S, Chawla-Sarkar M, Chakraborty N, Basak M, Naik TN. (2009). Prevalence of respiratory syncytial virus group B genotype BA-IV strains among children with acute respiratory tract infection in Kolkata, Eastern India. J Clin Virol. 45(4):358-61. Epub 2009 Jun 30.

Akhter J, Al Johani S, Dugaishm F, Al Hefdhi R (2008). Etiology of Respiratory Viral Infections using Rapid Virus Isolation Methods at a Tertiary Care Center in Riyadh, Saudi Arabia. Saudi Pharm J 17(2):177-80

Aldous , WK., Gerber K., Taggart, EW., Thomas, J., Tidwell, D., Daly, JA. (2004). A comparison of fluorescent assay testing for respiratory syncytial virus. Diagn Microbiol Infect Dis 49: 265-8.

Al Hajjar, S., Akhter, J., Al Jumaah, S., Hussain Qadri, SM. (1998). Respiratory viruses in children attending a major referral centre in Saudi Arabia. Ann Trop Paediatr 18(2):87-92.

Al-Muhsen, AZ. (2010). Clinical profile of Respiratory Syncytial Virus (RSV) bronchiolitis in the intensive care unit at a Tertiary Care Hospital. Curr Pediatr Res 14 (2): 75-80

Al Shehri, MA., Sadeq, A. and Quli, K (2005). Bronchiolitis in Abha, Southwest Saudi Arabia:viral etiology and predictors for hospital admission. West Afr J Med 24(4):299-304.

Al Toum, R., Bdour, S., and Ayyash, H. (2006). Epidemiology and clinical characteristics of respiratory syncytial virus infections in Jordan. J Trop Pediatr 52(4):282-7.

Bakir TM, Halawani M, Ramia S. (1998). Viral Aetiology and Epidemiology of Acute Respiratory Infections in Hospitalized Saudi Children J Trop Pediatr 44(2): 100-103 doi:10.1093/tropej/44.2.100

Beck, ET., and Henrickson KJ (2010). Molecular Diagnosis of Respiratory Viruses. Future Microbiology 5(6):901-16.

Belderbos ME, Houben ML, Wilbrink B, Lentjes E, Bloemen EM, Kimpen JL, Rovers

M,Bont, L. (2011). Cord blood vitamin d deficiency is associated with respiratory syncytial virus bronchiolitis. Pediatrics. ;127(6):1513-20.

Boonyasuppayakom, S., Kowitdamrong, E., and Bhattarakosol P. (2007). Molecular and demographic analysis of respiratory syncytial virus infection in patients admitted to King Chulalongkorn Memorial Hospital, Thailand, 2007. Influenza Other Respi Viruses 4(5):313-23.

Borg, I., Rohde, G., Löseke, S., Bittscheidt, J., Schultze-Werninghaus, G., Stephan, V. and Bufe A. (2003). Evaluation of a quantitative real-time PCR for the detection of respiratory syncytial virus in pulmonary diseases. Eurpean Respiratory J 21 (6):944-951

Casiano-Colon, AE., Hulbert, BB., Mayer, TK. (2003). Lack of sensitivity of rapid antigen tests for the diagnosis of respiratory syncytial virus infection in adults. J Clin Virol 28:169-74.

Centers for Disease Control (2010). Respiratory syncytial virus activity-United States, July 2008-December 2009. MMWR 59(08):230-233.

Dawson-Caswell, M and Muncie, HL.Jr., (2011). Respiratory syncytial virus in children. Am Fam Physician 83(2):141-6.

Falsey, AR., Formica, MA., Walsh, EE. (2003). Diagnosis of respiratory syncytial virus: comparison of reverse transcription PCR to viral culture and serology in adults with respiratory illness. J Clin Microbiol 40:817-20.

Ghildyal, R., Baulch-Brown, C., Mills, J. and Meanger, J. (2003). The matrix protein of Human respiratory syncytial virus localises to the nucleus of infected cells and inhibits transcription. Archives of Virology 148:1419-29

Gleaves, CA., Smith, TF., Shuster, EA., and Pearson, GR.(1984). Rapid detection of cytomegalovirus in MRC-5 cells inoculated with urine specimens by using low-speed centrifugation and monoclonal antibody to an early antigen. J. Clin. Microbiol 19:917-919.

Guney, C., kubar, A., Yapar, M., Besirbellioglu, AB., and Doganci, L. (2004). An outbreak of respiratory infection due to respiratory syncytial virus subgroup B in Ankara, Turkey. Jpn J Infect Dis 57(4):178-80.

Hall, CB.. (2001). Respiratory syncytial virus and parainfluenza virus. N Engl J Med 334:1917-28.

Hamze, M., Hais, S., Rachkidi, J., Lichaa, Z., and Zahab N. (2010). Infections with respiratory syncytial virus in North Lebanon-prevalence during winter 2008. East Mediter Health J 16(5):539-45.

Henrickson JK. (2004). Advances in the laboratory diagnosis of viral respiratory disease. Pediatr Infect Dis J 23(1s).

Hijazi , Z., Pacsa, A., El-Gharbawy, F., Chugh, TD., Essa, S., El Shazli, A., and Abd El-Salam, R. (1997). Acute lower respiratory tract infections in children in Kuwait. Ann Trop Paediatr 17(2):127-34.

Jafri, H. (2003). Treatment of respiratory syncytial virus:antiviral therapies. Pediatr Infect Dis J 22:s89-95

Jamjoom GA., Al-Semran AM., Board, A., Al-Frayh AR., Artz, F., and Al-Mobaireek, KF. (1993). Respiratory syncytial virus infection in young children hospitalized with respiratory illness in Riyadh.

Kanra G, Tezcan S, Yilmaz G; Turkish National Respiratory Syncytial Virus (RSV) Team. 2005. Respiratory syncytial virus epidemiology in Turkey. Turk J Pediatr. 47(4):303-8.

Khadadah, M., Essa, S., Higazi, Z., Behbehani, N and Al-Nakib, W. (2010). Respiratory syncytial virus and human rhinoviruses are the major causes of severe lower respiratory tractinfections in Kuwait. J Med Virol 82(8):1462-7.

Kilani, RA (2002). Respiratory syncytial virus (RSV) outbreak in the NICU: description of eight cases. J Trop Pediatr 48(2):118-22.

Khuri-Bulos, N., Williams JV., Shehabi AA., Faori, S., Al jundi, E., Abushariah, O., Chen, Q., Ali, SAA., Vermund S., and Halasa NB. (2010). Burden of respiratory syncytial virus in hospitalized infants and young children in Amman, Jordan. Scand J Infect Dis 42(5):368-74.

Lapena, S., Robles, MB., Castenon, L., Martinez, JP., Reguero, S., Alonslo, MP., Fernandez, I., (2005). Climactic factors and lower respiratory tract infection due to respiratory syncytial virus in hospitalised infants in Northern Spain. European J Epidemiology 20:271-276

Leland D S and Ginocchio CC. (2007). Role of Cell Culture for Virus Detection in the Age of Technology. Clinical Microbiology Reviews, Vol. 20.(1) :49-78,

Lieberthal, AS., Bauchner, H., Hall, CB., Johnson, DW., Kotagal, U., Light, MJ., Mason, W., Meissner, HC., Phelan, KJ., Zorc, JJ. (2006). Diagnosis and management of bronchiolitis. Pediatrics 118(4): 1775-93.

Meqdam, MM. and Subaih, SH. (2006). Rapid detection and clinical features of infants and young children with acute lower respiratory tract infection due to respiratory syncytial virus. FEMS Immunol Med Microbiol47(1):129-33.

Milinaric-Galinovic, G., Welliver, RC., Vilibic-Cavlek, T., Ljubin-Starnak, S., Drazenovic, V., Galinovic, I., and Tomic, V. (2008). The biennial cycle of respiratory syncytial virus outbreaks in Croatia. Virology J 5:18

Miller MB.and Tang YW. (2009). Basic Concepts of Microarrays and Potential Applications in Clinical Microbiology. Clinical Microbiology Reviews 22. (4) :611-633,

Mullins, JA., Lamonte, AC., Bresee, JS., Anderson LJ. (2003). Substantial variability in community RSV season timing. Paediatr Infect Dis 22:857-62.

Nair, H., Nokes, DJ., Gessner, BD., et al. (2010). Global burden of acute lower respiratory infections due to respiratory syncytial virus in young children: a systematic review and meta-analysis. Lancet 375:1545–1555).

Nair, H., Verma, VR., Theodoratou, E., Zgaga, L., Huda, T., Simoes, EA., Wright, PF., Rudan, I., Campbell, H. (2011). An evaluation of the emerging interventions against respiratory syncytial virus (RSV)-associated acute lower respiratory virus infections in children. BMC Public Health 13(11):suppl3 s30.

Nicholson KG, Kent J, Hammersley V, Cancio E. 1997. Acute viral infections of upper respiratory tract in elderly people living in the community: comparative, prospective, population based study of disease burden. BMJ. 25;315(7115):1060-4.

Pankovics P, Szabó H, Székely G, Gyurkovits K, Reuter G. 2009. Detection and molecular epidemiology of respiratory syncytial virus type A and B strains in childhood respiratory infections in Hungary. Orv Hetil. Jan 18;150(3):121-7

Ramirez, JA (2008). RSV infection in the adult population. Man Care 17(11):13-5

Rechsteiner, J and Winkler, KC. (1969). Inactivation of Respiratory Syncytial Virus in Aerosol. J Gen Virol 5:405-410

Robertson, SE., Roca, A., Sinoes, EAF., Kartasasmita, CB., Olaleye, DO., Odaibo, GN., Collinson, M., Venter, M., and Wright PF. (2004). Respiratory syncytial virus infection: denominator-based studies in Indonesia, Mozambique, Nigeria and South Africa. Bulletin of the World Health Organization 82(12):914-22.

Sato, M., Saito, R., Sakai, T., Sano, Y., Nishikawa, M., Sasaki, A., Shobugawa, Y., Gejyo, F., Suzuki, H. (2005). Molecular epidemiology of respiratory syncytial virus infections among children with acute respiratory symptoms in a community over three seasons. J Clin Microbiol. 43(1):36-40

Shay, DK., Holman, RC., Newman, RD., Liu, LL., Stout, JW., Anderson LJ. (1999). Bronchial associated hospitalizations among U.S. children, 1980-1996. JAMA 282:1440-6.

Shobugawa Y, Saito R, Sano Y, Zaraket H, Suzuki Y, Kumaki A, Dapat I, Oguma T, Yamaguchi M, Suzuki H. 2009 . Emerging genotypes of human respiratory syncytial virus subgroup A among patients in Japan. J Clin Microbiol. Aug;47(8):2475-82. Epub 2009 Jun 24.

Simões, EAF., Mutyara K., Soh, S., Agustian, D., Hibberd, ML. ,Kartasasmita, C. 2011 The Epidemiology of Respiratory Syncytial Virus Lower Respiratory Tract Infections in Children Less than 5 Years of Age in Indonesia. Pediatric Infectious Disease Journal: Apr:

Stensballe, LF. (2002). An epidemiological study of respiratory syncytial virus associated hospitalizations in Denmark. Respiratory Research 3(1):s34-s39.

Stewart DL, Romero JR, Buysman EK, Fernandes AW, Mahadevia PJ.(2009). Total healthcare costs in the US for preterm infants with respiratory syncytial virus lower respiratory infection in the first year of life requiring medical attention. Curr Med Res Opin. 25(11):2795-804.

Takahashi, H., Norman S A., Mather E L., and Patterson B K. (2008). Evaluation of the NanoChip 400 System for Detection of Influenza A and B, Respiratory Syncytial, and Parainfluenza Viruses. Journal of Clinical Microbiology 46.(5): 1724-1727

Uduman, SA., Ijaz, MK., Kochiyil, J., Mathew, T and Hossam MK. (1996). Respiratory syncytial virus infection among hospitalized young children with acute lower respiratory illnesses in Al Ain, UAE. J Commun Dis 28(4):246-52.

Wahab, AA., Dawood ST., and Raman HM. (2001). Clinical characteristics of resiratory syncytial virus infection in hospitalised healthy infants and young children in Qatar. J Trop Pediatr 47(6):363-46.

Waness, A, El-Sameed, Y, Mahboub, B, Noshi, M, Al-Jahdali, H, Vats, M, Mehta, Ac (2011). Respiratory Disorders In The Middle East: A Review. Respirology 16(5), Pages 755–766,

Weber, MW., Mulholland, BK., and Greenwood BM. (1998). Respiratory syncytial virus infection in tropical and developing countries. Tropical and international Health 3:268-80.

Weir E., Fisman, DN. (2004). Canadian Medical Assoc J 170(2):141

Whiley, Dm., Syrmis, MW., Mackay, MM., and Sloots, TP. (2002). Detection of human respiratory syncytial virus by lightcycler reverse transcriptase PCR. J Clin Microbiol 40(12):4418-22.

Welliver, R. (2009). The relationship of meteorological conditions to the epidemic activity of respiratory syncytial virus. Paediatric Respiratory Reviews 10 Suppl 1 (2009) 6-8

Wong, CW., Wah Heng, C L, Yee, LW., Soh, SWL., Kartasasmita, CB., Simoes, EAF., Hibberd, ML., Sung W K. and Miller, LD. (2007). Optimization and clinical validation of a pathogen detection Microarray. Genome Biology, 8:R93

Wu, W., Tang, YW a(2009). Emerging molecular assays for detection and characterization of respiratory viruses. Clini Lab Med. 29(4):673-93

Part 3

Treatment and Prophylaxis of Human RSV Disease

9

Anti-Respiratory Syncytial Virus Agents from Phytomedicine

Damian Chukwu Odimegwu[1,2], Thomas Grunwald[1]
and Charles Okechukwu Esimone[3]
[1]*Department of Molecular and Medical Virology, Ruhr University Bochum*
[2]*Division of Pharmaceutical Microbiology, Department of Pharmaceutics*
University of Nigeria Nsukka
[3]*Faculty of Pharmaceutical Sciences, Nnamdi Azikiwe University, Awka*
[1]*Germany*
[2,3]*Nigeria*

1. Introduction

Although the global importance of RSV as a respiratory pathogen has been recognized for over 40 years, suitable prophylactic and therapeutic interventions have not been truly available. Vaccine development, unfortunately, has been fraught with spectacular failure and with difficult obstacles, and there are only limited therapeutic options for treatment of this disease. Currently, the only approved prophylactic options available involve the use of Palivizumab and its derivative Motivizumab (currently under trial) which are both monoclonal antibodies directed against RSV surface fusion protein. Ribavirin, a broad-spectrum anti-viral agent, is the only therapeutic option employed as adjunctive therapy for the sickest patients; however, its efficacy has been called into question by multiple studies, and most institutions no longer use it. Moreover, the use of both agents has been shown to be costly and difficult to handle. Therefore, the search for novel anti viral inhibitors of RSV has become more intensive. It could be recalled that potent anti-viral agents have previously been harnessed from medicinal plants. Since medicinal plants have consistently served as suitable lead sources for potent anti-viral agents, efforts have also been made by several investigators in developing anti-RSV compounds from phytomedicine. In this present research paper, we present a review of the past to present activities involving the discovery and development of novel and effective anti-RSV compounds from phytomedicine. First, we begin by briefly describing the problem of the global disease burden of RSV as well as efforts and approaches so far adopted to contain the viral menace. In the next section we introduce the subject of phytomedicine and anti-RSV therapeutic products originating from various reported medicinal plants. Straightforward and discreet description is made of investigations carried out by our workgroup in our attempt to develop anti-RSV compounds from medicinal plants especially *Ramalina farinaceae* and *Aglaia ignea*. Here also in this section, we present and discuss published results from other investigators regarding compounds from other medicinal plant sources. The importance of the process and techniques leading to their identification and isolation is highlighted. Attention is drawn to some common markers that characterize their discovery. We devote tables to give comprehensive listings and profile of these agents and also discuss other relevant results. Attempt is made to shed adequate light on the therapeutic efficacy to safety profile of promising compounds since the overall relevance of the compounds and their derivatives should depend largely on their efficacy-safety characteristics. Additionally, space is devoted to discuss the proffered or validated mechanistic bases of the observed the anti-viral and disease inhibitory activities of the phytoconstituents and compounds. The importance of structural modifications is equally reflected where applicable to grant a quick and early preview on the more likely positive alteration direction that could possibly select for enhancement of efficacy and cellular compatibility. Lastly, we discuss in the next section the promises and the crucial position occupied by anti-RSV compounds and phyto-constituents harnessed form phytomedicines in the treatment and control of RSV infection and disease. In conclusion, we comment on the future of RSV infection and disease control; the role that should expectedly be occupied by chemotherapy, especially phytomedicines-derived. In answering the questions of discovering and developing the tomorrow's effective anti-RSV compounds, we make some concluding remarks on some key performance indicators that should characterize the phytocompounds of desirable anti-RSV activity.

1.1 Respiratory syncytial virus

Respiratory syncytial virus (RSV) which belongs to the *Pneumovirus* genus of the Paramyxoviridae family is the most important cause of viral lower respiratory tract illness (LRI) in infants and children worldwide (Collins *et al.* 1996; Hall, 1994). Amongst children in the US, up to 125,000 RSV-associated hospitalizations and 500 RSV-associated deaths respectively could occur each year (Langley and Anderson, 2011). RSV was, on average, responsible for 17% of acute respiratory infections in children admitted to hospital in the developing countries (Martins *et al. 1998*), and studies from Africa have equally reported the influence of malnutrition on the prevalence of RSV (Adegbola *et al.* 1994; Nwankwo *et al.* 1994). In Nigeria it is reported that RSV infections occur all year round with a peak during the rainy season (Nwankwo *et al.* 1994). Infants who are premature (Berkovich, 1964; Cunningham *et al.* 1991) or have chronic lung disease (Groothuis *et al.* 1988) or congenital heart disease (MacDonald *et al.* 1982) are at particular risk for severe RSV disease. Although traditionally regarded as a pediatric pathogen, RSV can also cause life-threatening pulmonary disease in bone marrow transplant recipients (Fouillard *et al.* 1992) and the elderly (Dowell *et al.* 1996; Falsey *et al.* 1992, 1995, 2005; Falsey and Walsh, 1998). Although the global prevalence of RSV infection especially among infants and young children is on the increase, vaccine development, unfortunately, has been fraught with spectacular failure and with difficult obstacles, and there are only limited therapeutic options for treatment of this disease (Collins *et al.*, 1996; Wright *et al.*, 2000; Kohlmann et al., 2009; Tregoning and Schwarze *et al.*, 2010). Therefore, the search for novel anti-viral inhibitors of RSV has become more intensive.

1.2 Phytomedicine and anti-viral agents

Natural products from plants traditionally have provided the pharmaceutical industry with one of its most important sources of lead compounds and up to 40% of modern drugs are derived from natural sources, using either the natural substance or a synthesized version. Currently, over a 100 new products are in clinical development, particularly as anti-cancer agents and anti-infectives (Gautam *et al.*, 2007; Harvey, 2008; Jassim and Naji, 2003). This has influenced many of pharmaceutical companies to produce new antimicrobial formulations extracted from plants or herbs. The bioactive molecules occur in plants as secondary metabolites and as defense mechanisms against predation, herbivores, fungal attack, microbial invasion and viral infection. During the past decade, potent agents have become available against viral infections. Therefore, extracts of plants and phytochemicals are getting more important as potential sources for viral inhibitors during the recent decade. Extensive studies have shown that medicinal plants of several parts of the world contain compounds active against viruses that cause human diseases (Kott *et al.*, 1999; Semple *et al.*, 1998; Sindambiwe *et al.*, 1999). Correspondingly, several potent agents against the respiratory virus- RSV have been reported. The aim of this review is to give a comprehensive outlook on the available and emerging promising phyto-constituents effective against RSV and an overview of the reported associated researches done so far. This review encompassed introduction, methodology, outcomes, and overall promises of the discovered putative anti-RSV agents. Furthermore, useful guiding components for future discovery and analysis of promising anti-RSV candidates are equally highlighted.

2. Plant species possessing anti-respiratory syncytial virus anti-viral activities

2.1 Aglaia species

Aglaia represents the largest genus within the family Meliaceae and contains more than 100 species (Bohnenstengel *et al.* 1999; Pannell 1992). It is a woody small or medium- sized tree found mostly in Southeast Asia. Extracts or pure compounds from the various species have been shown to display diverse biological activities ranging from anti-proliferation, anti-inflammatory, fungicidal, bactericidal, anthelminthic and anti-viral activity (Bohnenstengel *et al.* 1999; Lipipun *et al.* 2003; Perry 1980; Poehland *et al.* 1987). Although *Aglaia species* are traditionally used in Southeast Asia and Indo-China for the treatment of various diseases, including ailments related to lower respiratory tract infection and inflammation (Lipipun *et al.* 2003; Perry 1980), anti-viral screening with Aglaia species has essentially been limited to Herpes Simplex Virus types 1 and 2 (Lipipun *et al.* 2003; Poehland *et al.* 1987). Given that RSV infection has a strong bearing with inflammation of the lower respiratory tract, we decided to explore various compounds from these species for possible anti-RSV activities *in vitro*.

Our investigation (Esimone *et al.*, 2008) involving the isolation and screening of eighteen (18) compounds from various species of Aglaia (*A. ignea, A. duppereana, A. cucculata, A. euphoroides and A. tsangii*) showed only ignT1 (dammarenolic acid), dupT1 (aglaiol) and cucT1 (niloticin) exhibited selective anti-RSV activity. Time-of-addition studies revealed that both ignT1 and dupT1 inhibit RSV replication at a post-entry stage, with ignT1 being significantly more potent than dupT1. This post-entry inhibition of viral replication could suggest that the inhibitors possibly target the viral replicative enzyme, the RNA polymerase. The compound IgnT1 demonstrated favorable cellular safety when compared to reference plant derived diterpenoid compound (aphidicolin), which was at the concentration used about twice as cytotoxic as ignT1 while demonstrating virtually no anti-RSV activity. Besides, ribavarin which is the only currently approved anti-RSV therapeutic agent exhibits much more toxicity resulting from its effect on cellular RNA and DNA polymerases (Lafeuillade *et al.* 2001; Prince 2001; Seetharama and Narayana 2005). Moreover, we also observed that methylation of ignT1 resulted in a complete loss of anti-RSV as well as cytotoxicity. This remarkable loss of activity could be related to an interaction of the polar carboxylic group of dammarenolic acid with a potential target molecule of the virus. In the case of the methylated derivative this group is chemically masked and hence the interaction is nullified. However, this hypothesis needs to be further confirmed. Thus anti-RSV compounds from *Aglaia species* present useful sources of lead compounds against RSV.

Code	Name	Isolated from	[a]IC_{50} [μg/ml]	[b]TC_{50} [μg/ml]	[c]S.I.
[ignT1]	Dammarenolic acid	*A. ignea* – bark	0.1	2.9	29
[ignT1A]	Methyldammarenolate	*A. ignea* – bark	>40	>40	[d]ND
[ignT2]	(20*S*,24*S*)-20,24-Dihydroxy-3,4-secodammara-4(28),25-diene-3-carboxylic acid	*A. ignea* – bark	>40	10.4	[d]ND
[ignT4]	(20*S*,23*E*)-20,25-Dihydroxy,3,4-secodammara-4(28),23-diene-carboxylic acid	*A. ignea* – bark	>40	70.4	[d]ND
[ignT3]	(23*E*)-(20*S*)-20-hydroxy-25-methoxy-3,4-secodammara-4(28),23-diene-3-carboxylic acid	*A. ignea* – bark	>40	68.4	[d]ND
[ignT5]	Methylester of 20*S*,24-epoxy-25,26,27-trisnor-24-oxo-3,4-seco-4(28)-dammaren-3-carboxylic acid	*A. ignea* – bark	>40	14	[d]ND
[dupT4AB]	Mixture of epimers eichlerianic acid (24(*S*) [8a]) and shoreic acid (24(*R*) [8b])	*A. duppereana* – roots	39.6	12.3	0.3
[dupT5AB]	Mixture of epimers cabraleone (24(*S*)) and ocotillone (24(*R*))	*A. cucculata*- twigs	7.2	7.9	1.1
[dupT1]	Aglaiol	*A. duppereana* – leaves	11.8	168.8	14.3
[dupT2]	24,25-Epoxy-dammar-20-ene-3-one	*A. duppereana* – leaves	21.7	>40	[d]ND
[dupT3]	24,25-Dihydroxy-5α-dammar-20-ene-3-one	*A. duppereana* – leaves	25.5	52.1	2.0
[eupT1]	31-Nor-cycloartenol (29-nor-cycloartenol)	*Aglaia euphoroides* – leaves	>40	>40	[d]ND
[tsaT4]	4α,14-Dimethyl-9,19-cyclocholestan-3β,24α,25-triol	*Aglaia tsangii* – leaves	18.4	19.6	1.1
[tsaT3]	24,25-epoxy-cycloartan-3-ol	*Aglaia tsangii* – leaves	30.1	63.2	2.1
[cucT1]	Niloticin	*A. cucculata* – twigs	15.8	66.8	4.2
[cucT2]	Piscidinol A	*A. cucculata* – twigs	12.8	17.7	1.4
[tsaT1]	Lupeol	*Aglaia tsangii* – leaves	21.2	25.7	1.2
[tsaT2]	Lupeone	*Aglaia tsangii* – leaves	18	14.8	0.8

[a] Concentration of compound (μg/ml) that inhibits RSV infectivity by 50%
[b] Concentration of compound (μg/ml) that inhibits viability of target cells (HEp2) by 50%
[c] Selectivity index (SI) = TC_{50}/IC_{50}
[d] Not determined (ND), because observed activity was not dose-dependent
Experiments were performed at least thrice
Reproduced from Esimone *et al.*, 2008

Table 1. Summary of anti-RSV screening of purified compounds from *Aglaia spp*

2.2 *Ramalina farinaceae*

Some lichens and lichen-derived substances have been shown to possess anti-viral activities (Cohen *et al.*, 1996; Pengsuparp *et al.*, 1995; Neamati *et al.*, 1997). *Ramalina farinacea*, a lichen found to Nigeria but also available in other isolated places, has earlier been shown to possess broad anti-retro-viral (including lentiviruses) and anti-adenoviral principles (Esimone *et al.*, 2005). Depsides and depsidones have been previously identified as antimicrobial active phytochemicals from *R. farinaceae* (Esimone and Adikwu, 1999; 2002; Esimone *et al.*, 1999; 2006). In another related screening studies for active constituents against the respiratory syncytial virus, the ethylacetate fraction (*ET4*) of the plant was effective against RSV (IC_{50}= 3.65μg/ml). Mechanistic studies suggested that *ET4* targets an entry rather than a post-entry step by inhibiting the RSV fusion protein (Esimone *et al.*, 2009). Further screening exercises and isolation studies are ongoing.

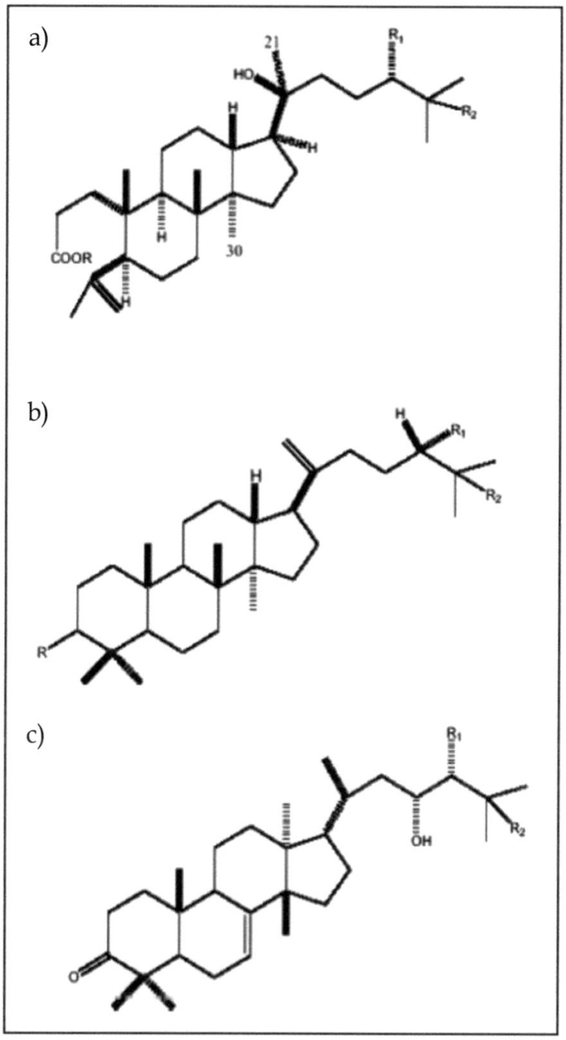

a) ignTl (Dammarenolic acid, isolated from the bark of *Aglaia ignea*)
b) dupTl (Aglaiol, isolated from the twigs of *Agliaia duppereana*)
c) cucTl (Niloticin, isolated from the twigs of *Aglaia cucculata*)
Reproduced from Esimone *et al.*, 2008

Fig. 1. Structual formulae of anti-RSV compounds isolated from *Aglaia* spp.

2.3 Anemarrhena asphodeloides

The rhizomes of *Anemarrhena asphodeloides* Bunge (Liliaceae) have been used as a traditional medicine for anti-diabetic, anti-phlogistic, anti-pyretic, asthma, cough, bronchitis, allergy, sedative, diuretic, and anodyne properties in Korea, China, and Japan (Duke *et al.*, 2002). Phytochemicals present in this species include xanthones (Pardo-Andreu *et al.*, 2006), norlignans (Iida *et al.*, 2000; Park *et al.*, 2003; Lim *et al.*, 2009), and steroidal saponins (Nakashima *et al.*, 1993; Sy *et al.*, 2008; Ren *et al.*, 2006; Wang *et al.*, 2010), associated with biological activities such as anti-diabetic (Nakashima *et al.*, 1993), anti-cancer (Sy *et al.*, 2008), anti-oxidant (Pardo-Andreu *et al.*, 2006), anti-fungal (Iida *et al.*, 2000; Park *et al.*, 2003), anti-depressant (Ren *et al.*, 2006), anti-inflammatory (Lim *et al.*, 2009) activity, and neuroprotective effects (Wang *et al.*, 2010). Nyasol and its derivatives isolated from the ethyl acetate fraction of *A. asphodeloides* rhizomes had potent RSV inhibitory potential (IC_{50}= 0.39 to 0.89 µM) (Bae *et al.*, 2007). Thus, these three known phenolic compounds, (-)-(R)-nyasol (= 4,4′-(1Z,3R)-Penta-1,4-diene-1,3 diyldiphenol; 1), its derivative (-)-(R)-4′-O-methylnyasol (2), and broussonin A (3) isolated from the rhizomes of *Anemarrhena asphodeloides* were for the first time identified as the active principles capable of efficient respiratory syncytial virus (RSV) inhibition. Later on, Youn and coworkers (Youn *et al.*, 2011) working with this plant to find novel inhibitors of plant origin against the RSV-A2 strain propagated in HEp-2 cells, the butanol extract of the rhizomes of *A. asphodeloides* showed significant inhibitory activity. Two steroidal saponins and two xanthone derivatives were isolated from the butanol extract of the rhizomes of *A. asphodeloides*. The structures of the isolated compounds were identified as timosaponin A-III (1) (Kawasaki *et al.*, 1963), anemarsaponin B (2) (Dong *et al.*, 1991), mangiferin (3) (Qin *et al.*, 2008), and neomangiferin (4) (Qin *et al.*, 2008) using 1D- and 2D-NMR techniques such as 1H-13C HSQC and 1H-13C HMBC experiments and by comparison with published values. All the isolates (1-4) were evaluated for their ability to inhibit RSV. Timosaponin A-III exhibited potential anti-viral activity against the RSV-A2 strain propagated in HEp-2 cells, with an IC_{50} of 1.00 µM, which is more potent than the positive control, ribavirin (IC_{50} = 1.15 µM). The remaining compounds anemarsaponin B (2) which has a furostanol skeleton, and xanthone glycosides (3 and 4) were inactive (IC_{50} > 5 µM). These results suggest that the spirostane skeleton (1) is more active than the furostanol structure (2) in the steroidal saponins. They envisaged that further study with more diverse compounds is needed to develop these structure-activity relationships.

2.4 *Ligustrum lucidum*

From Ma Shuang-Cheng and coworkers (2001) report is made about activities of six secoiridoid glucoside compounds, lucidumoside C, oleoside dimethylester, neonuezhenide, oleuropein, ligustroside and lucidumoside A, isolated from the fruits of *Ligustrum lucidum* (Oleaceae). They were examined *in vitro* for their activities against four strains of pathogenic viruses, namely herpes simplex type 1 virus (HSV-1), influenza type A virus (Flu A), respiratory syncytial virus (RSV) and parainfluenza type 3 virus (Para 3) with Oleuropein being the most potent (IC_{50} 23.4µg/ml) as well as possessing an overall large and best therapeutic window (TC_{50} 562.5µg/ml/IC_{50} 23.4µg/ml) comparable to that of ribavirin, an approved drug for the treatment of RSV infections in human. Oleuropein is known to possess a wide range of biological activities (Ma *et al.*, 2001), one of them being immune-modulatory activities (He *et al.*, 2001; Saija *et al.*, 1998; Visioli *et al.*, 1995; 1998;). The associated immune effects could enhance its anti-RSV benefit in the biological compartment.

2.5 *Hydroclathrus clathratus* and *Lobophora variegata*

Products from marine organisms show many interesting activities. Their constituents are more novel than those of many terrestrial plants. Seaweeds have long been recognized as rich and valuable natural resources of bioactive compounds because of their various biological properties (Mayer and Lehmann, 2000). The water-soluble extracts of seaweeds have been shown to exhibit anti-viral activity against a wide spectrum of viruses (Witvrouw and de Clercq, 1997). There are more than 200 species of seaweeds in Hong Kong coastal waters (Ang, 2005), but research on their anti-viral activity is very limited (Zhu *et al.*, 2003). Wang *et al.* (2008) in their study employed crude water extracts of six species of seaweeds *Colpomenia sinuosa* (Mertens ex Roth), *Dictyota dichotoma* (Hudson) J.V. Lamouroux, *Hydroclathrus clathratus*, *Lobophora variegata* (Lamouroux) Womersley ex Oliveira, *Padina australis* Holmes and *Sargassum hemiphyllum* (Turner) C. Agardh from Hong Kong coastal waters were examined for their cellular toxicity and anti-viral activities. *H. clathratus* and *L. variegate* showed potent anti-RSV activities with EC_{50} values of 25µg/ml and 100µg/ml respectively.

2.6 *Echinacea purpurea*

Several viruses associated with upper respiratory diseases have been shown to stimulate the secretion of pro-inflammatory cytokines, including chemokines, sometimes in the absence of viral cytopathology. Some plant natural products are known to hold potential of reversing the pro-inflammatory effects induced by these viruses, and hence the disease-associated symptoms due to their infections (such as cold and flu symptoms of respiratory viruses). One such candidate agent is the herbal medicine *Echinacea purpurea*, which has become one of the most popular commercial herbal preparations in North America and Europe (Brevoort, 1998; Barnes *et al.*, 2005). There have been numerous reports of immune modulatory properties in various preparations derived from different parts of several species of *Echinacea* (Gertsch *et al.*, 2004; Barnes *et al.*, 2005; Sharma *et al.*, 2006, 2008; Wang *et al.*, 2006), although the composition of these preparations is inconsistent, a fact that has made it difficult to propose a mechanism of action (Woelkart and Bauer, 2007). Widely varied anti-viral properties among different *Echinacea* species and component parts have been reported (Hudson et al., 2005; Vimalanathan *et al.*, 2005). Thus it is important to carry out research on *Echinacea* preparations that have been standardized and chemically characterized.

Sharma *et al.*, 2009 evaluated the ability of a standardized preparation of the popular herbal medicine *Echinacea* (Echinaforce®), an ethanol extract of herb and roots of *E. purpurea*, and containing known concentrations of marker compounds) to inhibit the viral induction of various cytokines in a line of human bronchial epithelial cells (BEAS-2B), and in two other human cell lines. They found *Echinacea* (Echinaforce® to inhibit respiratory syncytial virus (RSV)-induced IL-6 and IL-8 (CXCL8) secretion, in addition to several other chemokines. In every case however *Echinacea* inhibited this induction. The *Echinacea* preparation also showed substantial virucidal activity against RSV (MIC 2.5µg/ml) indicating the multi-functional potential of the herb. These results support the concept that certain *Echinacea* preparations can alleviate "cold and flu" symptoms, and possibly other respiratory disorders, by inhibiting viral growth and the secretion of pro-inflammatory cytokines.

2.7 *Dysoxylum gaudichaudianum*

The medicinal plant *Dysoxylum gaudichaudianum* Miq. (Meliaceae) is local to Papua New Guinea. The leaves and bark are used as a medicine by the indigenous people for treating rigid limbs, facial distortion in children, lumps under the skin, and other irritations, and as a remedy for sexually transmitted diseases (Weiner, 1984). They are also reportedly used as a remedy for fish poisoning and for convulsions (Cambie and Ash, 1994). A liquid drink made by adding boiling water to the chopped leaves is considered to be a cure for most aches and pains (Parham, 1943) and is used for lung hemorrhage (Donald *et al.*, 1975). Anti-RSV agents from *Dysoxylum gaudichaudianum* were described by Chen *et al.*, 2007. Both aqueous (water or 1:1 water-2-propanol) and organic (1:1 methylene chloride-2-propanol) extracts of *D. gaudichaudianum* bark showed inhibitory activity against the RSV strain A2 in *CPE* inhibition and plaque reduction assays. Using respiratory syncytial viral CPE inhibition and plaque reduction assays to guide bioactivity-directed fractionation, the active fraction was found to be present in the more lipophilic phase, following liquid-liquid partition (chloroform/ aqueous ethanol). Reversed-phase chromatography of the organic extract led to the complete separation and isolation of four structurally related new compounds. The four new compounds, belonging to the tetranortriterpenoid family, named dysoxylins A-D, which were found to exhibit potent anti-viral activity against RSV. NMR spectroscopic analysis of this fraction indicated the presence of complex structures. These new compounds showed significant anti-RSV activity in both the cytopathic effect (CPE) inhibition and plaque reduction assays (1 to 4 μg/ml).

2.8 *Caesalpinia minax*

Caesalpinia minax Hance, a member of the *Caesalpinia* genus, is a prickly shrub growing in the tropics and subtropics. The seeds of this plant, which is called 'ku-shi-lian', have long been used as Chinese folk medicine for the treatment of common cold, fever and dysentery (Jiangsu New Medical College, 1977). Jiang *et al.* (2001) working with the chloroform fraction of the ethanol (95%) extract of the seeds was found to show *in vitro* anti-RSV activity, and a subsequent bioassay-guided study led to the isolation of a novel rearranged vouacapane diterpenoid possessing a new carbon skeleton, now designated spirocaesalmin. Spirocaesalmin, a novel rearranged vouacapane diterpenoid that exhibits significant activity against respiratory syncytial virus, possesses a new carbon skeleton with a spiro-CD ring system. Spirocaesalmin has been found to exhibit significant activity against respiratory syncytial virus (IC_{50} = 19.5 ± 1.5 μg mL, TC_{50} = 126.9 ± 2.0 μg ml and SI = 6.5) in cell culture, and the corresponding values for the positive control (ribavirin) are 3.6 ± 0.2 μg ml, 62.5 ± 1.9 μg ml and 17.4, respectively. Thus isolation of spirocaesalmin with a novel spiro-heterocyclic ring skeleton and the first bioassay against RSV in the family of vouacapane diterpenoids provide a potentially useful lead to the search for anti-viral drugs.

2.9 *Lithraea molleoides*, *Polygonum punctatum* and *Myrcianthes cisplatensis*

The search for anti-viral agents against RSV among the province of Entre Rı´os in Argentina has led to the discovery of plants which are expected to lead to identification of promising hits. These plants include *Lithraea molleoides, Polygonum punctatum* and *Myrcianthes cisplatensis*.

The trees of the genus *Lithraea* Hook. et Arn. (Anacardiaceae) are traditionally known for their irritating effects, especially among woodcutters and carpenters. *Lithraea molleoides* (Vell.) Engler called 'a´rbol malo' (evil tree), common name 'chichita', or 'molle de Co´rdoba', produces discomfort, drowsiness, lack of strength, rash and swelling in exposed parts of the body to anyone approaching to the tree. A myth exists about the healing powers of this tree, which also provides good quality timber and has tanning and dyeing bark (Munoz, 1990). Fruits have a volatile oil believed to cause, according to the ancient tradition, very strong and disturbing irritation of the eyes and the skin (Storni, 1994). In the northwest of Argentina the fruits are used to make an alcoholic drink. The infusion of the leaves and fruits is said to be diuretic and stomachic (Cabrera, 1938). A decoction of the twigs is useful for breathing and digestive diseases (Ratera and Ratera, 1980). The tincture and the decoction are a good remedy for cough, bronchitis and phlegm. They are also hemostatic, stomachic, tonic and refreshing (Burgstaller Chiriani, 1974) and are used for arthritis (Martius, 1843).

The genus *Polygonum* L. is rich in medicinal species in the old as well as the new world. All of them are rich in tannins and some are occasionally used as foods (Lewis and Elvis-Lewis, 1977). *Polygonum punctatum* Elliot (Polygonaceae) is one of the most widely spread species of the genus in the province of Entre Rı´os, and is found in different habitats. It is considered poisonous to man and ocasionally fatal to livestock (Lewis and Elvis-Lewis, 1977). The acrid juice can cause both internal and external inflammation. It should be used only in professionally-made preparations and with medical supervision. It has astringent, diaphoretic, diuretic and rubefacient properties. A cold extract can be applied to skin problems, scabies, and hemorrhoids and as a gargle for toothache and problems in the larynx. The juice, pure or thinned with water, is effective in drawing pus out of sores (Lust, 1974). Infusion of the whole plant of *Polygonum punctatum* Elliot var., Aquatile (Martins) Fasset, also called 'erva do bicho' or 'caa-tai', 'ajicillo', is used in traditional medicine by the Toba indians of the northeastern region of Argentina, as a disinfectant and vulnerary in lavages of pimples, wounds and rash and as an antihemorrhoidal (Martı´nez Crovetto, 1964, 1965, 1981).

Many species of Argentine *Myrtaceae* are recognized as astringents and they are often mixed to potentiate their effects. The infusion of the leaves and the wood decoction of *Myrcianthes cisplatensis* (Camb.) Berg. (Myrtaceae) 'lapachillo', 'guayabo colorado' or 'palo pelado', is claimed to be astringent, tonic, stimulant, febrifuge and diuretic, and especially useful to wash and heal ulcers (Gonza´lez Torres, 1992). It is also a good remedy for lung and bronchial affections (Font Quer, 1988). It is a very common tree in the river-banks of the province of Entre Rı´os, easily recognizable by its clear bark and the strong odor of its leaves,which have contributed for its popularity.

The anti-RSV activities of *L. molleoides*, *P. punctatum* and *M. cisplatensis* extracts were reported by Kott *et al.*, 1998. They reported ED_{50} values ranging from 78 to 120μg/ml. Their preliminary work therefore validated the continued traditional utilization of these plants as anti-viral remedies especially against RSV, and concluded on the need to further purify to isolate active compounds for further developments as anti-RSV agents.

2.10 Anti-RSV herbs commonly used in traditional Chinese medicines

Ma *et al.* (2002) described about 44 Chinese herbs commonly used in treatment of RSV disease. Traditional Chinese medicinal herbs have long been used as remedies against infectious diseases in China. Traditional medicines in the form of hot water extracts have been used orally for the treatment of various diseases. It is very likely that hot water extracts of some herbs would exhibit direct anti-viral activity *in vitro* at the concentration used for therapy. In this study Ma and coworkers assayed 44 medicinal herbs, which are currently used for the treatment of respiratory tract infectious diseases in China, to test anti-viral activities against RSV *in vitro* by cytopathic effect assay. The extracts of *Sophora flaescens* Ait.

and *Scutellaria baicalensis* Georgi with anti-viral properties were further investigated to identify their anti-viral components against RSV.

Aqueous extracts from these traditional Chinese medicines were also studied to detect anti-viral activity against RSV. Of all the 44 herbs tested, 41 showed anti-RSV activities with the following 25 herbs showing the strongest potency (IC_{50}= 6.3 to 52.1µg/ml) and also largest selective index (SI= 4.0 to 32.1): *Andrographis paniculata, Artemisia capillaries, Bupleurum chinense, Callicarpa nudiflora, Dendranthema morifolium, Forsythia suspensa, Ipomoea cairica, Gardenia jasminoides, Isatis indigotica, Lonicera japonica, Paeonia suffruticosa, Patrinia _illosa, Perilla frutescens, Phragmites communis, Platycodon grandiflorum, Polygonum cuspidatum, Polygonum multiflorum, Prunella _ulgaris, Pueraria lobata, Sarcandra glabra, Schizonepeta tenuifolia, Scutellaria baicalensis, Selaginella sinensis, Sophora flaescens* and *Tinospora* capillipes. All of these traditional Chinese medicines extracts were considered active, and of interest for further investigation. Further purification of 2 of the herbs (*Sophora flavescens* and *Scutellaria baicalensis*) led to the isolation of potent anti-viral compounds. *Sophora flaescens* and of *Scutellaria baicalensis* were further investigated and led to the identification from these two herbs anagyrine, oxymatrine, sophoranol, wogonin, and oroxylin A as the most potent anti-viral compounds against RSV; their IC_{50} values ranged from 7.4 to 14.5 µg/ml.

2.11 *Narcissus tazetta*, *Youngia japonica* and *Flos lonicerae*

Ooi *et al.*, 2010 investigated the inhibitory effect of a novel mannose-binding lectin NTL isolated, purified and cloned from the bulbs of the Chinese daffodil, *Narcissus tazetta* var. *chinensis,* against human RSV, and various strains of influenza A (H1N1, H3N2, H5N1) and influenza B viruses. NTL was obtained after FPLC-gel filtration followed by desalting with a PD-10 column, and its purity was analysed by SDS-PAGE. It was determined to have a molecular mass of about 26 kDa by gel filtration and 13 kDa by SDS–PAGE. NTL is suggested to be a mannose-binding homodimer with two identical subunits of about 13 kDa. Molecular cloning revealed that the deduced amino acid sequence of the full-length cDNA encoding NTL contained a mature polypeptide consisting of 105 amino acids and a C-terminal peptide extension beyond the C-terminal amino acids Thr-Gly. NTL could effectively inhibit RSV-induced plaque formation (IC_{50}= 2.30 µg/ml). Its cytotoxicity against HEp-2 cells was low (CC_{50}= 325.4 µg/ml) and thus it had a high SI value of 141.36.

In another related earlier study, Ooi together with other investigators (Ooi et al., 2006) reported the anti-RSV activity of the ethanol extract of a biannual medicinal herb, *Youngia japonica* (commonly known as Oriental hawk's beard). Two potent anti-RSV compounds namely 3,4-dicaffeoylquinic acid and 3,5-dicaffeoylquinic acid, were subsequently purified and chemically characterized from the ethanol extract of *Youngia japonica*. The two dicaffeoylquinic acids exhibited prominent anti-RSV with an IC_{50} of 0.5µg/ml and there was no sign of cytotoxicity up to 100µg/ml concentration.

CJ 4-16-4 is a promising potent inhibitor of RSV isolated from *Flos lonicerae* using bioassay-guided fractionation. The drug inhibits of RSV in Hep-2 cells maintained in tissue culture at a very low concentration (~0.07 µM) with cell toxicity >400 µM (SI > 5880). In a cotton rat model of RSV infection, the drug was able to reduce viral titers by ~1 log at dose 12.5 and 25 mg/kg/day, and by >2 log at 100 mg/kg/day. This antiviral activity was specific as influenza A and B and herpes simplex 1 and 2 viruses were not inhibited (Ojwang *et al.*, 2005).

Scientific name of Plant	Promising isolated compounds	References
Aglaia ignea	Dammarenolic acid	Esimone *et al.*, 2008
Aglaia duppereana	Aglaiol	Esimone *et al.*, 2008
Aglaia cucculata	Niloticin	Esimone *et al.*, 2008
Anemarrhena asphodeloides	(-)-(R)-Nyasol* (-)-(R)-4′-O-methylnyasol* Broussonin A* timosaponin A-III*	Bae *et al.*, 2007; Youn *et al.*, 2011; Kawasaki *et al.*, 1963
Dysoxylum gaudichaudianum	Dysoxylins A-D*	Chen *et al.*, 2007
Sophora flavescens	Allmatrine Anagyrine Cytisine Isomatrine Matrine *N*-methylcytisine Oxymatrine Oxysophocarpine Sophocarpine Sophoranol Sophoridine	Ma *et al.*, 2002
Scutellaria baicalensis	Wogonin Oroxylin A Baicalein Scutellarein Baicalin	Ma *et al.*, 2002
Caesalpinia minax	Spirocaesalmin	Jiang *et al.*, 2001
Ligustrum lucidum	Oleuropein	Ma *et al.*, 2001
Narcissus tazetta	NTL	Ooi et al., 2010
Youngia japonica	Dicaffeoylquinic acids	Ooi et al., 2006
Flos lonicerae	CJ 4-16-4	Ojwang et al., 2005

Key: Promising isolated compounds determined on the basis of S.I index ≥ 4
*SI index not reported

Table 2. Promising anti-RSV compounds isolated from phytomedicines

3. Potential usefulness of anti-RSV compounds and phyto-constituents harnessed from phytomedicines in the treatment and control of RSV infection and disease

Complementary and alternative medicines have been used effectively by humans over several centuries for treating various diseases and can therefore be effectively employed to target the host response during RSV infection. Currently, no effective vaccine or therapeutic drug is available against RSV. Although ribavirin, a broad-spectrum anti-viral agent, is being marketed under approval, its clinical benefits are small and limited coupled, with the high cost and toxicity associated with it (Kneyber *et al.* 2000; Lafeuillade *et al.* 2001; Seetharama and Narayana 2005). New therapies designed to combat moderate to severe RSV infection and disease are clearly needed. Anti-RSV compounds from phytomedicines could fill this gap. Although there have been several reports on natural anti-RSV agents, including some flavans (Li *et al.*, 2006), caffeoylquinic acid (Li *et al.*, 2005), and some alkaloids such as anagyrine, oxymatrine, and sophoranol (Ma *et al.*, 2002). However, more anti-RSV drug candidates from phytomedicines need to be discovered for future development. A number of synthetic organic compounds have also received attention as anti-RSV agents however some are too cytotoxic to develop as clinically useful agents (Golankiewicz *et al.*, 1995). Given the foregoing therefore, the potential usefulness of medicinal plants - either as suitable sources for the development of potent anti-viral anti-RSV agents or as effective tools in alternative medical practice, cannot be in question. Medicinal plants remain sources of cost-effective and accessible anti-viral remedies for use in developing and developed countries (Chen *et al.*, 2008; Cowan, 1999; De Clercq, 1995; Jassim and Naji, 2003; Vlietinck and Vanden, 1991; Williams, 2001). They also could reduce time to be spent synthesizing new molecules. Moreover, reports of some strains of RSV developing resistance to currently administered therapeutic agents such as Ribavirin further underscore the need for effort for the development of new and more effective anti-viral agents to be undertaken. Finally, the screening of plants as a possible source of anti-viral in the ethnopharmacological approach enhances the probability of identifying new bioactive plant compounds (Vlietinck and Vanden, 1991; Baker *et al.*, 1995). It is therefore hoped that anti-viral compounds from phytomedicines against RSV would greatly serve diverse usefulness in the management of RSV infection and disease.

4. Conclusion

Historically, plants have provided a source of inspiration for novel drug compounds, as plant derived medicines have made large contributions to human health and well-being. Their role is twofold in the development of new drugs: first, they may become the base for the development of a medicine, a natural blueprint for the development of new drugs, or; second: a phytomedicine to be used for the treatment of disease. There are numerous illustrations of plant derived drugs. It is estimated that today, plant materials are present in, or have provided the models for at least 50% Western drugs (Schuster, 2001). Many commercially proven drugs used in modern medicine were initially used in crude form in traditional or folk healing practices, or for other purposes that suggested potentially useful biological activity. The primary benefits of using plant derived medicines are that they are relatively safer than synthetic alternatives, offering profound therapeutic benefits and more affordable treatment.

Currently, investigations into the anti-RSV virus activities of numerous plant species are ongoing. A sense of urgency accompanies the search as the pace of species extinction continues. More of these compounds should be subjected to animal and human studies to determine their effectiveness in whole-organism systems, including in particular toxicity studies. It would be advantageous to standardize methods of extraction and *in vitro* testing so that the search could be more systematic and interpretation of results would be facilitated. Also, alternative mechanisms of infection prevention and treatment should be included in initial activity screenings. Disruption of adhesion is one example of an anti-infection activity not commonly screened for currently. Attention to these issues could usher in a badly needed new era of chemotherapeutic treatment of infection by using plant-derived principles.

5. References

Adegbola RA, Falade AG, Sam BE *et al.* (1994) The etiology of pneumonia in malnourished and well-nourished Gambian children. Pediatric Infectious Disease Journal 13, 975–982.

Ang PO (2005) Studies of Marine Algae in Hong Kong. *In*: Critichley AT, Ohno M, Largo D. (Eds.), World Seaweed Resources. ETI Information Services Ltd., Wokingham, Berkshire, UK, Part 3. 04.

Bae G, Yu JR, Lee J, Chang J, Seo EK (2007). Identification of nyasol and structurally related compounds as the active principles from *Anemarrhena asphodeloides* against respiratory syncytial virus (RSV). Chem. Biodivers., 4: 2231-2235.

Baker, T., Borris, R., Carte, B., Cragg, G., Gupta, M., Iwu, M., Madulid, D., Tyler, V., 1995. Natural product drug discovery and development: new perspectives on international collaboration. Journal of Natural Products 58, 1325–1357.

Barnes J, Anderson LA, Gibbons S, Phillipson JD (2005) *Echinacea* species (*Echinacea angustifolia* (DC.) Hell. *Echinacea pallida* (Nutt.) Nutt., *Echinacea purpurea* (L.) Moench: a review of their chemistry, pharmacology and clinical properties. J. Pharm. Pharmacol. 57: 929-954.

Berkovich, S. 1964. Acute respiratory illness in the premature nursery associated with respiratory syncytial virus infections. Pediatrics 34:753–760.

Bohnenstengel FI, Steube KG, Meyer C, Nugroho BW, Hung PD, Kiet LC, Proksch P (1999) Structure activity relationships of antiproliferative rocaglamide derivatives from Aglaia species (Meliaceae). Z Naturforsch. 54: 55–60.

Brevoort P (1998) The booming US botanical market. HerbalGram 44: 33–48.

Burgstaller Chiriani CH (1974) La vuelta a los vegetales, 5th edn. La Prensa Me´dica Argentina, Buenos Aires.

Cambie RC, Ash J (1994) *Fijian Medicinal Plants;* CSIRO: Collingwood, Victoria, Australia.

Chen JL, Kernan MR, Jolad SD, Stoddart CA, Bogan M, Cooper R (2007) Dysoxylins A-D, Tetranortriterpenoids with Potent Anti-RSV Activity from *Dysoxylum gaudichaudianum. J. Nat. Prod.* 70: 312-315.

Cheng HY, Huang HH, Yang CM, Lin LT, Lin CC (2008) The in vitro anti-herpes simplex virus type-1 and type-2 activity of Long Dan Xie Gan Tan, a prescription of traditional Chinese medicine. Chemotherapy. 54: 77-83.

Cohen PA, Hudson JB, Towers GH (1996) Anti-viral activities of anthraquinones, bianthrones and hypericin derivatives from lichens. Experientia. 52: 180-183.

Collins, P. L., K. McIntosh, and R. M. Chanock. 1996. Respiratory syncytial virus, p. 1313-1351. *In* B. N. Fields (ed.), Fields virology. Raven Press, New York, N.Y.

Cowan MM (1999) Plant products as antimicrobial agents. Clin Microbiol Rev. 12: 564-582.De Clercq E (1995) Anti-viral therapy for human immunodeficiency virus infections. Clin Microbiol. Rev. 8: 200-239.

Donald C, Artney L, Innes H (1975) *Medicines of the Maori;* Collins: Auckland, pp 1-6.

Dong J, Han G (1991). A new active steroidal saponin from *Anemarrhena asphodeloides*. Planta Med., 57: 460-462.

Dowell, S. F., L. J. Anderson, H. E. Gary, Jr., D. D. Erdman, J. F. Plouffe, T. M. File, Jr., B. J. Marston, and R. F. Breiman (1996) Respiratory syncytial virus is an important cause of community-acquired lower respiratory infection among hospitalized adults. J. Infect. Dis. 174:456–462.

Duke JA, Bogenschutz-Godwin MJ, duCellier J, Duke PAK (2002). Handbook of Medicinal Herbs, 2th ed, CRC Press, New York, p. 27.

Esimone CO, Adikwu MU (1999) Antimicrobial activity and cytotoxicity of *Ramalina farinacea*. Fitoterapia. 70: 428-431.

Esimone CO, Adikwu MU (2002) Susceptibility of some clinical isolates of *Staphylococcus aureus* to bioactive column fractions from the lichen *Ramalina farinacea* (L) Ach. Phytother Res. 16: 494-496.

Esimone CO, Adikwu MU, Ebi GC, Anaga A, Njoku C (1999) Physicochemical evaluationsand bioactive properties of column fractions from the lichen *Ramalina farinacea* (L) Ach. Boll Chim Farm. 138: 19-25.

Esimone CO, Grunwald T, Nworu CS, Kuate S, Proksch P, Uberla K (2009) Broad Spectrum Anti-viral Fractions from the Lichen *Ramalina farinacea* (L.) Ach. Chemotherapy. 55:119-126.

Esimone CO, Nwodo NJ, Iroha, IR and Ogbuefi NR (2006) Antifungal screening of the methanolic extract of the Lichen *Ramalina farinacea* (L) Ach. Afric J Pharm Res Dev. 2: 1-6.

Esimone, C. O., Eck, G., Duong, T. N., Uberla, K., Proksch, P., Grunwald, T. 2008. Potential anti-respiratory syncytial virus lead compounds from Aglaia species. *Pharmazie.* 63: 1-6.

Falsey AR, Patricia AH, Maria AF, Christopher C, and Walsh EE. 2005. Respiratory Syncytial Virus Infection in Elderly and High-Risk Adults. N. Engl. J. Med. 352: 1749-1759.

Falsey, A. R. and E. E. Walsh. 1998. Relationship of serum antibody to risk of respiratory syncytial virus infection in elderly adults. J. Infect. Dis. 177: 463–466.

Falsey, A. R., C. K. Cunningham, W. H. Barker, R. W. Kouides, J. B. Yuen, M. Menegus, L. B.

Falsey, A. R., J. J. Treanor, R. F. Betts, and E. E. Walsh. 1992. Viral respiratory infections in the institutionalized elderly: clinical and epidemiologic findings. J. Am. Geriatr. Soc. 40:115–119.

Font Quer, P., 1988. Plantas Medicinales. El Diosco´ rides Renovado. Labor, Barcelona.

Fouillard, L., L. Mouthon, J. P. Laporte, F. Isnard, J. Stachowiak, M. Aoudjhane, J. C. Lucet, M. Wolf, F. Bricourt, L. Douay, M. Lopez, C. Marche, A. Najman, and N. C. Gorin. 1992. Severe respiratory syncytial virus pneumonia after autologous bone marrow transplantation: a report of three cases and review. Bone Marrow Transplant. 9:97–100.

Gautam R, Saklani A, Jachak SM (2007) Indian medicinal plants as a source of antimycobacterial agents. J Ethnopharmacol. 110: 200-34.

Golankiewicz B, Januszczyk P, Ikeda S, Balzarini J, DeClercq E (1995) Synthesis and anti-viral activity of benzyl-substituted imidazo [1,5-a]-1,3,5-triazine (5,8-diaza-7,9 dideazapurine) derivatives. *J. Med. Chem.* 38: 3558-3565.

Gonza´lez Torres, D.M., 1992. Cata´logo de Plantas Medicinales usadas en Paraguay. Asuncio´n.Groothuis, J. R., K. M. Gutierrez, and B. A. Lauer. 1988. Respiratory syncytial virus infection in children with bronchopulmonary dysplasia. Pediatrics 82:199–203.

Harvey AL (2008) Natural products in drug discovery. Drug Discov Today. 13: 894-901.

He ZD, But PPH, Chan TWD, Dong H, Xu HX, Lau CP, Sun HD (2001) Antioxidative glucosides from the fruits of *Ligustrum lucidum*. *Chem. Pharm. Bull.*, 49, 780–784 (2001).

Hudson J, Vimalanathan S, Kang L, Treyvaud Amiguet V, Livesey J, Arnason JT (2005) Characterization of anti-viral activities in *Echinacea* root preparations. Pharmacol. Biol. 43: 790-796.

Iida Y, Oh KB, Saito M, Matsuoka H, Kurata H (2000). *In vitro* synergism between nyasol, an active compound isolated from *Anemarrhena asphodeloides*, and azole agents against *Candida albicans*. Planta Med., 66: 435-438.

Jassim SAA, Naji MA (2003) Novel anti-viral agents: a medicinal plant perspective. J Appl Microbiol. 95: 412-27.

Jiang R, Ma S, But PP, Mak TCW (2001) Isolation and characterization of spirocaesalmin, a novel rearranged vouacapane diterpenoid from Caesalpinia minax Hance. *J. Chem. Soc., Perkin Trans. 1.* 2920-2923.

Jiangsu New Medical College (1977) *Dictionary of Chinese Traditional Medicine*, Shanghai People's Publishing House, P. R. China, p. 1289.

Kawasaki T, Yamauchi T (1963). Saponins of Timo (Anemarrhenae Rhizoma). II. Structure of timosaponin A-III. Chem. Pharm. Bull., 11: 1221-1224.

Kneyber MCJ, Moll HA, de Groot R (2000) Treatment and prevention of respiratory syncytial virus infection. *Eur. J. Pediatr.* 159 (6): 399-411.

Kohlmann R, Schwannecke S, Tippler B, Ternette N, Temchura V, Tenbusch M, Überla K and Grunwald T. 2009. Protective Efficacy and Immunogenicity of an Adenoviral Vector Vaccine Encoding the Codon-Optimized F Protein of Respiratory Syncytial Virus. 83 (23): 12601-12610.

Kott V, Barbini L, Cruanes M, *et al.* (1999) Anti-viral activity in Argentine medicinal plants. J. Ethnopharmacol. 64: 79-84.

Lafeuillade A, Hattinger G, Chadapaud S (2001) Increased mitochondrial toxicity with ribavirin in HIV/HCV coinfection. Lancet 357: 280–281.

Langley GF and Anderson LJ. 2011. Epidemiology and Prevention of Respiratory Syncytial Virus Infections Among Infants and Young Children. Pediatr. Infect. Dis. J. 30: 510–517.

Lewis WH, Elvis-Lewis MP (1977) Medical Botany. John Wiley and Sons, New York.

Li Y, But PP, Ooi VE (2005) Anti-viral Res. 68: 1.

Li Y, Leung K, Yao F, Ooi LS, Ooi VE (2006) J. Nat. Prod. 69: 833.

Lipipun V, Kurokawa M, Suttisri R, Taweechotipatr P, Pramyothin P, Hattori M, Shiraki K (2003) Efficacy of Thai medicinal plant extracts against herpes simplex virus type 1 infection *in vitro* and *in vivo*. Antivir Res 60 : 175–180.

Lust J (1974) The Herb Book. Bantam Books, New York.

Ma S, Du J, But PP, Deng X, Zhang Y, Ooi VE, Xu H, Lee SH, Lee SF (2002) Anti-viral Chinese medicinal herbs against respiratory syncytial virus. *Journal of Ethnopharmacology*. 79: 205-211.

Ma S, He Z, DENG X, But PP, Ooi VE, Xu H, Lee SH, Lee S (2001) *In Vitro* Evaluation of Secoiridoid Glucosides from the Fruits of *Ligustrum lucidum* as *Antiviral Agents*. *Chem. Pharm. Bull.* 49 (11): 1471-1473.

MacDonald, N. E., C. B. Hall, S. C. Suffin, C. Alexson, P. J. Harris, and J. A. Manning. 1982. Respiratory syncytial viral infection in infants with congenital heart disease. N. Engl. J. Med. 307:397–400.

Martı´nez Crovetto R (1964) Estudios Etnobota´nicos I. Bonplandia. 4: 270-333.

Martı´nez Crovetto, R., 1965. Estudios etnobota´nicos II. Nombres de plantas y su utilidad segu´n los indios tobas del estedel Chaco. Bonplandia. 4: 279-333.

Martı´nez Crovetto, R., 1981. Las plantas utilizadas en medicina popular en el Noroeste de Corrientes. Repu´ blica Argentina. Fundacio´n M. Lillo. Tucuma´n, Argentina.

Martin W.Weber1, E. Kim Mulholland and Brian M. Greenwood. (1998) Respiratory syncytial virus infection in tropical and developing countries. Tropical Medicine and International Health. 3 (4): 268–280.

Martius FP (1843 Systema Material Madicae Vegetabilis Brasiliensis. Fleischer, Leipzig and Beck, Vienna.

Mayer AMS, Lehmann VKB, (2000) Marine pharmacology in 1998: marine compounds with antibacterial, anticoagulant, antifungal, anti-inflammatory, anthelmintic, antiplatelet, antiprotozoal, and anti-viral activities; with actions on the cardiovascular, endocrine, immune, and nervous systems, and other miscellaneous mechanism of action. *The Pharmacologist*. 42: 62-69.

Munoz J de D (1990) Usos principales de la especies de Anacardiaceae, particularmente de Paraguay. Candollea. 45: 671-680.

Nakashima N, Kimura I, Kimura M (1993). Isolation of pseudoprototimosaponin AIII from rhizomes of *Anemarrhena asphodeloides* and its hypoglycemic activity in streptozotocin-induced diabetic mice. J. Nat. Prod., 56: 345-350.

Neamati N, Hong H, Mazumder A., Wang S, Sunder S, Nicklaus MC, Milne GW, Proksa B, Pommier Y (1997) Depsides and depsidones as inhibitors of HIV-1 integrase: discovery of novel inhibitors through 3D database searching. J Med Chem. 40: 942-951.

Nwankwo MU, Okuonghae HO, Currier G and Schuit KE (1994) Respiratory syncytial virus in malnourished children. *Annals of Tropical Paediatrics* 14, 125–130.

Ojwang JO, Wang Y, Wyde PR, Fischer NH, Schuehly W, Appleman JR, Hinds S, Shimasaki CD. 2005. A novel inhibitor of respiratory syncytial virus isolated from ethnobotanicals. Antiviral research. 68 (3): 163-172.

Ooi LSM, Ho W, Ngai KLK, Tian L, Chan PKS, Sun SSM, Ooi VEC. 2010. *Narcissus tazetta* lectin shows strong inhibitory effects against respiratory syncytial virus, infl uenza A (H1N1, H3N2, H5N1) and B viruses. J. Biosci. 35(1): 95–103.

Ooi LSM, Wang H, He Z, Ooi VEC. 2006. Antiviral activities of purified compounds from *Youngia japonica* (L.) DC (Asteraceae, Compositae). Journal of Ethnopharmacology. 106: 187–191

Pannell CM (1992) A taxonomic monograph of the genus Aglaia Lour. (Meliaceae). Kew Bulletin Additional Series XVI, Royal Botanic Gardens, Kew. HMSO, London, p. 1–379.

Pardo-Andreu GL, Sanchez-Baldoquin C, Avila-Gonzalez R, Delgado R, Naal Z, Curti C (2006). Fe(III) improves antioxidant and cytoprotecting activities of mangiferin. Eur. J. Pharmacol., 547: 31-36.

Parham HBR (1943) *Polynesian Soc. Mem. 16*, 1-4.

Park HJ, Lee JY, Moon SS, Hwang BK (2003). Isolation and antioomycete activity of nyasol from *Anemarrhena asphodeloides* rhizomes. Phytochem., 64: 997-1001.

Pengsuparp T, Cai L, Constant H, Fong HH, Lin LZ, Kinghorn AD, Pezzuto JM, Cordell GA, Ingolfsdottir K, Wagner H, Hughes SH (1995) Mechanistic evaluation of new plant-derived compounds that inhibit HIV-1 reverse transcriptase. J Nat Prod. 58: 1024-1031.

Perry LM (1980) Medicinal plants of East and Southeast Asia. MIT Press, Cambridge, MA.

Poehland BL, Carte BK, Francis TA, Hyland LJ, Allaudeen HS, Troupe N (1987) In vitro anti-viral activity of dammar resin triterpenoids. J Nat Prod 50: 706–713.

Preceding Mitochondria-Mediated Apoptosis in HeLa Cancer Cells. Cancer Res., 68: 10229-10237.

Prince GA (2001) An update on respiratory syncytial virus anti-viral agents. Expert Opin Investig Drugs 10: 297–308.

Qin L, Han T, Zhang Q, Cao D, Nian H, Rahman K, Zheng H (2008). Antiosteoporotic chemical constituents from Er-Xian Decoction, a traditional Chinese herbal formula. J. Ethnopharmacol., 118: 271- 279.

Ratera E, Ratera M (1980) Plantas de la flora argentina empleadas en medicina popular. Edicio´n hemisferio sur, Buenos Aires.

Ren LX, Luo YF, Li X, Zuo DY, Wu YL (2006). Antidepressant-like effects of sarsasapogenin from *Anemarrhena asphodeloides* BUNGE (Liliaceae). Biol. Pharm. Bull., 29: 2304-2306.

Saija A, Trombetta D, Tomaino A, Lo Cascio R, Princi P, Uccella N, Bonina F, Castelli F (1998) In vitro evaluation of the antioxidant activity and biomembrane interaction of the plant phenols Oleuropein and hydroxytyrosol. *Int. J. Pharmaceut.*, 166: 123-133.

Schuster BG (2001) A new integrated program for natural product development and the value of an ethnomedical approach. J. Altern. Complement Med. 7 (Suppl 1): S61-72.

Seetharama RKS, Narayana K (2005) In vivo chromosome damaging effects of an inosine monophosphate dehydrogenase inhibitor: Ribavirin in mice. Indian J Pharmacol 37: 90–95.

Semple SJ, Reynolds GD, O'Leary GD, Flower RLP (1998) Screening of Australian medicinal plants for anti-viral activity. J. Ethnopharmacol. 60: 163-72.

Sharma M, Anderson SA, Schoop R, Hudson JB (2009) Induction of multiple pro-inflammatory cytokines by respiratory viruses and reversal by standardized *Echinacea*, a potent anti-viral herbal extract. Anti-viral Research. 83: 165–170.

Sharma M, Arnason JT, Burt A, Hudson,JB (2006) Echinacea extracts modulate the pattern of chemokine and cytokine secretion in rhinovirus-infected and uninfected epithelial cells. Phytother. Res. 20: 147-152.

Sharma M, Schoop R, Hudson JB (2008) Echinacea as an anti-inflammatory agent: the influence of physiologically relevant parameters. Phytother. Res. doi:10.1002/ptr.2714.

Sindambiwe JB, Calomme M, Cos P, *et al.* (1999) Screening of seven selected Rwandan medicinale plants for antimicrobial and anti-viral activities. J. Ethnopharmacol. 65: 71-7.

Storni J (1994) Hortus guaranensis. Flora. Universidad Nacional de Tucuma´n. Publicacio´n Nu´mero, 354.Sy LK, Yan SC, Lok CN, Man RYK, Che CM (2008). Timosaponin A-III Induces Autophagy

Tregoning JS, Schwarze J. 2010. Respiratory viral infections in infancy: causes, clinical symptoms, virology, and immunology. *Clinical Microbiology Reviews* 23: 74–98.

Tucuman TH, Shihman CR, Smith K (1989) Isolation, purification and partial characterization of prunellin, an anti-HIV component from aqueous extracts of *Prunella vulgaris*. *Antiviral Research* 11, 263-274.

Vimalanathan S, Kang L, Treyvaud Amiguet V, Livesey J, Arnason JT, Hudson J (2005) *Echinacea purpurea* aerial parts contain multiple anti-viral compounds. Pharmacol. Biol. 43: 740-745.

Visioli F, Bellasta S, Galli C (1998) Oleuropein, the bitter principle of olives, enhances nitric oxide production bymousemacrophages. *Life Sci.* 62: 541-546.

Visioli F, Bellomo G, Galli C (1998) Free radical-scavenging properties of olive oil polyphenol. *Biochem. Biophys. Res. Commun.* 247 (1): 60-4.

Visioli F, Bellomo G, Montedoro GF, Galli C (1995) Low density lipoprotein oxidation is inhibited in vitro by olive oil constituents. *Atherosclerosis.* 117 (1): 25-32.

Vlietinck A, Vanden BD (1991) Can ethnopharmacology contribute to the development of anti-viral drugs. Journal of Ethnopharmacology. 32: 141-153.

Wang CY, Chiao MT, Yen PJ, Huang WC, Hou CC, Chien SC, Yeh KC, Yang WC, Shyur LF, Yang NS (2006) Modulatory effects of *Echinacea purpurea* extracts on human dendritic cells: a cell- and gene-based study. Genomics. 88: 801-808.

Wang H, Ooi EV, Ang PO Jr (2008) Anti-viral activities of extracts from Hong Kong seaweeds. Journal of Zhejiang University SCIENCE B. 9 (12): 969-976.

Wang WJ, Li DJ, Li J, Zhou WJ (2010). An *in vitro* study on neuroprotective effects of serum containing Gengnianchun decoction and its main monomers against amyloid beta protein-induced cellular toxicity. J. Chin. Integr. Med., 8: 67.

Weiner MA (1984) *Secrets of Fijian Medicine*; University of California: Berkely, CA, pp 65-67.

Weiner, C. A. Bonville, and R. F. Betts. 1995. Respiratory syncytial virus and influenza A infections in the hospitalized elderly. J. Infect. Dis. 172:389–394.

Williams JE (2001) Review of anti-viral and immunomodulating properties of plants of the Peruvian rainforest with a particular emphasis on Una de Gato and Sangre de Grado. Altern Med. Rev. 6: 567-579.

Witvrouw M, de Clercq E (1997) Sulfated polysaccharides extracted from sea algae as potential anti-viral drugs. *Gen. Pharmacol.* 29 (4): 497-511.

Woelkart K, Bauer R (2007) The role of alkamides as an active principle of Echinacea. Planta Med. 73: 615-623.

Wright PF, Karron RA, Belshe RB, Thompson J, Crowe JE Jr, Boyce TG, Halburnt LL *et al.* 2000. Evaluation of a live, cold-passaged, temperature-sensitive, respiratory syncytial virus vaccine candidate in infancy. *J. Infect. Dis.* 182 (5): 1331-42.

Youn UJ, Jang J, Nam J, Lee YJ, Son YM, Shin HJ, Han A, Chang J, Seo E (2011) Anti-respiratory syncytial virus (RSV) activity of timosaponin A-III from the rhizomes of *Anemarrhena asphodeloides*. Journal of Medicinal Plants Research.. 5 (7): 1062-1065.

Zhu W, Ooi VEC, Chan PKS, Ang PO Jr (2003) Isolation and characterization of a sulfated polysaccharide from the brown alga *Sargassum patens* and determination of its anti-herpes activity. *Biochem. Cell Biol.* 81 (1): 25-33.

10

Treatment of Respiratory Syncytial Virus Infection: Past, Present and Future

Dirk Roymans and Anil Koul
Tibotec-Virco Virology BVBA
Belgium

1. Introduction

Respiratory syncytial virus (RSV) has emerged since its isolation from infected children in 1957 as an important respiratory pathogen (Falsey et al, 2005; Hall et al, 2009; Nair et al, 2010; Ruuskanen et al, 2011). Generally, infection is restricted to the upper respiratory tract and not associated with long-term pathology, but progression to a more severe lower respiratory tract infection is frequent.

In developed countries, there are well-defined high-risk groups in whom infection with RSV is more likely to progress into severe acute lower respiratory tract infection (ALRI) (Simoes, 1999) (Fig. 1). Infants that are born prematurely or close to the RSV season and/or suffering from bronchopulmonay dysplasia or congenital heart disease are at the highest risk to develop severe ALRI because of RSV (Feltes et al, 2007; Hall et al, 1986; Weisman, 2003). Additional high-risk groups include immunosuppressed patients or patients with underlying disorders of cellular immunity, individuals living in institutions and the elderly. In developing countries, host-related risk factors are less well defined although some environmental factors like low socioeconomic status, malnutrition, crowded living conditions and indoor smoke pollution likely attribute also to the development of more severe disease. This seems to be reflected in the fact that although age distribution of RSV infection in children in countries with poor socioeconomic status is similar to that seen in developed countries, older children are more severely affected in developing countries (Law et al, 2002; Simoes, 1999; Weber et al, 1998).

Today the virus is considered as the most important virus causing ALRI and a major cause of hospital admissions and death in young children worldwide (Nair et al, 2010; Rudan et al, 2008; Simoes, 1999). More than 90% of the children are infected at least once by the time they reach the age of two. RSV-associated ALRIs in children under five were recently estimated at around 34 million cases globally, accounting for 22% of all ALRIs, with a mortality rate of approximately 3 to 9% (Nair et al, 2010). In addition, a growing body of evidence suggests that RSV infection results in substantial morbidity among adults with underlying chronic illnesses and the elderly (Falsey et al, 2005). Current data indicate that RSV is the causative agent of approximately 3% of all community-acquired pneumonia cases in adults (reviewed in Ruuskanen et al, 2011). Roughly 2-9% of elderly patients admitted to hospital with pneumonia in the USA have infection associated with this virus (Han et al, 1999) and in this age group, mortality linked to RSV infection is substantial (Thompson et al, 2003). Limited research exists on the economic impact of

RSV-associated ALRI among vulnerable patient populations, but the excess first-year healthcare cost per patient in late-preterm infants was calculated to be roughly $17,000 - $22,000 and $2,000 - $4,000 for inpatient and outpatient RSV ALRI, respectively (Palmer et al, 2010; Stewart et al, 2009); resulting in an annual additional healthcare cost exceeding $650 million among children in the US alone (Paramore et al, 2004).

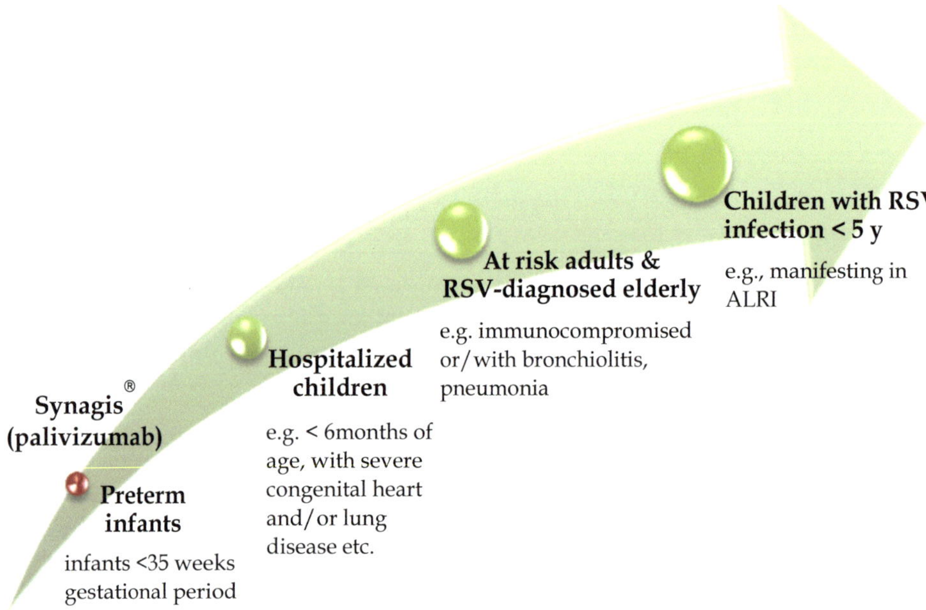

Fig. 1. Stratification of the total respiratory syncytial virus patient population. Groups of RSV patients who may seek specific RSV therapy are indicated by 4 bullets in the arrow, with the relative number of patients in each group increasing in the direction of the arrow. Current therapeutic options are limited to passive immunization of premature infants with palivizumab. Preemies are less than 35 weeks of gestational age and include infants at high risk for developing severe RSV disease. At-risk adults present immunocompromised patients including those with underlying pulmonary or cardiac disease. Elderly patients are more than 65 years of age.

Despite the huge medical and economical burden that is associated with severe RSV infection, no licensed vaccine is available today, and there are only very limited options to treat RSV-associated bronchiolitis (Wainwright, 2009). Chest physiotherapy for acute bronchiolitis in children less than 2 years of age seems not efficacious (Perrotta et al, 2007), although alternative supportive therapy including oxygenation remains a major treatment (Wainwright, 2009; American academy of pediatrics subcommittee on diagnosis and management of bronchiolitis, 2011). Prophylaxis is limited to passive immunization with the humanized monoclonal antibody Synagis®. However, administration of Synagis® is restricted to at-risk infants below the age of two and does not address disease burden in infants with no apparent underlying risk factors. Presently, there is no clear evidence that supports the routine use of ribavirin (Ventre and Randolph, 2007), corticosteroids (Blom et al, 2007; Ermers et al, 2009; Patel et al, 2004), or bronchodilators (Gadomski and Bhasale, 2006) as mainstays of acute therapy. The usage of ribavirin is limited due to its problematic mode of aerosolic administration, limited efficacy and teratogenicity. Corticosteroids do not seem to improve acute symptoms nor post-bronchiolitic wheezing, while the usage of bronchodilators is not recommended for routine management because of the high-cost, associated adverse events and the questionable efficacy. Clearly, new measures are demanded to decrease the medical burden associated with RSV infection.

2. Pathogenesis and clinical manifestation

RSV infects the upper respiratory tract particularly via the nasopharynx and the eyes, and appears to be spread via large droplets or through fomite contamination. Spread requires either close contact with infected individuals or contact of contaminated hands with nasal or conjunctival mucosa (Collins and Crowe, 2007). The incubation period usually is 3-5 days. RSV infection is associated with a large variety of disease symptoms, many of them related to the age of infection. For instance, neonatal RSV infection is often associated with non-specific symptoms such as failure to thrive, periodic breathing or apnea, and feeding difficulties (Bem et al, 2011), but in older children or adults, nasopharyngeal virus replication leads to rhinitis, cough and sometimes low-grade fever. In cases of severe apnea, mechanical ventilation may be required despite the absence of respiratory failure (Simoes, 1999). Croup also occurs with RSV infection, but especially in susceptible hosts, the virus can spread rapidly to the lower respiratory tract, causing bronchiolitis or pneumonia a few days after the onset of rhinorrhea. Virus likely spreads from the upper to the lower respiratory tract primarily by aspiration of secretions. Some cell-cell fusion may occur, but the rapid kinetics of viral spread suggests that this is not the major route of transmission. The virus is believed to replicate primarily in the superficial layer of the respiratory epithelium and is being shed from the apical surface into the lumen of the respiratory tract (Gardner et al, 1970; Neilson and Yunis, 1990; Zhang et al, 2002). Immunohistochemical sections of airway tissues from infected patients demonstrate a patchy distribution of the infection, with only superficial cells expressing viral antigen. Pathological specimens often demonstrate antigen-positive material in the airway, likely representing sloughing of dead infected cells into the airway. During bronchiolitis, wheeze may be audible on auscultation, and tachypnea and crackles are characteristic (Bem et al, 2011; Simoes, 1999). Air trapping and obstructive atelectasis often result in severe bronchiolitis involving alveolar hypoventilation. As a consequence, RSV-infected infants are at risk for respiratory failure associated with bilateral lung infiltrates, severe bronchospasm, moderate to severe hypoxemia and hypercapnia. In about two thirds of the severe cases bronchiolitis is observed, while in the remainder of cases a restrictive pattern (pneumonia) is observed. Most of the latter patients tend to be younger, have more predisposing underlying disease, and require longer ventilation (Simoes, 1999). In case of interstitial pneumonia, there is widespread inflammation and necrosis of lung parenchyma, and severe lesions of the bronchial and bronchiolar mucosa as well (Aherne et al, 1970). In addition to the acute symptoms, young children may also suffer from delayed sequelae of RSV disease. Recurrent wheezing and airway hyperreactivity have been reported later in childhood (Peebles, 2004; Simoes et al, 2007, 2010), and infant age at the time of initial RSV infection seems to be associated with the potential to develop asthma later in childhood (Sigurs et al, 2005; Wu et al, 2008). In adults, particularly in the elderly, RSV-associated upper or lower respiratory tract infection may promote exacerbations of asthma and/or chronic obstructive pulmonary disease (Falsey et al, 2005; Falsey, 2007).

3. Disease drivers

Because the pathogenesis of RSV disease is not very well understood, different concepts are prevailing about which are the primary disease drivers. This controversy has major implications for the development of prophylactic or therapeutic strategies for RSV. A first concept places a dominant focus on the host's immune response in causing severe RSV disease (Graham et al, 2002; Openshaw and Tregoning, 2005; Ostler et al, 2002; Pinto et al, 2006). It postulates that RSV disease is a result from an exaggerated Th_2 cellular response with contributions of bystander killing effects caused by cytotoxic T lymphocytes (CTLs) (Aung et al, 2001; Legg et al, 2003). The concept is influenced heavily by the previous experiences with formalin-inactivated RSV vaccines in the 1960s. However, it may be incomplete and may need adjustment. For instance, RSV disease progression is different in different patient groups. While in immunocompetent individuals RSV disease is more characterized by obstruction of the airway, often accompanied by alveolar sparing (Wohl and Chernick, 1978), RSV-related illness in immunocompromised patients presents more as a progressive pneumonia with alveolar infiltrate and fluid, and with less frequent or less degree of wheezing (Englund et al, 1988; Whimbey et al, 1995). In addition, a study evaluating the immune responses in a collection of autopsy specimens from Chilean infants that unfortunately had suffered from a fatal RSV infection, failed to provide evidence for a predicted pathogenic cytotoxic immune response (Welliver et al, 2007). Instead, massive RSV antigen was detected in the lungs accompanied by a lot of apoptotic sloughing of respiratory cells and an absence of cytotoxic T cells. Moreover, deaths were reported at day 4 after onset of disease. This timing essentially eliminates the possibility that an exaggerated immune response would have contributed substantially to the dramatic outcome. Instead of assuming that severe forms of RSV disease are the result of an hyperresponsive immune response, severe disease might be more a consequence of an inadequate response. The study from Welliver et al. (2007) has indicated an important role of the virus to progress RSV disease. In addition, several studies in children and adults have demonstrated a positive correlation between viral load and RSV disease severity. Infant RSV pathogenesis seems to be driven mainly by a rapid and profound viral replication and the ineffectiveness of an adaptive immune response to limit the infection. Moreover, treatment of RSV disease in infants with corticosteroids seems to be ineffectual (Buckingham et al, 2002; Ermers et al, 2009), and a correlation has been demonstrated between the quantity of RSV in the respiratory tract of infants and disease severity (Buckingham et al, 2000; DeVincenzo et al, 2005). A recent study in experimentally infected adults with RSV demonstrated a close correlation between viral load and manifestation of disease symptoms (DeVincenzo et al, 2010). Symptoms appeared near the time of initial virus detection, peaked in severity near the peak of viral load and decreased concomitantly with a decline in viral load. For drug developers and clinicians it is imperative that such aspects of RSV pathology are well studied and understood in all patient populations because they ultimately drive the decision how preventive measures will have the greatest impact on RSV disease and what type of RSV therapeutics will need to be developed. In addition, understanding the disease pathology may also provide insight on whether patients will benefit most from treatment with direct antivirals, immunomodulators or a combination of both.

4. Prevention

Clinicians and health care agencies for many years have been advocating the need for a safe and effective vaccine against RSV (Crowe, 1995; DMID, 2002). Especially infants in their first few months of life are considered the preferred patient population for vaccination (Chang, 2011; Langley and Anderson, 2011; Simoes, 1999). The first clinical trials with a formalin-inactivated vaccine that was immunogenic and showing high rates of seroconversion, were already performed in the 1960s. However, developing a vaccine for very young RSV-naïve infants seems particularly challenging for a number of reasons (Haas, 2009; Murata, 2009; Nokes et al, 2008). Despite the immunogenicity of the formalin-inactivated vaccine, vaccinated children were not protected from subsequent RSV infections. The immature immune system of these infants and the presence of circulating maternal anti-RSV antibodies may attenuate a robust immune response following vaccination (Crowe, 2001; Schmidt, 2007). It is well-recognized now that natural infection and maternally acquired antibodies only induce partial protection against subsequent infections - even in sequential years - and consequently, there have been concerns about the ability of vaccine candidates to induce protective immunity (Langley & Anderson, 2011). Repeated vaccinations may be required because immune protection after natural infection is only limited in time and re-infection with RSV is common in all stages of life. Vaccine strategies therefore need to elicit an immune response which is more robust and prolonged than the immune response against the natural virus. Strain coverage of candidate vaccines may be limited by the genetic variability and the post-translational processing of some of the viral proteins. In addition, RSV-naïve patients who received the formalin-inactivated vaccine, were more likely than placebo recipients to develop severe RSV disease in the lower respiratory tract than when they were naturally infected with RSV later. The mechanism behind this enhanced disease is not completely clear, although failure of the immunogen to elicit an antibody response with effective neutralizing capacity [due to lack of recognition of the immunogen by pattern recognizing receptors like Toll-like receptors (TLRs)] as well as a RSV-specific CD8+ T cell response and induction by the immunogen of an aberrant CD4+ T cell response, is likely to contribute (Delgado et al, 2009; Kapikian et al, 1969; Kim et al, 1969; Murphy and Walsh, 1988). Analysis of lung tissue from two vaccine recipients who later died of RSV infection demonstrated immunopathology not characteristic of naturally occurring RSV lower respiratory tract infection (Neilson and Yunis, 1990). This experience with vaccine-enhanced disease has probably been the main reason why the development of new RSV-vaccines for RSV-naïve infants has been so cautious. The safety profile of vaccine candidates will have to be monitored very closely during development mainly because a RSV vaccine should elicit an appropriate balance between attenuation and immunogenicity and it should not reduce the safety or efficacy of other vaccines that are routinely administered in infants. Effective clearance of the virus may require the induction of a balanced Th_1/Th_2 adaptive immune response, able to promote production of RSV neutralizing antibodies together with an induction of interferon γ-secreting cytotoxic CD8+ T cells (Bueno et al, 2008; Welliver et al, 2007). Therefore, novel vaccine strategies may include addition of TLR-stimulating adjuvants that may help to find a vaccine that elicits an appropriate immune response which is more robust and prolonged than the immune response against the natural infection. To avoid the challenges described above, an alternative vaccine strategy may be to target healthy children between six months and five years of age or at risk adults in order to promote herd immunity and to eventually indirectly lower the risk of RSV infection in very young infants.

Various strategies have been or are being pursued to develop a safe and effective vaccine against RSV (reviewed in Chang, 2011; Murata, 2009) (Table 1). A major approach is the usage of live-attenuated RSV strains to create a vaccine with the capacity to elicit a protective immune response while avoiding significant disease. Several of such strains, developed using cold passage and/or chemical mutagenesis or reverse genetics, have already been evaluated in clinical trials (Karron et al, 2005; Pringle et al, 1993; Wright et al, 2000, 2006). Vaccination of RSV-naïve infants with cpts248/404, a cold-passaged and mutagenesis-selected live-attenuated RSV strain, resulted in more than 80% infection rate and an approximately 4-fold increase in RSV-specific IgA levels following challenge. The majority of infants that received the vaccine were resistant to infection with a second dose of the vaccine. However, more than 70% of the vaccine recipients developed nasal congestion at the time of peak viral titer, deeming the strain as insufficiently attenuated for use in very young RSV-naïve infants (Wright et al, 2000). This result highlights that finding an appropriate balance between attenuation and immunogenicity is a major challenge for live-attenuated RSV-vaccine candidates. Second-generation live-attenuated RSV strains like rA2cp248/404/1030ΔSH (MEDI-559) and derivatives bearing deletions in the NS2 gene (i.e. rA2cpΔNS2, rA2cp248/404ΔNS2 or rA2cp530/1009ΔNS2) are currently undergoing clinical evaluation in young infants or adults. MEDI-559, now developed by Medimmune, has been demonstrated to elicit an approximately 4-fold increase in anti-RSV antibodies in 44% of previously RSV-naïve patients that received a first vaccine dose (Karron et al, 2005). The results also showed that protective immunity was achieved in a majority of RSV-naïve vaccine recipients. Unfortunately, MEDI-559 shows some genetic and phenotypic instabilities necessitating further improvement of this vaccine candidate (Karron et al, 2005; Murata, 2009).

The immunogenicity and safety of a new nanoemulsion-adjuvanted, inactivated mucosal RSV vaccine in mice was reported recently (Lindell et al, 2011). The water-miscible emulsion droplets (<400 nm size) are believed to inactivate viruses by the physical disruption of the viral envelope. Results showed that the immunization with the vaccine induced durable, RSV-specific humoral responses, both systemically and in the lungs. Vaccinated mice exhibited increased protection against subsequent live viral challenge, which was associated with an enhanced Th_1/Th_{17} response. In these studies, vaccinated mice displayed no evidence of Th_2 mediated immunopotentiation, as has been previously described for other inactivated RSV vaccines. One advantage of this approach may be that these types of vaccines can be kept at ambient temperature before administration. Especially in remote areas of developing countries this could represent a significant logistic benefit. NanoBio, the company that is developing this vaccine candidate announced that a phase I clinical trial is planned.

Initial preclinical studies in rodents immunized with subunit vaccines based on RSV F and G protein have resulted in antibody immune responses and lung pathology comparable to those observed with formalin-inactivated RSV (Murphy et al, 1989, 1990). Because these studies have demonstrated that the use of subunit vaccines may have the potential for disease exacerbation, they have since then been considered inappropriate for the very young RSV-naïve pediatric population. Despite the possibility that the usage of adjuvants (e.g; those recognized by specific TLRs) could improve immunogenicity and

Experimental approach	Company/Institution	Vaccine description	Development stage
Inactivated/ attenuated/ genetically engineered virus	AstraZeneca/MedImmune	MEDI-559	Phase II
	NanoBio/NIH	inactivated virus incorporating a nanoemulsion adjuvant	Preclinical
	Merck	Attenuated strains	Preclinical
	Seattle Children's Research Institute	Inactivated mucosal RSV vaacine, nano-emulsion adjuvated	Preclinical
Subunit-based	Novavax/University of Massachusetts	F-targeting VLP-based	Phase I
	Mymetics/MedImmune	Virosome-based	Preclinical
	ImmunoBiosciences	IPN-1	Preclinical
	TI Pharma	T4-214	Preclinical
	Artificial Cell Technologies	Nanofilm carrier	Preclinical
	iBioPharma	RSV subunits produced by non-engineered plants	Preclinical
	LigoCyte	VLP-based	Preclinical
	TechnoVax	VLP-based	Preclinical
	Pevion Biotech	PEV-4 (virosome-based)	Preclinical
	US Government	G-derived immunogenic peptides	Preclinical
	GlaxoSmithKline/ID Biomedical Corporation of Quebec	F protein polypeptides	Preclinical
	Crucell/Janssen	F protein based	Preclinical
	Mucosis BV	Particles expressing viral antigen and containing *Lactococcus lactis* as adjuvant	Preclinical
	Novartis	F protein derived	Preclinical
	University of Groningen	VLP-based vaccine ± pam3csk4	Preclinical
Vector-based	AstraZeneca/MedImmune	MEDI-534	Phase II
	Bavarian Nordic	MVA-BN RSV (vaccinia-based)	Preclinical
	GenVec/NIAID	Adenovector-based	Preclinical
	AlphaVax	Alphavector-based, producing virus-like replicon particles	Preclinical
	Okairon	Adenovector-based	Preclinical
	Crucell/Janssen	Adenovector-based	Preclinical
DNA-based	Inovio Pharmaceuticals/University of Pennsylvania	IL-12 cytokine gene vaccine adjuvant and DNA vaccine	Preclinical

Table 1. Overview of the different companies/institutions currently running active programs in the development of RSV vaccines and the different vaccine approaches applied. Information was obtained from following sources: Thomson Pharma Partnering, ADIS R&D Insight, Citeline Pipeline, and a variety of public domain sources like scientific literature, patents and press releases.

diminish the adverse effects of protein subunit vaccines, a very cautious approach is being followed in the development of such vaccine candidates. Nevertheless, several subunit vaccines have been evaluated already in the clinic (Table 1). Two preparations were evaluated in phase III clinical trials but were finally discontinued. The first, a purified F protein series (PFP-1, 2 and 3) of vaccines underwent the most extensive clinical evaluation in either RSV-seropositive children (Paradiso et al, 1994; Tristram et al, 1993), children with bronchopulmonary dysplasia (Groothuis et al, 1998) or cystic fibrosis (Piedra et al, 1996, 2003), elderly adults (Falsey and Walsh, 1996, 1997) or pregnant women (Munoz et al, 2003). Although in a majority of the pediatric patients a more than 4-fold increase was observed in RSV-neutralizing titre, the rate of re-infection after vaccination was not different between vaccinees and control subjects. Eventually, the lack of efficacy among the different patient groups resulted in the discontinuation of this vaccine series. BBG2Na, a bacterially expressed protein consisting of an amino acid stretch of subgroup A RSV G protein fused to the albumin-binding domain of streptococcal protein G. This vaccine candidate was discontinued because of some unexpected safety observations in the phase III clinical trial and because of anti-RSV serum antibody titers that dropped significantly within four weeks after vaccination in adults (Power et al, 2001). Currently, several other efforts with subunit vaccines that include the use of F and/or G-derived peptides or virus-like particles (VLPs) are undergoing (pre)clinical evaluation, but limited data are available (Table 1). One exception is a prophylactic VLP-based vaccine candidate from Novavax of which the safety, immunogenicity and tolerability is currently being evaluated in a blinded, placebo-controlled, escalating-dose study in 100 healthy adults between 18 and 49 years old. Novavax recently announced that it expects to report the interim top-line data from this trial in October 2011, and they expect to initiate a phase II trial with their vaccine candidate in the beginning of 2012. In addition, data recently presented on a VLP RSV vaccine that consists of a reconstituted viral envelope with or without incorporated the TLR-2 ligand Pam3CSK4, showed that in the presence of adjuvant, virus-specific serum IgG and IgG2a was increased in mice. Moreover, in cotton rats, the vaccine induced virus neutralizing antibodies and did not predispose for enhanced disease (Stegmann et al, 2010). Some of the peptide-derived vaccines have been struggling with immunogenicity and protective efficacy at least in animal models (Singh et al, 2007a, 2007b; Trudel et al, 1991b). Despite an inefficient neutralizing response, protection against RSV was observed in mice with a RSV G-derived peptide vaccine (Bastien et al, 1999; Trudel et al, 1991a).

Already in the 1990s, different live virus vectors including vaccinia- and adenovirus-derived vectors expressing RSV F and/or G protein, have been designed as vector-based RSV vaccines. Some of these vaccine candidates were abandoned because there was no significant immunogenicity nor protective immunity in primates (Collins et al, 1990; Crowe et al, 1993; de Waal et al, 2004), but others are still actively pursued (Table 1). The current candidates seem to be promising in terms of being sufficiently immunogenic and generating protection against RSV in animal challenge studies, but currently limited clinical evaluation of these vaccine candidates is ongoing. MEDI-534, an intranasal recombinant vaccine which expresses the F proteins of RSV and human parainfluenza 3 together with the hemagglutinin-neuraminidase protein of human PIV-3 in a bovine PIV3 virus genomic backbone, is the only exception, and has been shown to be immunogenic and efficacious in RSV challenge studies in primates (Tang et al, 2004). Recently, results of a phase I trial studying viral take, serum antibody response and safety were encouraging and at the moment, the vaccine is undergoing phase II clinical evaluation in 2-24 month children (van Bleeck et al, 2011). A big advantage of such chimeric vaccine candidates is that they can be developed as a bivalent RSV/PIV vaccine for the pediatric population (Schmidt et al, 2001, 2002; Tang et al, 2003).

Finally, immunization of the host with DNA plasmids that encode for the RSV F or G protein have also been explored, and experiments in rodents have demonstrated that these plasmids are immunogenic and protective to a certain extent (Bembridge et al, 2000a,b; Kumar et al, 2002; Li et al, 1998, 2000). For instance, Inovio Pharmaceuticals recently announced on their company website that they are developing a vaccine that combines an IL-12 cytokine gene vaccine adjuvant and DNA vaccine technology for multiple indications including RSV. The vaccine technology was licensed from the university of Pennsylvania, and is currently undergoing preclinical evaluation (Table 1). The advantages of using this strategy is that the viral proteins can be expressed in the host in their native conformation in the context of the immature immune system of babies, and therefore may overcome the maternal antibody-associated immunosuppression of anti-RSV response (Murata, 2009). However, this technique is far from mature and several technical challenges need to be overcome before this technology can be applied broadly in the clinical setting.

In summary, the development of a RSV vaccine remains a high priority in view of the high disease burden. Considering past experiences with formalin-inactivated vaccine candidates and a limited understanding of the immunopathology of RSV, the way forward to develop a safe and effective vaccine will be a cautious one, and considering the incomplete immune response against natural infection in very young RSV-naïve babies, it may be that two different vaccines need to developed - one for RSV-naïve infants and another for RSV-infected adults. Many different approaches are currently applied to develop a safe and effective vaccine, although only a limited number of vaccine candidates are actually under clinical evaluation. The two most advanced candidate vaccines are MEDI-559 and MEDI-534, currently in phaseI/II of clinical development. However, approval of the first RSV vaccine is not expected before the end of this decade.

5. Immunoprophylaxis

In 1985, two studies reported the protection of cotton rats and primates against subsequent RSV infection by parenteral administration of RSV-neutralizing antibodies (Hemming et al, 1985; Prince et al, 1985). These studies, together with experiences in vaccine trials, initiated the development of a successful strategy of passive immunoprophylaxis against RSV (Table 2).

Approximately one decade later, the first immunoprophylactic agent - RSV immunoglobulin for intravenous administration (RSV-IVIG) - was approved by the US Food and Drug Administration (FDA). Marketed as RespiGam®, the product was licensed for premature infants and children with/without bronchopulmonary dysplasia, and reduced the RSV hospitalization rate in these patients with 41% (PREVENT study group, 1997). In a second trial, performed in patients with congenital heart disease, only a 31% fewer cases of RSV lower respiratory tract infection were observed in the infused group versus the control group, but specifically in those under 6 months of age, a significant 56% reduction of the number of cases was reported (Simoes et al, 1998). Moreover, administration of RespiGam® was also associated with fewer cases and episodes per child of otitis media (PREVENT study group, 1997; Simoes et al, 1996). However, the product was difficult to administer and the infusion had a high volume and high protein content. It also had the potential to interfere with other childhood vaccinations because of the presence of antibodies specific for other pathogens. Moreover, it was not recommended for use in children with congenital heart disease because it had been shown that children with cyanotic heart disease are more likely to experience adverse events upon cardiac surgery if they received RespiGam® (Simoes et al, 1998). The drug was taken of the market in 2004.

After the withdrawal from RespiGam®, the use of RSV-IVIG was replaced by the humanized murine monoclonal antibody palivizumab (Synagis®). This drug (approved by the FDA in 1998) is to be used for prophylaxis in those infants most at risk for developing RSV-associated severe ALRI. A multicenter, randomized trial with 15 mg/kg palivizumab given intramuscularly to children every month during the RSV season, resulted in a 55% reduction of laboratory-confirmed RSV hospitalizations (IMpact-RSV study group, 1998; Johnson et al, 1997). Subgroup analysis further demonstrated a significant reduction in hospitalizations of children with (7.9 % vs. 12.8 %, $P = 0.04$) or without (1.8 % vs. 8.1 %, $P < 0.001$) bronchopulmonary dysplasia compared to the control group. In infants born between 32 and 35 weeks of gestational age, the reduction in hospital admissions (80%) was similar between those with and without bronchopulmonary dysplasia. There was a reduction in hospitalization days and the number of intensive care unit (ICU) admissions among individuals that received palivizumab. Palivizumab was not effective in decreasing the incidence of acute otitis media or non-RSV related admissions. In another study, a 45% reduction in hospitalization rate was observed in children with congenital heart disease that received palivizumab versus individuals that received placebo (Feltes et al, 2003). No significant differences were observed in number of deaths, number of ICU admissions, length of stay in ICU, need for mechanical ventilation or length of mechanical ventilation, although it has to be mentioned that the study was not powered to differences in these outcomes. In the clinical trials, the antibody was found safe and well tolerated with less than 3% of antibody recipients showing injection site reactions (IMpact-RSV study group, 1998). Pre- and postlicensure monitoring have not revealed any excess mortality or significant safety problems with palivizumab (Mohan, et al, 2004; Romero, 2003). However, the high cost of the product restricts the use of palivizumab to very young pediatric patients in the developed world, and serious questions are currently being raised about the cost-benefit balance of the product (Hampp et al, 2011; Morris et al, 2009; Smart et al, 2010; Wang et al, 2011). Palivizumab patents will begin to expire from 2015 onwards, and the entrance of biogenerics is expected because of the worldwide market potential. Availability of cheaper biogenerics may represent a game changer, although their potential market impact remains unclear for the moment. For instance, will generic palivizumab ever be cheap enough for use in resource-poor countries?

In an effort to improve immunoprophylactic therapy, next-generation antibodies are being developed and some of them are already progressing through clinical development. A second-generation monoclonal antibody, motavizumab (MedImmune), has completed phase III noninferiority clinical evaluation. Motavizumab is an affinity-matured variant of palivizumab which gives improved protection to the upper respiratory tract and aims to reduce the number of treatment failures that are associated with palivizumab (Wu et al, 2007, 2008). In a randomized, double-blind Phase III trial in at risk infants, the primary endpoint of noninferiority of motavizumab was met by demonstrating a 26% reduction of hospital admission relative to palivizumab (Carbonell-Estrany et al, 2010). The overall occurance of adverse or serious adverse events did not differ between the 2 groups, but on June 2, 2010, the FDA's Antiviral Drugs Advisory Committee panel voted not to recommend motavizumab for licensure, raising concerns about hypersensitivity issues (allergic skin rash occurring within two days of dosing) as a primary safety alarm during the risk-benefit assessment of motivizumab (Young, 2010). In December last year, MedImmune withdrew its application for licensure of motavizumab and announced that the product will not be further developed for immunoprophylaxis of severe RSV infection. Nevertheless, the antibody has been explored in two randomized, double-blind, placebo-controlled Phase II trials both to evaluate the therapeutic potential in children up to 12 months of age, but no results have been published so far.

ADMA Biologics Inc. has recently evaluated RI-001, a new high-titer RSV-IVIG, in a Phase II trial in immunosuppressed patients with a confirmed upper respiratory RSV infection and at risk for developing severe ALRI. Primary outcome of the study was circulating RI-001 and secondary outcome was the incidence of progression from URTI to LRTI, but no results have been made public.

One other antibody is currently undergoing Phase I clinical evaluation. MEDI-557, a third-generation monoclonal antibody derived from motavizumab, contains a triple mutation known as YTE that extents the half-life of the antibody. A randomised, double-blind phase I study is currently underway in the US to evaluate the safety, tolerability and pharmacokinetics of a single intravenous dose of MEDI-557, although the FDA's decision on motavizumab may impact the development of MEDI-557.

Finally, several antibodies are currently progressed through the preclinical pipeline (Table 2). One of the antibodies, ALX-0171 has recently been shown to reduce RSV viral load in cotton rats, even when administered two days after infection (van Bleeck, 2011). ALX-0171 was also found superior to palivizumab in a plaque-reduction assay of a panel of 51 out of 61 recent clinical RSV isolates. The molecule is a trivalent anti-RSV nanobody consisting of three identical epitopes, based on the smallest functional fragments of heavy chain-only antibodies found in camels and llamas. Ablynx announced on their company website that the program is on track to enter Phase I clinical trials in healthy volunteers during the course of 2011. Evaluation of ALX-0171 as a therapeutic agent may reveal the efficiency of this novel approach.

In summary, many different programs are ongoing to develop new immunoprophylactic agents. Palivizumab today remains the only available agent to prevent severe RSV infection, and although it has been shown to significantly reduce the hospitalization rate in high-risk pediatric patients, more data are needed to demonstrate whether immunoprophylaxis could have a significant impact also on outcomes like death rate, need for mechanical ventilation or reduction of long-term symptomology associated with RSV, like long-term wheezing or asthma development. Moreover, palivizumab treatment is expensive and economic analyses suggest that the use of palivizumab is only cost effective in the highest risk children. For these reasons palivizumab is not broadly available to the general RSV population. The major challenge for the immunoprophylactic agents will be to use them in a cost-effective and judicious manner. The potential appearance of biogenerics or cheaper production processes may present as potential game changers.

Company/Institution	Antibody description	Development stage
AstraZeneca/MedImmune	RespiGam® (RSV-IVIG)	Launched
AstraZeneca/MedImmune	Synagis® (palivizumab)	Launched
ADMA Biologics	RI-001	Phase II
AstraZeneca/MedImmune	MEDI-557	Phase I
Ablynx	ALX-0171®	Preclinical
AstraZeneca/MedImmune	F protein monoclonal antibodies	Preclinical
Symphogen	Polyclonal antibodies against F and G protein	Preclinical
Symphogen	Sym-003 (fully humanized Mab)	Preclinical
Medarex/MedImmune	Mabs using HuMab-Mouse technology	Preclinical
Intracel	HumaRESP (fully humanized Mab)	Preclinical
Kenta Biotech	KBRV-201 (series of human Mabs)	Preclinical
Bioresponse	Polyclonal antibodies against F and G	Preclinical

Table 2. Overview of the different companies/institutions currently active in the development of RSV immunoprophylactic therapy and the different approaches applied.

6. Treatment

Ribavirin (Virazole®) was approved in 1986 in the US for treatment of RSV infection, and is currently the only approved agent for this indication (Ventre & Randolph, 2007). Ribavirin is a nucleoside analog that seems to act by mutagenic incorporation into the viral genome, although the mechanism of action is not fully known. The drug is administered as a small-particle aerosol, 6-18 hrs daily for a period of 3-7 days. Although initial clinical studies in a limited number of subjects indicated a modest beneficial effect on viral load and clinical symptoms, follow-on studies only provided questionable evidence of benefit upon treatment of severe infections (Hall et al, 1983; Ventre & Randolph, 2007). In addition, potential for toxic effects in health care workers (Virazole package insert), and high cost (Glanville et al, 2005) have led to a situation in which ribavirin is not routinely used by most centers to treat RSV in otherwise healthy children. Currently, the American Academy of Pediatrics does not generally recommend ribavirin treatment for RSV infections (American Academy of Pediatrics, 2006).

RSV therapy will likely extend to patient groups other than at risk infants over the next decade (e.g. the at risk adults or children suffering from an acute RSV-confirmed upper respiratory tract infection to prevent severe ALRI), not only because therapeutic options with antibodies may expand beyond the very young infants, but also because of ongoing development programs of small-molecules and small interfering RNA (siRNA) agents that may be more suitable for treating patient groups not eligible for prophylactic antibody therapy (Roymans and Koul, 2010).

6.1 Antivirals

6.1.1 N-protein inhibitors

Two investigational agents targeting the nucleocapsid (N) protein, critical to viral replication of RSV, are currently in Phase II clinical evaluation (Table 3). ALN-RSV01 (Alnylam), a siRNA with the potential to be a new class of drugs to treat human disease, and the small molecule RSV-604 (Arrow Therapeutics/Novartis). In a first randomized, placebo-controlled Phase IIa trial, intranasally administered ALN-RSV01 was evaluated in healthy adults challenged with RSV (DeVincenzo et al, 2010). Patients were treated once daily for two days before and three days after RSV inoculation with a nasal spray containing either ALN-RSV01 or placebo, resulting in an approximately 38% decrease in the number of infections detected by quantitative culture of patients that received the investigational agent as compared to patients receiving placebo. In a second randomized, placebo-controlled Phase IIb trial, the safety and efficacy of the product was evaluated in lung transplant patients with a confirmed RSV infection (Zamora et al, 2011). ALN-RSV01 was reported to be well tolerated, with no drug-related serious adverse events or post-inhalation perturbations in lung function. Despite the observation that viral AUC on days 0 to 6

Company/Institution	Therapeutic description	Development stage
Valeant/Shering Plough	Virazole® – Rebetol® (ribavirin)	Launched
Alnylam/Kyowa	ALN-RSV01	Phase II
Alnylam/Kyowa/cubist	ALN-RSV second generation	Phase II
Arrow Therapeutics/Novartis	RSV-604	Phase II
Clarassance	CG-100	Phase II
Microdose Therapeutx	MDT-637 (VP-14637)	Phase I
AstraZeneca/MedImmune	motavizumab	Phase I
Alnylam	Intranasally administered siRNA molecules	Preclinical
Sirnaomics	STP-92 (siRNA delivered through nanoparticle based delivery systems)	Preclinical
Inhibikase	iKT-041 (small molecule RSV inhibitor)	Preclinical
Biota/MedImmune	Second generation small-molecule F inhibitors	Preclinical
Shared Research/University of Tokyo/Todai TLO	siRNA delivered by cationic polyamino acids	Preclinical
Chimerix	Small-molecule nucleoside analogs	Preclinical
AstraZeneca/Trellis Bioscience	Monoclonal antibodies	Preclinical
Mapp Biopharmaceutical	Monoclonal antibodies	Preclinical
AIMM Therapeutics	Monoclonal antibodies	Preclinical

Table 3. Overview of the different companies/institutions currently active in the development of RSV therapeutics and the different approaches applied.

trended lower in the ALN-RSV01 group, no statistically significant antiviral effect could be shown. Interpretation of the viral load data was reported to be confounded by baseline differences between the two groups and by time from symptom onset to first dose (Zamora et al, 2011). However, mean daily symptom scores were lower in individuals that received ALN-RSV01, and the mean cumulative daily total symptom score over a time period of 14 days was significantly lower with ALN-RSV01 (114.7 ± 63.13 vs. 189.3 ± 99.59, P = 0.035). The rate of new or progressive bronchiolitis obliterans syndrome (BOS) was significantly lower (6.3 % vs. 50 %, P = 0.027) in patients who received the study drug relative to the control group, raising the possibility that ALN-RSV01 may be able to lower the risk of late serious clinical sequelae associated with RSV infection like BOS or morbidity and mortality that originate from loss of lung function. Alnylam is also developing second-generation siRNA molecules against RSV. It is expected that a phase IIb pediatric study with the second-generation molecule will start soon.

RSV-604 (Arrow Therapeutics), an oral benzodiazepine with submicromolar potency against RSV A and B subfamilies (Chapman et al, 2007), is being developed in collaboration with Novartis. The safety and efficacy of this compound was tested in a multi-center trial that included RSV-infected adult bone marrow transplant patients. Although initiated in 2005, the study was only completed in the beginning of this year and data from the trial are still expected to be released. In addition, RSV-604 is also undergoing Phase I evaluation with pediatric formulations.

6.1.2 Entry inhibitors

Another interesting strategy to tackle RSV infection is to disturb the virus entry process. Enveloped viruses like RSV, HIV-1 or influenza virus need to attach and fuse with a host cell in order to deposit their genome and to initiate their replication cycle (Lamb and Jardetzky, 2007). In RSV, attachment and fusion are facilitated by the attachment (G) and fusion (F) protein, although it has been shown that the F protein is sufficient to lead to productive viral replication (Karron et al, 1997; Techaarpornkul et al, 2001). It is thought that either G and/or F bind to a specific host cell receptor in order to initiate the entry process, but how exactly this happens remains largely unknown. Binding to glycosaminoglycans containing heparin sulphate has been reported as a potential receptor candidate since addition of heparin blocks virus attachment in vitro (Hallak et al, 2000; Krusat and Streckert, 1997). Recently, evidence was reported strongly suggesting that nucleolin may be a cellular receptor for RSV (Tayyari et al, 2011; van Bleeck et al, 2010). The results were validated via several different strategies. It was shown for instance that nucleolin antibody neutralization and RNAi knock-down of nucleolin was able to inhibit RSV infection, turning nucleolin into a potential target for development of anti-RSV therapeutics (Tayyari et al, 2011).

MBX 300 (NMSO-3), a sulphated sialyl lipid, has been under development by Microbiotix as an attachment inhibitor since it seems to target the G protein (Table 3). The compound has an EC_{50} of approximately 0.2-0.3 μM and appears to be a specific inhibitor for RSV (Douglas, 2004; Kimura et al, 2000). In cotton rats, lung viral titers were reduced significantly when animals were treated intraperitoneally with a daily dose of 100 mg/kg/day (Douglas, 2004). MBX 300 was reported by Microbiotix to display potent oral anti-RSV efficacy and safety in preclinical evaluation, including primates, but no further development activities were announced recently.

The market approval of palivizumab has validated F as a clinically relevant target. Since then, drug research has been focusing on this protein as a target for developing next-generation therapeutics including antibodies and small-molecule inhibitors (Bonfanti and Roymans, 2009; Roymans and Koul, 2010). The availability of structural information on how small-molecules can inhibit the virus-host fusion process has helped in understanding this process better and also helped in identifying potential drug binding pockets in the F protein (Cianci et al, 2004b; Roymans et al, 2010).

RSV-IVIG and palivizumab have also been clinically evaluated as potential therapeutic agents, but the studies have resulted in a mixed outcome. A first randomized, double-blind, placebo-controlled trial with RSV-IVIG in previously healthy children less than 2 years of age hospitalized with a proven RSV lower tract infection, reported some beneficial effect of RSV-IVIG treatment in a subgroup of children with more severe disease, but no evidence was found in the total study cohort for reduced hospitalization or reduced ICU stay when patients were treated with RSV-IVIG compared to placebo recipients (Rodriguez et al, 1997a). A second trial with RSV-IVIG in hospitalized children younger than 2 years at high risk for severe RSV infections did not show any efficacy (Rodriguez et al, 1997b). In addition, two randomized, double-blind, placebo-controlled multicenter trials in previously healthy children less than 2 years of age hospitalized with acute RSV infection demonstrated no difference in disease severity or clinical outcome between patients treated with a single intravenous dose of palivizumab or placebo, albeit that a reduction in tracheal viral load was observed in one study (Malley et al, 1998; Sáez-Llorens et al, 2004).

Despite these mixed outcomes , some programs aim to maximize the therapeutic potential of antibodies to treat RSV (Table 3). Companies like AIMM Therapeutics, Symphogen, Trellis Bioscience or Mapp Biopharmaceutical in collaboration with Vanderbilt University are developing monoclonal antibodies targeting the envelope proteins of RSV. Especially when extracellular (viral) proteins are targeted, therapeutic use of antibodies can be envisioned to limit the infection, provided the antibody is properly delivered in the lung.

In 2003, a very potent series against RSV of substituted benzimidazoles was reported by Johnson & Johnson (Andries et al, 2003). Exemplified by JNJ-2408068, selected as a candidate for clinical evaluation, the series was putatively shown to target the F protein on the basis of in vitro selection of resistance associated mutations and time-of-addition experiments. JNJ-2408068 has an EC_{50} = 0.16 nM and SI > 625 x 10^3, and was demonstrated to be active against both A and B sybtypes of RSV as well as a panel of clinical isolates. Although the compound reduced lung viral titers in cotton rats to undetectable levels when administered by aerosol shortly prior to or after virus challenge (Wyde et al, 2003), it showed an unfavorable PK profile in terms of tissue retention (Bonfanti et al, 2007). The aminoethylpiperidine moiety was identified as being responsible for the long elimination half-life from several tissues. The subsequent back-up program was focused on the modulation of this basic part of the molecule. The objectives were to reduce the elimination half-life from tissues while keeping the high activity level. This lead optimization program resulted in the discovery of TMC353121 as a clinical candidate (Bonfanti et al, 2008). The in vivo efficacy of this new antiviral was demonstrated in the cotton rat model by different routes of administration: inhalation (1.25 mg/mL solution in the reservoir of the nebulizer) and IV (10 mg/kg dose) lead to >90% inhibition versus control, and oral (40 mg/kg dose) lead to > 80% inhibition versus control. Recent PK-PD modeling of this compound indicated that in order to reach

50% inhibition of the viral load in the cotton rat, a plasma concentration of 200 ng/ml is required, a concentration much higher than the 50% inhibitory concentration observed in vitro in HeLaM cells (0.07 ng/ml)(Rouan et al, 2010). In addition, it was shown in a RSV infectious mouse model that TMC353121 can be used either prophylactically or therapeutically to decrease RSV lung infection and virus-associated lung inflammation and histopathology (Olszewska et al, 2011). Single-dose intravenous administration up to 48 hours after infection reduced the RSV viral load with 1 to 2 log_{10} at the peak of infection (day 4 post-RSV inoculation in the mouse model), indicating that the window between onset of infection and onset of treatment has a practical utility for RSV infections in the clinical setting (Hegele, 2011). Moreover, investigation of lung histopathology, measurement of inflammatory cells and chemical mediators in bronchoalveolar lavage fluids also demonstrated that host immune and inflammatory responses were attenuated significantly.

A series of benzotriazole benzimidazoles was reported by researchers from Brystol-Myers Squibb as a class of inhibitors that prevent fusion of RSV with the host cell membrane (Meanwell and Krystal, 2007). BMS433771, an azabenzimidazolone derivative, binds to a hydrophobic pocket situated in the central trimeric coiled-coil formed upon refolding of F after initiation of the viral fusion process (Cianci et al, 2004b). The compound was shown to be active against multiple strains and clinical isolates from both A and B subfamilies of RSV with an EC_{50} of approximately 20 nM (Cianci et al, 2004c). In addition, rodent models were used to assess the in vivo activity of BMS-433771 after oral administration. The maximum effect observed was > 1 log_{10} reduction in viral load at doses of ≥ 5mg/kg in BALB/c mice and ≥ 50 mg/kg in cotton rats (Cianci et al, 2004a).

Wyeth-Ayerst discovered RFI-641, a biphenyl triazine cationic compound that inhibits both A and B subfamilies of RSV with EC_{50} values around 20 nM and with 417 < SI < 2500 (Huntley et al, 2002; Nikitenko et al, 2001). The compound is an analog of CL-309623, a previously identified dendrimer-like stilbene-containing inhibitor with anti-RSV activity (Gazumyan et al, 2000). RFI-641 was shown to inhibit fusion and to interact directly with the RSV F protein (Razinkov et al, 2002). The in vivo potency of RFI-641 was evaluated in different animal model systems (Huntley et al, 2002; Weiss et al, 2003). RFI-641 administered intravenously did not exhibited efficacy in vivo, and therefore, this route of administration was not pursued. However, 1.3 mg/kg intranasally delivered compound 2h prior virus challenge in mice reduced virus lung titers by 1.5 log_{10}, and in cotton rats a dose of 10 mg/kg reduced the lung viral titer by 2.6 to 3.2 log_{10} when given at a same prophylactic dosing regimen. In the African Green Monkey model, RFI-641-treated monkeys exhibited a 3.4 log_{10} reduction in viral load. At the 6 mg dose, viral titers were significantly lower on days 4 to 9 (peak viral load) with a 1.8 to 3.4 log_{10} reduction. In addition, daily therapeutic intranasal administration of RFI-641, initiated 24 h after RSV infection in monkeys, also reduced viral titers.

In 2005, Biota Holdings Ltd. published a patent claiming the discovery of imidazoisoindolone derivatives as a new class of fusion inhibitors of RSV (Bond et al, 2005). BTA9881, was selected as a clinical candidate. The compound is orally bioavailable and has been shown to demonstrate favorable pharmacokinetics in phase I clinical trials (Bond, 2007). However, the clinical development of BTA9881 was stopped because the compound failed to develop an acceptable safety profile. Rights to the compound have been returned by AstraZeneca to Biota, which will attempt to develop more attractive derivatives. In this respect, Biota announced that they discovered a new series of orally bioavailable RSV fusion inhibitors and they recently published a patent application claiming a new series of fused imidazopyrazinones as RSV fusion inhibitors, with the most potent compounds having a single digit nM in vitro antiviral activity (Mitchell et al, 2011).

Multiple compounds have been in development as a specific RSV fusion inhibitor. However, the attrition rate during pharmaceutical development has been high, and none of the above described compounds are in clinical development today; either as a result of strategic decisions taken by the developing companies or because of unfavorable pharmaceutical properties of the compounds. The only small-molecule fusion inhibitor under clinical evaluation today is MDT-637, developed by MicroDose Therapeutx. MDT-637 was previously reffered to as VP-14637, a bis-tetrazole-benzhydrylphenol derivative, with an EC_{50} = 0.001 μM against RSV in vitro (Douglas et al, 2003). In addition, cotton rats that received as little as 126 μg drug/kg by divided-dose aerosol starting 1 day after viral challenge with either a RSV A or B subtype had significantly lower mean pulmonary RSV titers and reduced histopathology scores than control animals (Wyde et al, 2005). VP-14637 was in Phase I trials prior to a decision from ViroPharma not to develop it further as an aerosol, partly because of excessive organic solvent content of the aerosol, partly because of strategic reasons. In 2009, MicroDose Therapeutx acquired the assets from ViroPharma and they re-formulated MDT-637 as a dry powder for inhalation. Preclinical results have demonstrated that the product can be effectively delivered in both the upper and lower respiratory tract (van Bleeck, 2010), and a Phase I trial assessing the safety, tolerability and pharmacokinetic profile of MDT-637 in 48 healthy adult volunteers is initiated.

6.1.3 RNA-dependant RNA polymerase inhibitors

Two different classes of compounds that target the polymerase complex of RSV have been reported. Screening of a large chemical library resulted in the discovery of benzazepines as inhibitors of RSV (Sudo et al, 2005). YM-53403 was selected as an interesting candidate, and exhibited an EC_{50} = 0.2 μM in a RSV plaque reduction assay. Time-of-addition experiments suggested inhibition to be maximal around 8 h after virus exposure and mutant viruses with single point mutations in the polymerase (L) protein were resistant to inhibition with YM-53403, indicating the compound to be an inhibitor of the RSV L protein. The discovery of a second inhibitor of RSV polymerase through screening of a chemical library with a poly(A) capture assay was reported in 2004 by researchers from Boehringer Ingelheim (Mason et al, 2004). Shortly after, a series of imidazo[4,5-h]isoquinoline-7,9-dione inhibitors were synthesized that target the 5′ capping of viral mRNA transcripts (Liuzzi et al, 2005). The most potent compound, compound D, exhibited an antiviral EC_{50} = 0.021 μM (polymerase IC_{50} = 0.089 μM) with a SI ≤ 400. Lung virus titers in a mouse model were reduced upon intranasal administration of the compounds 3 and 6h post-viral challenge, and then three times daily for 3 days at 0.4-4.1 mk/kg/day. Today none of these compounds are actively developed as a therapeutic.

6.2 Bronchodilators

RSV bronchiolitis resembles asthma in that both conditions cause air trapping and wheezing because of increased airway resistance. Therefore, several drugs that are being used to treat reversible airway smooth muscle constriction in asthma have also been tested in children with RSV infection. However, multiple clinical trials suggest that treatment with β2-

adrenoreceptor agonists like albuterol, only offer a modest short-term improvement (Gadomski and Bhasale, 2010). Racemic epinephrine treatment has been shown to relieve some respiratory distress, but no effect on length of hospitalization could be demonstrated (Langley et al, 2005). Epinephrine stimulates both α- and β-adrenergic receptors, but it is thought that its α-adrenoreceptor stimulation of the sympathetic nervous system could be expected to reduce mucosal edema and to increase airway caliber (Barr et al, 2000). However, a recent study could not demonstrate a difference in effectivity between high volume normal saline alone and nebulized salbutamol-normal saline, epinephrine-normal saline, or 3% saline in mild bronchiolitis (Anil et al, 2010). The reason for the observed discrepancies in the clinical trial results may be that RSV bronchiolitis is caused by a fixed high resistance of the bronchioles due to their small size - potentially further facilitated by sloughed cells and high mucous content - rather than it being caused by reversible smooth muscle constriction, but another reason for the persisting controversy about bronchodilator responsiveness in bronchiolitis could be the lack of sufficiently sensitive methods for assessing lung function in young children (Modl et al, 2000, 2005). A thorough investigation of such factors may help to settle this controversy, and consequently may contribute on how to properly treat RSV infection.

6.3 Anti-inflammatory agents

After adverse responses to formalin-inactivated RSV vaccination were reported, a believe derived that RSV disease following infection is driven by an exuberant pathogenic immune response (Aung et al, 2001; Kapikian et al, 1969; Kim et al, 1969; Legg et al, 2003). Attempts have been made to develop anti-inflammatory therapy to reduce RSV respiratory distress. Although corticosteroids are commonly used by physicians as anti-inflammatory therapy, a review of more than a dozen clinical trials in both outpatient and hospitalized settings indicated that the drug is of no benefit on its own (Patel et al, 2004). Systemic administration of prednisolone and topical application of fluticasone, budesonide, and deoxiribonuclease I were ineffective (Bulow et al, 1999; Cade et al, 2000; Nasr et al, 2001; Wong et al, 2000). Intravenous dexamethasone had little effect, although when the drug was received by inhalation, patients hospital stay seemed to be reduced (Bentur et al, 2005; Buckingham et al, 2002). Recent data however illustrate that, at least in children, severe forms of RSV disease are related to inadequate rather than hyperresponsive immune reactions (DeVincenzo, 2007; Welliver et al, 2007; Welliver, 2008). Since these compounds only have an effect on the hyper-inflammatory response and not on the virus directly, a more effective treatment might be the combination of an antiviral and an anti-inflammatory compound. A combination of palivizumab and a glucocorticosteroid significantly reduced the RSV viral load in lungs from cotton rats over 3 $\log_{10}$ and reduced pulmonary histopathology significantly (Prince et al, 2000).

A clinical trial reported in 2003 with montelukast, a selective and competitive antagonist of cysteinyl leukotrienes, indicated a possible general reduction of lung symptoms and an improvement in persistent wheezing after RSV-induced bronchiolitis (Bisgaard, 2003). Although cysteinyl leukotrienes seem to contribute to the pathophysiology of RSV-induced bronchiolitis and thus may represent an interesting therapeutic target (Dimova-Yaneva et al, 2004; Oh et al, 2005; Wedde-Beer et al, 2002), the trial results were confounded by the included patient population and conclusions made on improvement of post-bronchiolitis reactive airway disease considering the 4 week therapy window (López-Andreu et al, 2004; Szefler and Simoes, 2003). As the patient population included both very young infants and children up to 36 months of age, the study effects may have been biased towards effects in the older children; i.e. children that did experience RSV infection in the 1 or 2 previous seasons, and at the time of study, presented with post-RSV reactive airway disease that responds to montelukast (Stein et al, 1999; Szefler and Simoes, 2003). Unfortunately, results from 3 prospective randomized, double-blind, placebo-controlled follow-on trials in children less than 24 months of age were not consistent, leaving a potential benefit of montelukast treatment on post-RSV bronchiolitis symptoms unclear. A first study in 979 patients randomized to placebo or to montelukast treatment at 4 or 8 mg/day for 4 or 20 weeks did not show a significant difference in the percentage of symptom-free days (SFD) over a treatment period of 4 weeks (Bisgaard et al, 2008). In both groups, % SFD was approximately 29%. Post hoc analyses of patients with persistent symptoms (SFD ≤ 30% over weeks 1-2) resulted in slight differences in % SDF over weeks 3 to 24 of 5.7 to 5.9 for montelukast (4 or 8 mg/day, respectively) versus placebo groups. A second study in 58 pediatric patients hospitalized with a first episode of RSV bronchiolitis seemed to confirm the conclusions of the previous study, and concluded that montelukast treatment did not reduce symptoms of cough and wheeze (Proesmans et al, 2009). During the three month trial period, no differences between the treatment and control groups were observed for symptom-free days and nights, and during the one year follow-up, no significant differences were observed in the number of exacerbations or time to first exacerbations, number of unscheduled visits and need to start inhaled steroids. However, a third study performed in 200 children treated with or without 4 mg/day of montelukast for 3 months showed a significantly decreased level of serum eosinophil-derived neurotoxin in treated patients versus placebo controlled patients that remained significantly different for the entire 12-month follow-up period. In addition, cumulative recurrent wheezing episodes at 12 months were significantly lower in the montelukast-treated group (Kim et al, 2010).

Leflunomide (Arava®, Aventis Pharmaceuticals) (Table 4), an immunosuppressive agent approved for treatment of patients with rheumatoid arthritis and currently evaluated in Phase I clinical trials in transplant patients (Williams et al, 2002), has previously been shown to exert a powerful antiviral activity against several viruses like cytomegalovirus and herpes simplex virus (Chong et al, 2006; Knight et al, 2001; Waldman et al, 1999). Recently, it has been demonstrated that the A77 active metabolite of leflunomide dose-dependently inhibits RSV in cell cultures and in vivo (Dunn et al, 2011). Pulmonary viral load in RSV-inoculated cotton rats was reduced > 3 $\log_{10}$ in leflunomide-treated animals versus controls, even when treatment was delayed until day 3 post-challenge.

CG-100 is an intratracheal formulation of recombinant human CC10 (Clara cell 10 kD protein; uteroglobin) under development by Clarassance for the treatment of severe RSV infections and other respiratory indications (Table 4). CC10 protein has several clinical applications in inflammatory, fibrotic, and autoimmune diseases, particularly respiratory diseases. More recently, CC10 has been found to reduce viral titers for influenza and RSV. Two Phase 1/2 clinical trials have been completed with CC10. The first trial was conducted in premature infants with respiratory distress syndrome who were at risk of developing bronchopulmonary dysplasia. These patients are deficient in their own CC10 supply due to extreme prematurity and underdevelopment of the lungs. In this study, CC10 was safe and well-tolerated and demonstrated powerful anti-inflammatory effects in the short term and profound protective effects in keeping infants out of the hospital for respiratory causes over the long term (6 to 12 months after a single dose). The second trial was performed in healthy adult volunteers with seasonal allergies. CC10 was also safe and well tolerated in these patients. Furthermore, no drug interactions between CC10 and other drugs such as antibiotics, diuretics, decongestants, antihistamines were observed in either trial.

Synairgen and the Jewesh Children Hospital are applying other strategies to tackle RSV infection (Table 4). Synairgen is developing SYN-11, an inhalable interferon beta, in an effort to improve the innate immune respons against RSV. The Jewesh Children Hospital has a program in preclinical development evaluating the efficacy of POPG, palmitoyl-oleoyl-phosphatidylglycerol, one of several lipids in the fluid that lines the air sacs of the lungs. POPG, together with other lipids and proteins in the surfactant fluid, is known to prevent collapse of the air sacs and to contribute to innate immunity. Gilead is developing small-molecule TLR7 agonists with broad-spectrum antiviral activity including RSV. Interferon-alpha production in human peripheral blood mononuclear cells could be induced with a minimum effective concentration of 1 nM.

Company/Institution	Anti-inflammatory/broad-spectrum description	Development stage
Functional Genetics	FGI-101-1A6	Phase I
Respivert/Centocor Ortho Biotech	RV 568	Phase I
Clarassance	CG-100 (Clara cell 10 kD protein or uteroglobin)	Phase I
Synairgen	SYN-11 (inhaled interferon beta)	Preclinical
Jewesh Children Hospital	POPG (palmitoyl-oleoyl-phosphatidylglycerol)	Preclinical
Functional Genetics	FGI-110 (an anti-Nedd4 monoclonal antibody)	Preclinical
Functional Genetics	FGI-103723 (small-molecule caspase 2 inhibitor)	Preclinical
Functional Genetics	FGI-102100 (small-molecule TSG101 inhibitor)	Preclinical
Gilead	Small-molecule TLR7 agonists	Preclinical
Summit	Imino sugars for treatment of CMV, HSV, RSV & VZV	Preclinical
Ohio State University Medical Center	Leflunomide (Arava®, Aventis Pharmaceuticals)	Preclinical
Pathfinder Pharmaceuticals	Compounds restoring host cell defense	Preclinical
Kineta	rOAS-1 (natural human protein for treatment of HCV, RSV & influenza A)	Preclinical
Emory University	JMN3-003 (small-molecule RdRp inhibitor against influenza A, RSV, PIV-3, …	Preclinical

Table 4. Overview of the different companies/institutions currently active in the development of anti-inflammatory compounds against RSV and broad-spectrum antivirals, and the different approaches applied.

In summary, clinical trial results with anti-inflammatory agents are somewhat conflicting but have up to now resulted in modest short-term benefits at best. However, studies with new anti-inflammatory compounds show promise as a potential treatment for RSV disease (Table 4). It will be interesting to see whether anti-inflammatory compounds have the potential as a single drug solution or whether they are most effective in a combination therapy with antiviral compounds.

6.4 Broad-spectrum antivirals

Targeting of a host cell factor is an antiviral strategy that has received considerable interest the last couple of years (Table 4). This approach is expected to increase the barrier for spontaneous viral escape from inhibition, since the loss of a host factor is less likely compensated by viral mutations than the high-affinity binding of a pathogen-directed antiviral with its viral target site. Because of some overlap in the host cell pathways used by different viruses to successfully replicate, this strategy offers potential to discover agents with broad-spectrum antiviral activity, and to move beyond the 'one-bug-one-drug' paradigm. A potential downside of the strategy is the higher potential for undesirable side effects induced by these drugs, although short-term treatment of acute infections like RSV may render drug-induced side effects tolerable to some extent.

In 2007, several micromolar hits were reported from a RNase L target-based high-throughput screen with the two most active compounds exhibiting EC_{50}s of 26 and 22 μM (Thakur et al, 2007). RNase L is a principal mediator of innate immunity to viral infections in vertebrates, and is required for a complete interferon antiviral response against certain RNA viruses (Malathi et al, 2007). Compounds were shown to bind to the 2-5A binding domain of RNase L, thereby inducing RNase L dimerization and activation. Interestingly, broad-spectrum antiviral activity against different types of RNA viruses was demonstrated, including human parainfluenza virus 3 (hPIV-3), but unfortunately, activity against RSV was not tested in this study.

In the same year, a paper appeared that reported the potential of arbidol as a broad-spectrum antiviral. The compound was found antivirally active in cellular infection assays of influenza A, RSV, human rhinovirus type 14, coxsackie virus B3 and adenovirus type 7, with EC_{50}s ranging from 2.7 to 13.8 μg/ml (Shi et al, 2007). Orally administered arbidol at 50 or 100 mg/kg/day starting at 24h before virus exposure and continuing for 6 days, reduced mean lung influenza A titers significantly as well as mortality.

Recently, JMN3-003 has been optimized from a class of compounds that was identified from a high-throughput screening campaign that aimed for discovering compounds with acceptable antiviral activity and selectivity index against a number of viruses (Krumm et al, 2011). JMN3-003 indeed demonstrates activity against members of both the ortho- and paramyxoviridae like influenza, RSV and hPIV-3, with EC_{50}-values ranging from 0.01 to 0.08 μM. The compound was found metabolically stable after incubation with S9 hepatocyte subcellular fraction, and viral escape attempts failed to induce resistance after prolonged exposure to JMN3-003. Extensive experimentation to elucidate the mechanism of action of the compound revealed that it blocks a host factor that is required for viral RNA-dependent RNA polymerase activity.

In addition to the examples above, many similar programs, targeting host factors like caspases (Kinch and Goldblatt, 2009a), TSG101 (Kinch and Goldblatt, 2009b), EGFR (jung,

2010; Monick et al, 2005), or kinases (Kalman, 2008) are currently in different stages of preclinical development (Table 4). The most advanced programs today are in Phase I clinical development. For instance, RV 568 is a small-molecule, narrow-spectrum phosphotransferase inhibitor under development by RespiVert (Centocor Ortho Biotech) as an inhaled therapy for lung and airway disorders such as asthma, chronic obstructive pulmonary disease, and allergic rhinitis. Moreover, efficacy studies in BALB/c mice infected with RSV, demonstrated a 83% and 67% inhibition of lung viral titer on days 3 and 5, respectively, when animals were treated with 2 μg/20 μl intratracheally, once daily for days -1 till 5 post infection (Anderson et al, 2011). In the meantime, a randomised, single-blind, placebo-controlled, phase I trial to investigate the effects of intranasal RV 568 on inflammation caused by infection of RSV has been completed but no results have been reported.

FGI-101-1A6 is a fully human monoclonal antibody that targets a host protein, TSG101, which is uniquely exposed on the surface of virus-infected cells. FGI-101-1A6 targets and eliminates infected cells via induction of normal host defense mechanisms. Functional Genetics Inc. has demonstrated that FGI-101-1A6 can selectively identify and eliminate cells that have been infected with many virus types, including RSV. They are currently recruiting for a randomized-placebo controlled Phase I trial to show the safety and tolerability of intravenously administered FGI-101-1A6. In addition to this, Functional Genetics focuses also on the development of antibodies against additional targets. For instance, FGI 110, an anti-Nedd4 monoclonal antibody is in preclinical development for HIV-1, RSV and influenza (Table 4).

Despite the fact that all programs are in the early (pre)clinical stages of development, this area seems to be very dynamic in terms of new initiatives to develop broad-spectrum antiviral therapies, and much more of these programs are expected to initiate clinical evaluation in the next few years.

6.5 Antibiotics

Bronchiolitis occurs most often during the first year of life and has most commonly a viral cause. RSV is the most common aethiological agent causing bronchiolitis, although it is recognized now that other viruses like human metapneumovirus, parainfluenza virus, adenovirus or rhinovirus may contribute significantly to the number of cases (Hall et al, 2009; Nair et al, 2010; Rudan et al, 2008; Simoes, 1999; Williams, 2004). A recent updated review of five randomized controlled trials comparing antibiotics to placebo in a total of 543 children less than 2 years of age diagnosed with bronchiolitis found minimal evidence to support the use of antibiotics to treat bronchiolitis (Spurling et al, 2011). The 2011 update included four randomized controlled trials investigating the use of macrolides for bronchiolitis. Macrolides are thought to have anti-inflammatory activities as well as antibiotic activity (Culic et al, 2001), and so are thought to have potential benefit for treating bronchiolitis. Of the five studies included in the review, one smaller study including 21 children found that clarithromycin treatment may reduce hospital admission (8% clarithromycin versus 44% placebo, $P = 0.081$), but this study was associated with a potential higher risk of performance, detection and reporting bias (Kabir et al, 2009). One other study found mixed results for the effects of antibiotics on wheeze, but did not identify any difference for other symptom measures (Mazumder et al, 2009). Four included studies did not find any difference between antibiotics and placebo for their primary outcomes of length of illness (Field et al, 1966) or lengt of hospital stay (Kabir et al, 2009; Kneyber et al, 2008; Mazumder et al, 2009). Despite these results, antibiotics are commonly used in 34% to 99% of hospitalized infants, even in those that do not require mechanical ventilation (Kabir et al, 2003; Vogel et al, 2003). The use of antibiotics is often associated with adverse reactions and community acquired bacterial resistance (Brook, 1998). On the other hand, severe bronchiolitis is commonly associated with bacterial co-infection (Bezerra et al, 2011). For these reasons, it is currently advised that antibiotics are used cautiously when treating bronchiolitis. Although no anti-inflammatory effects may be expected from the use of certain antibiotics, their use may be justified in cases when there is concern about secondary bacterial co-infections, particularly in very sick infants that require intensive care admission.

7. Conclusions

Despite the huge medical burden which is associated with RSV infection in different patient populations worldwide, no effective vaccine is available today. Several different approaches to design new vaccine candidates, i.e. live attenuated vaccines, subunit-based vaccines, or vector- or DNA-based vaccines, are being applied, but because of host-related challenges and limitations associated to each of the vaccine approaches, it will probably take another couple of years before the first vaccines will be approved. Likely, different vaccines may be required for RSV-naïve and experienced patients. Despite the many therapy failures with palivizumab, the use of it will remain the main therapy in the near future in the very young infants to provide protection against severe ALRI development due to RSV. However, new antibodies for RSV prophylaxis with improved efficacy and a more amenable route of administration or dosing regimen over palivizumab are currently being developed. The therapeutic potential of such antibodies is also being evaluated. Cost will nevertheless remain an important determinant for the generalisability of antibody treatment, especially in underdeveloped countries and adult patients. The potential appearance of biogenerics in this area may represent a potential game changer. In the meantime, several programs are ongoing to develop specific RSV and broadly-active antivirals. While several RSV viral targets have been clinically validated, attrition rate has been high during compound development, and as a consequence, first approval of such compounds will likely not happen in the near future. The area of broadly-active antiviral development has gained much interest the last couple of years, but the programs are still in early stages of pharmaceutical development, and because of the higher potential for drug-related adverse effects due to the targeting of host factors, it remains to be seen how high the attrition rate will be. Therefore, the first approval of a new RSV therapeutic agents will likely only take place in 2015-2016 at best.

8. References

Aherne, W., Bird, T., Court, S.D., Gardner, P.S. & McQuillin, J. (1970). Pathological changes in virus infections of the lower respiratory tract in children. *J. Clin. Pathol.* Vol. 23(1): 7-18.

American Academy of Pediatrics Subcommittee on Diagnosis and Management of Bronchiolitis. (2006). Diagnosis and management of bronchiolitis. *Pediatrics.* Vol. 118(4): 1774-1793.

Anderson, G., Cass, L., Dousha, L., Ferdinando, O., Gualano, R., Hansen, M., Ito, K., Jones, J., Langenbach, S., Lilja, A. & Wong, Z. (2011). Anti-Viral Effects Of RV568, A Narrow Spectrum Kinase Inhibitor (NSKI), In Respiratory Syncytial Virus (RSV) Infected Mice. Available at: https://myats2011.zerista.com/event/member?item_id=996168.

Andries, K., Moeremans, M., Gevers, T., Willebrords, R., Sommen, C., Lacrampe, J., Janssens, F. & Wyde, P.R. (2003). Substituted benzimidazoles with nanomolar activity against respiratory syncytial virus. *Antiviral Res.* Vol. 60(3): 209-219.

Anil, A.B., Anil, M., Saglam, A.B., Cetin, N., Bal, A. & Aksu, N. (2010). High volume normal saline alone is as effective as nebulized salbutamol-normal saline, epinephrine-normal saline, and 3% saline in mild bronchiolitis. *Pediatr. Pulmonol.* Vol. 45(1):41-47.

Aung, S., Rutigliano, J.A. & Graham, B.S. (2001). Alternative mechanisms of respiratory syncytial virus clearance in perforin knockout mice lead to enhanced disease. *J. Virol.* Vol. 75(20): 9918-9924.

Bastien, N., Trudel, M. & Simard, C. (1999). Complete protection of mice from respiratory syncytial virus infection following mucosal delivery of synthetic peptide vaccines. *Vaccine* Vol. 17(7-8): 832-836.

Barr, F.E., Patel, N.R. & Newth, C.J. (2000). The pharmacologic mechanism by which inhaled epinephrine reduces airway obstruction in respiratory syncytial virus-associated bronchiolitis. *J. Pediatr.* Vol. 136(): 699-700.

Bem, R.A., Domachowske, J.B. & Rosenberg, H.F. (2011). Animal models of human respiratory syncytial virus disease. *Am. J. Physiol. Lung Cell Mol. Physiol.* Vol. 301(2): L148-L156.

Bembridge, G.P., Rodriguez, N., Garcia-Beato, R., Nicolson, C., Melero, J.A. & Taylor, G. (2000a). Respiratory syncytial virus infection of gene gun vaccinated mice induces Th2-driven pulmonary eosinophilia even in the absence of sensitization to the fusion (F) or attachment (G) protein. *Vaccine* Vol. 19(9-10): 1038-1046.

Bembridge, G.P., Rodriguez, N., Garcia-Beato, R., Nicolson, C., Melero, J.A. & Taylor, G. (2000b). DNA encoding the attachment (G) or fusion (F) protein of respiratory syncytial virus induces protection in the absence of pulmonary inflammation. *J. Gen. Virol.* Vol. 81(Pt 10): 2519-2523.

Bezerra, P.G., Britto, M.C., Correia, J.B., Duarte Mdo, C., Fonceca, A.M., Rose, K., Hopkins, M.J., Cuevas, L.E. & McNamara, P.S. (2011). Viral and atypical bacterial detection in acute respiratory infection in children under five years. *PLoS One.* Vol. 6(4): e18928.

Bisgaard, H. & Study Group on Montelukast and Respiratory Syncytial Virus. (2003). A randomized trial of montelukast in respiratory syncytial virus postbronchiolitis. *Am. J. Respir. Crit. Care Med.* Vol. 67(3): 379-383.

Bisgaard, H., Florez-Nunez, A., Goh, A., Azimi, P., Halkas, A., Malice, M.P., Marchal, J.L., Dass, S.B., Reiss, T.F. & Knorr, B.A. (2008). Study of montelukast for the treatment of respiratory symptoms of post-respiratory syncytial virus bronchiolitis in children. *Am. J. Respir. Crit. Care Med.* Vol. 178(8): 854-860.

Blom, D., Ermers, M., Bont, L., van Aalderen, W.M. & van Woensel, J.B. (2007). Inhaled corticosteroids during acute bronchiolitis in the prevention of post-bronchiolitic wheezing. *Cochrane Database Syst Rev* Vol. 1: CD004881.

Bond, S., Draffan, A., Lambert, J., Lim, C.-Y., Lin, B., Luttick, A., Mitchell, J., Morton, C., Nearn, R., Sanford, V. & Tucker, S. (2007). Discovery of a new class of polycyclic RSV inhibitors. *Antiviral Res.* Vol. 74(3): A30.

Bond, S., Sanford, V.A., Lambert, J.N., Lim, C.Y., Mitchell, J.P., Draftan, A.G. & Nearn, R.H. (2005). Polycyclic agents for the treatment of respiratory syncytial virus infections. WO-2005061513.

Bonfanti, J.-F. & Roymans, D. (2009). Prospects for the development of fusion inhibitors to treat human respiratory syncytial virus infection. *Curr. Opin. Drug Dev.* Vol. 12(4): 479-487.

Bonfanti, J.-F., Doublet, F., Fortin, J., Lacrampe, J., Guillemont, J., Muller, P., Queguiner, L., Arnoult, E., Gevers, T., Janssens, P., Szel, H., Willebrords, R., Timmerman, P., Wuyts, K., Janssens, F., Sommen, C., Wigerinck, P. & Andries, K. (2007). selection of a respiratory syncytial virus fusion inhibitor clinical candidate, part 1: improving the pharmacokinetic profile using the structure-property relationship. *J. Med. Chem.* Vol. 50(19): 4572-4584.

Bonfanti, J.F., Meyer, C., Doublet, F., Fortin, J., Muller, P., Queguiner, L., Gevers, T., Janssens, P., Szel, H., Willebrords, R., Timmerman, P., Wuyts, K., van Remoortere, P., Janssens, F., Wigerinck, P. & Andries, K. (2008). Selection of a respiratory syncytial virus fusion inhibitor clinical candidate. 2. Discovery of a morpholinopropylaminobenzimidazole derivative (TMC353121). *J. Med. Chem.* Vol. 51(4): 875-896.

Brook, I. (1998). Do antimicrobials increase the carriage rate of penicillin resistant pneumococci in children? Cross sectional prevalence study. *Primary Care* Vol. 25(3): 633-648.

Buckingham, S.C., Bush, A. & DeVincenzo, J.P. (2000). Nasal quantity of respiratory syncytial virus correlates with disease severity in hospitalized infants. *Pediatr. Infect. Dis. J.* Vol. 19(2): 113-117.

Buckingham, S.C., Jafri, H.S., Bush, A.J., Carubelli, C.M., Sheeran, P., Hardy, R.D., Ottolini, M.G., Ramilo, O. & DeVincenzo, J.P. (2002). A randomized, double-blind, placebo-controlled trial of dexamethasone in severe respiratory syncytial virus (RSV) infection: effects on RSV quantity and clinical outcome. *J. Infect. Dis.* Vol. 185(9): 1222-1228.

Bueno, S.M., Gonzâlez, P.A., Pacheco, R., Leiva, E.D., Cautivo, K.M., Tobar, H.E., Mora, J.E., Prado, C.E., Zúñiga, J.P., Jiménez, J., Riedel, C.A. & Kalergis, A.M. (2008). Host immunity during RSV pathogenesis. *Int. Immunopharmacol.* Vol. 8(10): 1320-1329.

Carbonell-Estrany, X., Simões, E.A., Dagan, R., Hall, C.B., Harris, B., Hultquist, M., Connor, E.M. & Losonsky, G.A.; Motavizumab Study Group. (2010). Motavizumab for prophylaxis of respiratory syncytial virus in high-risk children: a noninferiority trial. *Pediatrics* Vol. 125(1): e35-e51.

Cianci, C., Genovesi, E.V., Lamb, L., Medina, I., Yang, Z., Zadjura, L., Yang, H., D'Arienzo, C., Sin, N., Yu, K.L., Combrink, K., Li, Z., Colonno, R., Meanwell, N., Clark, J. & Krystal, M. (2004a). Oral efficacy of a respiratory syncytial virus inhibitor in rodent models of infection. *Antimicrob. Agents Chemother.* Vol. 48(7): 2448-2454.

Cianci, C., Langley, D.R., Dischino, D.D., Sun, Y., Yu, K.L., Stanley, A., Roach, J., Li, Z., Dalterio, R., Colonno, R., Meanwell, N.A. & Krystal, M. (2004b). Targeting a binding pocket within the trimer-of-hairpins: small-molecule inhibition of viral fusion. *Proc. Natl. Acad. Sci. USA* Vol. 101(42): 15046-15051.

Cianci, C., Yu, K.L., Combrink, K., Sin, N., Pearce, B., Wang, A., Civiello, R., Voss, S., Luo, G., Kadow, K., Genovesi, E.V., Venables, B., Gulgeze, H., Trehan, A., James, J., Lamb, L., Medina, I., Roach, J., Yang, Z., Zadjura, L., Colonno, R., Clark, J., Meanwell, N. & Krystal, M. (2004c). Orally Active Fusion Inhibitor of Respiratory Syncytial Virus. *Antimicrob Agents Chemother.* Vol. 48(2): 413-422.

Chang, J. (2011). Current progress on development of respiratory syncytial virus vaccine. *BMB Rep.* Vol. 44(4): 232-237.

Chapman, J., Abbott, E., Alber, D.G., Baxter, R.C., Bithell, S.K., Henderson, E.A., Carter, M.C., Chambers, P., Chubb, A., Cockerill, G.S., Collins, P.L., Dowdell, V.C., Keegan, S.J., Kelsey, R.D., Lockyer, M.J., Luongo, C., Najarro, P., Pickles, R.J., Simmonds, M., Taylor, D., Tyms, S., Wilson, L.J. & Powell, K.L. (2007). RSV604, a novel inhibitor of respiratory syncytial virus replication. *Antimicrob. Agents Chemother.* Vol. 51(9): 3346-3353.

Chong, A.S., Zeng, H., Knight, D.A., Shen, J., Meister, G.T., Williams, J.W. & Waldman, W.J. (2006). Concurrent antiviral and immunosuppressive activities of leflunomide in vivo. *Am. J. Transplant.* Vol. 6(1):69-75.

Collins, P.L. & Crowe, J.E., Jr. (2007). Respiratory syncytial virus and metapneumovirus, *in* Knipe, D.M. & Howley, P.M. (eds.), *Fields Virology*, Wolters Kluwer-Lippincott Williams & Wilkins, Philadelphia, pp. 1601-1646.

Crowe, J.E., Jr. (1995). Current approaches to the development of vaccines against disease caused by respiratory syncytial virus (RSV) and parainfluenza virus (PIV). A meeting report of the WHO programme for vaccine development. *Vaccine* Vol. 13(4): 415-421.

Crowe, J.E., Jr. (2001). Influence of maternal antibodies on neonatal immunization against respiratory viruses. *Clin. Infect. Dis.* Vol. 33(10): 1720-1727.

Culić, O., Eraković, V. & Parnham, M.J. (2001). Anti-inflammatory effects of macrolide antibiotics. *Eur. J. Pharmacol.* Vol. 429(1-3): 209-229.

Delgado, M.F., Coviello, S., Monsalvo, A.C., Melendi, G.A., Hernandez, J.Z., Batalle, J.P., Diaz, L., Trento, A., Chang, H.Y., Mitzner, W., Ravetch, J., Melero, J.A., Irusta, P.M. & Polack, F.P. (2009). Lack of antibody affinity maturation due to poor Toll-like receptor stimulation leads to enhanced respiratory syncytial virus disease. *Nat. Med.* Vol. 15(1): 34-41.

DeVincenzo, J.P. (2007). A new direction in understanding the pathogenesis of respiratory syncytial virus bronchiolitis: how real infants suffer. *J. Infect. Dis.* Vol. 195(8): 1084-1086.

DeVincenzo, J.P., El Saleeby, C.M. & Bush, A.J. (2005). Respiratory syncytial virus load predicts disease severity in previously healthy infants. *J. Infect. Dis.* Vol. 191(11): 1861-1868.

DeVincenzo, J., Lambkin-Williams, R., Wilkinson, T., Cehelsky, J., Nochur, S., Walsh, E., Meyers, R., Gollob, J. &, Vaishnaw, A. (2010). A randomized, double-blind, placebo-controlled study of an RNAi-based therapy directed against respiratory syncytial virus. *Proc. Natl. Acad. Sci. USA* Vol. 107(19): 8800-8805.

DeVincenzo, J.P., Wilkinson, T., Vaishnaw, A., Cehelsky, J., Meyers, M., Nochur, S., Harrison, L., Meeking, P., Mann, A., Moane, E., Oxford, J., Pareek, R., Moore, R.,

Walsh, E., Studholme, R., Dorsett, P., Alvarez, R. & Lambkin-Williams, R. (2010). Viral load drives disease in humans experimentally infected with respiratory syncytial virus. *Am. J. Respir. Crit. Care Med.* Vol. 182(10): 1305-1314.

Dimova-Yaneva, D., Russell, D., Main, M., Brooker, R.J. & Helms, P.J. (2004).Eosinophil activation and cysteinyl leukotriene production in infants with respiratory syncytial virus bronchiolitis. *Clin. Exp. Allergy.* Vol. 34(4): 555-558.

DMID (Division of Microbiology and Infectious Diseases). (2002). The Jordan Report 20th Anniversary: Accelerated development of vaccines. Available at: http://www.niaid.nih.gov/dmid/vaccines/jordan20/jordan20%5F2002.pdf

Douglas, J.L. (2004). In search of a small-molecule inhibitor for respiratory syncytial virus. *Expert Rev. Anti Infect. Ther.* Vol. 2(4): 625-639.

Douglas, J.L., Panis, M.L., Ho, E., Lin, K.Y., Krawczyk, S.H., Grant, D.M., Cai, R., Swaminathan, S. & Cihlar, T. (2003). Inhibition of respiratory syncytial virus fusion by the small molecule VP-14637 via specific interactions with F protein. *J. Virol.* Vol. 77(9): 5054-5064.

Dunn, M.C., Knight, D.A. & Waldman, W.J. (2011). Inhibition of respiratory syncytial virus in vitro and in vivo by the immunosuppressive agent leflunomide. *Antivir. Ther.* Vol. 16(3): 309-317.

Englund, J.A., Sullivan, C.J., Jordan, M.C., Dehner, L.P., Vercellotti, G.M. & Balfour, H.H., Jr. (1988). Community respiratory virus infections among hospitalized adult bone marrow transplant recipients. *Ann. Intern Med.* Vol. 109(3): 203-208.

Ermers, M.J., Rovers, M.M., van Woensel, J.B., Kimpen, J.L. & Bont, L.J.; RSV Corticosteroid Study Group. (2009). The effect of high dose inhaled corticosteroids on wheeze in infants after respiratory syncytial virus infection: randomised double blind placebo controlled trial. *BMJ* 338:b897.

Falsey, A.R. (2007). Respiratory syncytial virus infection in adults. *Semin. Respir. Crit. Care Med.* Vol. 28(2): 171-171.

Falsey, A.R., Hennessey, P.A., Formica, M.A., Cox, C. & Walsh, E.E. (2005). Respiratory syncytial virus infection in the elderly and high-risk adults, *N. Engl. J. Med.* Vol. 352(17): 1749-1759.

Falsey, A.R. & Walsh, E.E. (1996). Safety and immunogenicity of a respiratory syncytial virus subunit vaccine (PFP-2) in ambulatory adults over age 60. *Vaccine* Vol. 14(13): 1214-1218.

Falsey, A.R. & Walsh, E.E. (1997). Safety and immunogenicity of a respiratory syncytial virus subunit vaccine (PFP-2) in the institutionalized elderly. *Vaccine* Vol. 15(10): 1130-1132.

Feltes, T.F., Cabalka, A.K., Meissner, H.C., Piazza, F.M., Carlin, D.A., Top, F.H., Jr., Connor, E.M. & Sondheimer, H.M.; Cardiac Synagis Study Group. (2003). Palivizumab prophylaxis reduces hospitalization due to respiratory syncytial virus in young children with hemodynamically significant congenital heart disease. *J. Pediatr.* Vol. 143(4): 532-540.

Feltes, T.F. & Sondheimer, H.M. (2007). Palivizumab and the prevention of respiratory syncytial virus illness in pediatric patients with congenital heart disease. *Expert Opin. Biol. Ther.* Vol. 7(9): 1471-80.

Field, C.M., Connolly, J.H., Murtagh, G., Slattery, C.M. & Turkington, E.E. (1966). Antibiotic treatment of epidemic bronchiolitis--a double-blind trial. *Br. Med. J.* Vol. 1(5479): 83-85.

Gadomski, A.M. & Bhasale, A.L. (2010). Bronchodilators for bronchiolitis. *Cochrane Database Syst Rev* Vol. 12: CD001266.

Gardner, P.S., McQuillin, J. & Court, S.D. (1970). Speculation on pathogenesis in death from respiratory syncytial virus infection. *Br. Med. J.* Vol. 1(5692): 327-330.

Gazumyan, A., Mitsner, B. & Ellestad, G.A. (2000). Novel anti-RSV dianionic dendrimer-like compounds: design, synthesis and biological evaluation. *Curr. Pharm. Des.* Vol. 6(5): 525-546.

Graham, B.S., Rutigliano, J.A. & Johnson, T.R. (2002). Respiratory syncytial virus immunobiology and pathogenesis. *Virology* Vol. 297(1): 1-7.

Groothuis, J.R., King, S.J., Hogerman, D.A., Paradiso, P.R. & Simoes, E.A. (1998). Safety and immunogenicity of a purified F protein respiratory syncytial virus (PFP-2) vaccine in seropositive children with bronchopulmonary dysplasia. *J. Infect. Dis.* Vol. 177(2): 467-469.

Haas, M.J. (2009). Besieging RSV. *SciBX* Vol. 2(1), 1-3.

Hall, C.B., Powell, K.R., MacDonald, N.E., Gala, C.L., Menegus, M.E., Suffin, S.C. & Cohen, H.J. (1986). Respiratory syncytial virus infection in children with immunocompromised immune function. *N. Engl. J. Med.* Vol. 315(2): 77-81.

Hall, C.B., Weinberg, G.A., Iwane, M.K., Blumkin, A.K., Edwards, K.M., Staat, M.A., Auinger, P., Griffin, M.R., Poehling, K.A., Erdman, D., Grijalva, C.G., Zhu, Y. & Szilagyi, P. (2009). The burden of respiratory syncytial virus in young children. *N. Engl. J. Med.* Vol. 360(6): 588-598.

Hallak, L.K., Spillmann, D., Collins, P.L. & Peeples, M.E. (2000). Glycosaminoglycan sulfation requirements for respiratory syncytial virus infection. *J. Virol.* Vol. 74(22): 10508-10513.

Hampp, C., Kauf, T.L., Saidi, A.S. & Winterstein, A.G. (2011). Cost-effectiveness of respiratory syncytial virus prophylaxis in various indications. *Arch. Pediatr. Adolesc. Med.* Vol. 165(6): 498-505.

Han, L.L., Alexander, J.P. & Anderson, L.J. (1999). Respiratory syncytial virus pneumonia among the elderly: an assessment of disease burden. *J. Infect. Dis.* Vol. 179(1): 25-30.

Hegele, R.G. (2011). Respiratory syncytial virus therapy and prophylaxis: have we finally turned the corner? *Eur. Respir. J.* Vol. 38(2): 246-247.

Hemming, V.G., Prince, G.A., Horswood, R.L., London, W.J., Murphy, B.R., Walsh, E.E., Fischer, G.W., Weisman, L.E., Baron, P.A. & Chanock, R.M. (1985). Studies of passive immunotherapy for infections of respiratory syncytial virus in the respiratory tract of a primate model. *J. Infect. Dis.* Vol. 152(5): 1083-1087.

Huntley, C.C., Weiss, W.J., Gazumyan, A., Buklan, A., Feld, B., Hu, W., Jones, T.R., Murphy, T., Nikitenko, A.A., O'Hara, B., Prince, G., Quartuccio, S., Raifeld, Y.E., Wyde, P. & O'Connell, J.F. (2002). RFI-641, a potent respiratory syncytial virus inhibitor. *Antimicrob Agents Chemother.* Vol. 46(3): 841-847.

Impact-RSV Study Group. (1998). Palivizumab, a humanized respiratory syncytial virus monoclonal antibody, reduces hospitalization from respiratory syncytial virus infection in high-risk infants. *Pediatrics* Vol. 102(3 Pt. 1): 531-537.

Johnson, S., Oliver, C., Prince, G.A., Hemming, V.G., Pfarr, D.S., Wang, S.C., Dormitzer, M., O'Grady, J., Koenig, S., Tamura, J.K., Woods, R., Bansal, G., Couchenour, D., Tsao, E., Hall, W.C. & Young, J.F. (1997). Development of a humanized monoclonal antibody (MEDI-493) with potent in vitro and in vivo activity against respiratory syncytial virus. *J. Infect. Dis.* Vol. 176(5): 1215-1224.

Jung, B. (2010). Use of quinazoline derivatives for the treatment of viral diseases. WO2010026029.

Kabir, M.L., Haq, N., Hoque, M., Ahmed, F., Amin, R., Hossain, A., Khatoon, S., Akhter, S., Shilpi, T., Haq, R., Anisuzzaman, S., Khan, M.H., Ahamed, S. & Khashru, A. (2003). Evaluation of hospitalized infants and young children with bronchiolitis - a multi centre study. *Mymensingh Med. J.* Vol. 12(2): 128-133.

Kabir, A.R., Mollah, A.H., Anwar, K.S., Rahman, A.K., Amin, R. & Rahman, M.E. (2009). Management of bronchiolitis without antibiotics: a multicentre randomized control trial in Bangladesh. *Acta Paediatr.* Vol. 98(10): 1593-1599.

Kalman, D. (2008). Kinase inhibitors for preventing or treating pathogen infection and method of use thereof. WO2008079460.

Kapikian, A.Z., Mitchell, R.H., Chanock, R.M., Shvedoff, R.A. & Stewart, C.E. (1969). An epidemiologic study of altered clinical reactivity to respiratory syncytial (RS) virus infection in children previously vaccinated with an inactivated RS virus vaccine. *Am. J. Epidemiol.* Vol. 89(4), 405-421.

Karron, R.A., Buonagurio, D.A., Georgiu, A.F., Whitehead, S.S., Adamus, J.E., Clements-Mann, M.L., Harris, D.O., Randolph, V.B., Udem, S.A., Murphy, B.R. & Sidhu, M.S. (1997). Respiratory syncytial virus (RSV) SH and G proteins are not essential for viral replication in vitro: clinical evaluation and molecular characterization of a cold-passaged, attenuated RSV subgroup B mutant. *Proc. Natl. Acad. Sci. U S A.* Vol. 94(25): 13961-13966.

Karron, R.A., Wright, P.F., Belshe, R.B., Thumar, B., Casey, R., Newman, F., Polack, F.P., Randolph, V.B., Deatly, A., Hackell, J., Gruber, W., Murphy, B.R. & Collins, P.L. (2005). Identification of a recombinant live attenuated respiratory syncytial virus vaccine candidate that is highly attenuated in infants. *J. Infect. Dis.* Vol. 191(7): 1093-1104.

Kim, H.W., Canchola, J.G., Brandt, C.D., Pyles, G., Chanock, R.M., Jensen, K. & Parrott, R.H. (1969). Respiratory syncytial virus disease in infants despite prior administration of antigenic inactivated vaccine. *Am. J. Epidemiol.* Vol. 89(4), 422-434.

Kim, C.K., Choi, J., Kim, H.B., Callaway, Z., Shin, B.M., Kim, J.T., Fujisawa, T. & Koh, Y.Y. (2010). A randomized intervention of montelukast for post-bronchiolitis: effect of eosinophil degranulation. *J. Pediatr.* Vol. 156(5): 749-754.

Kimura, K., Mori, S., Tomita, K., Ohno, K., Takahashi, K., Shigeta, S. & Terada, M. (2000). Antiviral activity of NMSO3 against respiratory syncytial virus infection in vitro and in vivo. *Antiviral Res.* Vol. 47(1):41-51.

Kinch, M. & Goldblatt, M. (2009a). Methods of inhibiting viral infection. WO2009055524.

Kinch, M. & Goldblatt, M. (2009b). Methods of inhibiting viral infection. WO2009091435.

Kneyber, M.C., van Woensel, J.B., Uijtendaal, E., Uiterwaal, C.S. & Kimpen, J.L.; Dutch Antibiotics in RSV trial (DART) Research Group. (2008). Azithromycin does not improve disease course in hospitalized infants with respiratory syncytial virus

(RSV) lower respiratory tract disease: a randomized equivalence trial. *Pediatr. Pulmonol.* Vol. 43(2): 142-149.

Knight, D.A., Hejmanowski, A.Q., Dierksheide, J.E., Williams, J.W., Chong, A.S. & Waldman, W.J. (2001). Inhibition of herpes simplex virus type 1 by the experimental immunosuppressive agent leflunomide. *Transplantation.* Vol. 71(1): 170-174.

Krumm, S.A., Ndungu, J.M., Yoon, J.-J., Dochow, M., Sun, A., Natchus, M., Snyder, J.P. & Plemper, R.K. (2011). Potent host-directed small-molecule inhibitors of myxovirus RNA-dependent RNA-polymerases. *PLoS One* Vol. 6(5): e20069.

Krusat, T. & Streckert, H.J. (1997). Heparin-dependent attachment of respiratory syncytial virus (RSV) to host cells. *Arch. Virol.* Vol. 142(6): 1247-1254.

Kumar, M., Behera, A.K., Lockey, R.F., Zhang, J., Bhullar, G., De La Cruz, C.P., Chen, L.C., Leong, K.W., Huang, S.K. & Mohapatra, S.S. (2002). Intranasal gene transfer by chitosan-DNA nanospheres protects BALB/c mice against acute respiratory syncytial virus infection. *Hum. Gene Ther.* Vol. 13(12): 1415-1425.

Lamb, R.A. & Jardetzky, T.S. (2007). Structural basis of viral invasion: lessons from paramyxovirus F. *Curr. Opin. Struct. Biol.* Vol. 17(4): 427-436.

Langley, G.F. & Anderson, L.J. (2011). Epidemiology and prevention of respiratory syncytial virus infections among infants and young children. *Pediatr. Infect. Dis. J.* Vol. 30(6): 510-517.

Langley, J.M., Smith, M.B., LeBlanc, J.C., Joudrey, H., Ojah, C.R. & Pianosi, P. (2005). Racemic epinephrine compared to salbutamol in hospitalized young children with bronchiolitis; a randomized controlled clinical trial [ISRCTN46561076]. *BMC Pediatr.* Vol. 5(1): 7.

Law, B.J., Carbonell-Estrany, X. & Simoes, E.A. (2002). An update on respiratory syncytial virus epidemiology: a developed county perspective. *Respir. Med.* Vol. 96(Suppl. B): S1-S7.

Legg, J.P., Hussain, I.R., Warner, J.A., Johnston, S.L. & Warner, J.O. (2003). Type 1 and type 2 cytokine imbalance in acute respiratory syncytial virus bronchiolitis. *Am. J. Respir. Crit. Care Med.* Vol. 168(6): 633-639.

Li, X., Sambhara, S., Li, C.X., Ewasyshyn, M., Parrington, M., Caterini, J., James, O., Cates, G., Du, R.P. & Klein, M. (1998). Protection against respiratory syncytial virus infection by DNA immunization. *J. Exp. Med.* Vol. 188(4): 681-688.

Li, X., Sambhara, S., Li, C.X., Ettorre, L., Switzer, I., Cates, G., James, O., Parrington, M., Oomen, R., Du, R.P. & Klein, M. (2000). Plasmid DNA encoding the respiratory syncytial virus G protein is a promising vaccine candidate. *Virology* Vol. 269(1): 54-65.

Lindell, D.M., Morris, S.B., White, M.P., Kallal, L.E., Lundy, P.K., Hamouda, T., Baker, J.R., Jr. & Lukacs, N.W. (2011). A Novel Inactivated Intranasal Respiratory Syncytial Virus Vaccine Promotes Viral Clearance without Th2 Associated Vaccine-Enhanced Disease. *PLoS One* Vol. 6(7): e21823.

Liuzzi, M., Mason, S.W., Cartier, M., Lawetz, C., McCollum, R.S., Dansereau, N., Bolger, G., Lapeyre, N., Gaudette, Y., Lagacé, L., Massariol, M.J., Dô, F., Whitehead, P., Lamarre, L., Scouten, E., Bordeleau, J., Landry, S., Rancourt, J., Fazal, G. & Simoneau, B. (2005). Inhibitors of respiratory syncytial virus replication target cotranscriptional mRNA guanylylation by viral RNA-dependent RNA polymerase. *J. Virol.* Vol. 79(20): 13105-13115.

López-Andreu JA, Cortell-Aznar I, Ruiz-García V. (2004). Montelukast in respiratory syncytial virus postbronchiolitis. *Am. J. Respir. Crit. Care Med.* Vol. 169(11): 1255.

Malathi, K., Dong, B., Gale, M., Jr. & Silverman, R.H. (2007). Small self-RNA generated by RNase L amplifies antiviral innate immunity. *Nature* Vol. 448(7155): 816–819.

Malley, R., DeVincenzo, J., Ramilo, O., Dennehy, P.H., Meissner, H.C., Gruber, W.C., Sanchez, P.J., Jafri, H., Balsley, J., Carlin, D., Buckingham, S., Vernacchio, L. & Ambrosino, D.M. (2004). Reduction of respiratory syncytial virus (RSV) in tracheal aspirates in intubated infants by use of humanized monoclonal antibody to RSV F protein. *Pediatr Infect Dis J.* Vol. 23(8): 707-712.

Mason, S.W., Lawetz, C., Gaudette, Y., Dô, F., Scouten, E., Lagacé, L., Simoneau, B. & Liuzzi, M. (2004). Polyadenylation-dependent screening assay for respiratory syncytial virus RNA transcriptase activity and identification of an inhibitor. *Nucleic Acids Res.* Vol. 32(16): 4758-4767.

Mazumder, M., Hossain, M. & Kabir, A. Management of bronchiolitis with or without antibiotics - a randomized control trial. *J. Bangladesh Coll. Physic. Surg.* Vol. 27(2): 63-69.

Meanwell, N.A. & Krystal, M. (2007). Respiratory syncytial virus - the discovery and optimization of orally bioavailable fusion inhibitors. *Drugs Fut.* Vol. 32(5): 441-455.

Mitchell, J.P., Pitt, G., Draffan, A.G., Mayes, P.A., Andrau, L. & Anderson, K. (2011). Compounds for treating respiratory syncytial virus infections. WO2011094823.

Modl, M., Eber, E., Malle-Scheid, D., Weinhandl, E. & Zach, M.S. (2005). Does bronchodilator responsiveness in infants with bronchiolitis depend on age? *J. Pediatr.* Vol. 147(5): 617-621.

Modl, M., Eber, E., Weinhandl, E., Gruber, W. & Zach, M.S. (2000). Assessment of bronchodilator responsiveness in infants with bronchiolitis: A comparison of the tidal and the raised volume rapid thoracoabdominal compression technique. Am. J. Respir. Crit. Care Med. Vol. 161(3 Pt 1): 763-768.

Mohan, A.K., Braun, M.M., Ellenberg, S., Hedje, J. & Coté, T.R. (2004). Deaths among children less than two years of age receiving palivizumab: an analysis of comorbidities. *Pediatr. Infect. Dis. J.* Vol. 23(4): 342-345.

Monick, M.M., Cameron, K., Staber, J., Powers, L.S., Yarinovski, T.O., Koland, J.G. & Hunninghake, G.W. (2005). Activation of the epidermal growth factor receptor by respiratory syncytial virus results in increased inflammation and delayed apoptosis. *J. Biol. Chem.* Vol. 280(3): 2147-2158.

Morris, S.K., Dzolganovski, B., Beyene, J. & Sung, L. (2009). A meta-analysis of the effect of antibody therapy for the prevention of severe respiratory syncytial virus infection. *BMC Infect. Dis.* Vol. 5(9): 106.

Munoz, F.M., Piedra, P.A. & Glezen, W.P. (2003). Safety and immunogenicity of respiratory syncytial virus purified fusion protein-2 vaccine in pregnant women. *Vaccine* Vol. 21(24): 3465-3467.

Murata, Y. (2009). Respiratory syncytial virus vaccine development. *Clin. Lab. Med.* Vol. 29(4), 725-739.

Murphy, B.R. & Walsh, E.E. (1988). Formalin-inactivated respiratory syncytial virus vaccine induces antibodies to the fusion glycoprotein that are deficient in fusion-inhibiting activity. *J. Clin. Microbiol.* Vol. 26(8): 1595-1597.

Murphy, B.R., Sotnikov, A.V., Lawrence, L.A., Banks, S.M. & Prince, G.A. (1990). Enhanced pulmonary histopathology is observed in cotton rats immunized with formalin-inactivated respiratory syncytial virus (RSV) or purified F glycoprotein and challenged with RSV 3-6 months after immunization. *Vaccine* Vol. 8(5): 497-502.

Murphy, B.R., Sotnikov, A., Paradiso, P.R., Hildreth, S.W., Jenson, A.B., Baggs, R.B., Lawrence, L., Zubak, J.J., Chanock, R.M., Beeler, J.A., et al. (1989). Immunization of cotton rats with the fusion (F) and large (G) glycoproteins of respiratory syncytial virus (RSV) protects against RSV challenge without potentiating RSV disease. *Vaccine* Vol. 7(6):533-540.

Nair, H., Nokes, J.D., Gessner, B.D., Dherani, M., Madhi, S.A., Singleton, R.J., O'Brien, K.L., Roca, A., Wright, P.F., Bruce, N., Chandran, A., Theodoratou, E., Sutanto, A., Sedyaningsih, E.R., Ngama, M., Munywoki, P.K., Kartasasmita, C., Simões, E.A., Rudan, I., Weber, M.W. & Campbell, H. (2010). Global burden of acute lower respiratory infections due to respiratory syncytial virus in young children: a systematic review and meta-analysis. *Lancet* Vol. 375(9725): 1545-1555.

Neilson, K.A. & Yunis, E.J. (1990). Demonstration of respiratory syncytial virus in an autopsy series. *Pediatr. Pathol.* Vol. 10(4), 491-502.

Nikitenko, A.A., Raifeld, Y.E. & Wang, T.Z. (2001). The discovery of RFI-641 as a potent and selective inhibitor of the respiratory syncytial virus. *Bioorg. Med. Chem. Lett.* Vol. 11(8): 1041-1044.

Nokes, J.D., Cane, P.A. (2008). New strategies for control of respiratory syncytial virus infection. *Curr. Opin. Infect. Dis. Vol.* 21(6), 639-643.

Oh, J.W., Shin, S.A. & Lee, H.B. (2005). Urine leukotriene E and eosinophil cationic protein in nasopharyngeal aspiration from young wheezy children. *Pediatr. Allergy Immunol.* Vol. 16(5): 416-421.

Olszewska, W., Ispas, G., Schnoeller, C., Sawant, D., Van de Casteele, T., Nauwelaers, D., Van Kerckhove, B., Roymans, D., De Meulder, M., Rouan, M.C., Van Remoortere, P., Bonfanti, J.F., Van Velsen, F., Koul, A., Vanstockem, M., Andries, K., Sowinski, P., Wang, B., Openshaw, P. & Verloes, R. (2011). Antiviral and lung protective activity of a novel respiratory syncytial virus fusion inhibitor in a mouse model. *Eur. Respir. J.* Vol. 38(2): 401-408.

Openshaw, P.J.M. & Tregoning, J.S. (2005). Immune responses and disease enhancement during respiratory syncytial virus infection. *Clin. Microbiol. Rev.* Vol. 18(3): 541-555.

Ostler, T., Davidson, W. & Ehl, S. (2002). Virus clearance and immunopathology by CD8+ T cells during infection with respiratory syncytial virus are mediated by IFN_{γ}. *Eur. J. Immunol.* Vol. 32(8): 2117-2123.

Palmer, L., Hall, C.B., Katkin, J.P., Shi, N., Masaquel, A.S., McLaurin, K.K. & Mahadevia, P.J. (2010). Healthcare costs within a year of respiratory syncytial virus among Medicaid infants. *Pediatr. Pulmonol.* Vol. 45(8): 772-781.

Paradiso, P.R., Hildreth, S.W., Hogerman, D.A., Speelman, D.J., Lewin, E.B., Oren, J. & Smith, D.H. (1994). Safety and immunogenicity of a subunit respiratory syncytial virus vaccine in children 24 to 48 months old. *Pediatr. Infect. Dis. J.* Vol. 13(9): 792-798.

Paramore, L.C., Ciuryla, V., Ciesla, G. & Liu, L. (2004). Economic impact of respiratory syncytial virus-related illness in the US: an analysis of national databases. *Pharmacoeconomics* Vol. 22(5): 275-284.

Patel, H., Platt, R., Lozano, J.M. & Wang, E.E. (2004). Glucocorticoids for acute viral bronchiolitis in infants and young children. *Cochrane Database Syst Rev* Vol. 3: CD004878.

Peebles, R.S., Jr. (2004). Viral infections, atopy, and asthma: is there a causal relationship? *J. Allergy Clin. Immunol.* Vol. 113(1 Suppl): S15-S18.

Perrotta, C., Ortiz, Z. & Roque, M. (2007). Chest physiotherapy for acute bronchiolitis in paediatric patients between 0 and 24 months old. *Cochrane Database Syst. Rev.* Vol. 1:CD004873.

Piedra, P.A., Cron, S.G., Jewell, A., Hamblett, N., McBride, R., Palacio, M.A., Ginsberg, R., Oermann, C.M. & Hiatt, P.W.; Purified Fusion Protein Vaccine Study Group. (2003). Immunogenicity of a new purified fusion protein vaccine to respiratory syncytial virus: a multi-center trial in children with cystic fibrosis. *Vaccine* Vol. 21(19-20): 2448-2460.

Piedra, P.A., Grace, S., Jewell, A., Spinelli, S., Bunting, D., Hogerman, D.A., Malinoski, F. & Hiatt, P.W. (1996). Purified fusion protein vaccine protects against lower respiratory tract illness during respiratory syncytial virus season in children with cystic fibrosis. *Pediatr. Infect. Dis. J.* Vol. 15(1): 23-31.

Pinto, R.A., Arredondo, S.M., Bono, M.R., Gaggero, A.A. & Diaz, P.V. (2006). T helper 1/T helper 2 cytokine imbalance in respiratory syncytial virus infection is associated with increased endogenous plasma cortisol. *Pediatrics* Vol. 117(5): e878-e886.

Power, U.F., Nguyen, T.N., Rietveld, E., de Swart, R.L., Groen, J., Osterhaus, A.D., de Groot, R., Corvaia, N., Beck, A., Bouveret-Le-Cam, N. & Bonnefoy, J.Y. (2001). Safety and immunogenicity of a novel recombinant subunit respiratory syncytial virus vaccine (BBG2Na) in healthy young adults. *J. Infect. Dis.* Vol. 184(11): 1456-1460.

PREVENT study group. (1997). Reduction of respiratory syncytial virus hospitalization among premature infants and infants with bronchopulmonary dysplasia using respiratory syncytial virus immune globulin prophylaxis. *Pediatrics* Vol. 99(1): 93-99.

Prince, G.A., Mathews, A., Curtis, S.J. & Porter, D.D. (2000). Treatment of respiratory syncytial virus bronchiolitis and pneumonia in a cotton rat model with systemically administered monoclonal antibody (palivizumab) and glucocorticosteroid. *J. Infect. Dis.* Vol. 182(5): 1326-1330.

Prince, G.A., Horswood, R.L. & Chanock, R.M. (1985). Quantitative aspects of passive immunity to respiratory syncytial virus infection in infant cotton rats. *J. Virol.* Vol. 55(3): 517-520.

Pringle, C.R., Filipiuk, A.H., Robinson, B.S., Watt, P.J., Higgins, P. & Tyrrell, D.A. (1993). Immunogenicity and pathogenicity of a triple temperature-sensitive modified respiratory syncytial virus in adult volunteers. *Vaccine* Vol. 11(4): 473-478.

Proesmans, M., Sauer, K., Govaere, E., Raes, M., De Bilderling, G. & De Boeck, K. (2009). Montelukast does not prevent reactive airway disease in young children hospitalized for RSV bronchiolitis. *Acta Paediatr.* Vol. 98(11): 1830-1834.

Razinkov, V., Huntley, C., Ellestad, G. & Krishnamurthy, G. (2002). RSV entry inhibitors block F-protein mediated fusion with model membranes. *Antiviral Res.* Vol. 55(1): 189-200.

Rodriguez, W.J., Gruber, W.C., Groothuis, J.R., Simoes, E.A., Rosas, A.J., Lepow, M., Kramer, A. & Hemming, V. (1997a). Respiratory syncytial virus immune globulin treatment of RSV lower respiratory tract infection in previously healthy children. *Pediatrics*. Vol. 100(6): 937-942.

Rodriguez, W.J., Gruber, W.C., Welliver, R.C., Groothuis, J.R., Simoes, E.A., Meissner, H.C., Hemming, V.G., Hall, C.B., Lepow, M.L., Rosas, A.J., Robertsen, C. & Kramer, A.A. (1997b). Respiratory syncytial virus (RSV) immune globulin intravenous therapy for RSV lower respiratory tract infection in infants and young children at high risk for severe RSV infections: Respiratory Syncytial Virus Immune Globulin Study Group. *Pediatrics*. Vol. 99(3): 454-461.

Romero, J.R. (2003). Palivizumab prophylaxis of respiratory syncytial virus disease from 1998 to 2002: results from four years of palivizumab usage. Pediatr. *Infect. Dis. J.* Vol. 22(Suppl. 2): S46-S54.

Rouan, M.C., Gevers, T., Roymans, D., de Zwart, L., Nauwelaers, D., De Meulder, M., van Remoortere, P., Vanstockem, M., Koul, A., Simmen, K. & Andries, K. (2010). Pharmacokinetics-pharmacodynamics of a respiratory syncytial virus fusion inhibitor in the cotton rat model. *Antimicrob. Agents Chemother.* Vol. 54(11): 4534-4539.

Roymans, D., De Bondt, H.L., Arnoult, E., Geluykens, P., Gevers, T., Van Ginderen, M., Verheyen, N., Kim, H., Willebrords, R., Bonfanti, J.F., Bruinzeel, W., Cummings, M.D., van Vlijmen, H. & Andries, K. (2010). Binding of a potent small-molecule inhibitor of six-helix bundle formation requires interactions with both heptad-repeats of the RSV fusion protein. *Proc. Natl. Acad. Sci. USA* Vol. 107(1): 308-313.

Roymans, D. & Koul, A. (2010). Respiratory syncytial virus: a prioritized or neglected target? *Future Med. Chem.* Vol. 2(10): 1523-1527.

Rudan, I., Boschi-Pinto, C., Biloglav, Z., Mulholland, K. & Campbell, H. (2008). Epidemiology and etiology of childhood pneumonia. *Bull. World Health Organ.* Vol. 86(5): 408-416.

Ruuskanen, O., Lahti, E., Jennings, L.C. & Murdoch, D.R. (2011). Viral pneumonia. *Lancet* Vol. 377(9773): 1264-1275.

Sáez-Llorens, X., Moreno, M.T., Ramilo, O., Sánchez, P.J., Top, F.H., Jr. & Connor, E.M.; MEDI-493 Study Group. (1998). Safety and pharmacokinetics of palivizumab therapy in children hospitalized with respiratory syncytial virus infection. *J. Infect. Dis.* Vol. 178(6): 1555-1561.

Shi, L., Xiong, H., He, J., Deng, H., Li, Q., Zhong, Q., Hou, W., Cheng, L., Xiao, H. & Yang, Z. (2007). Antiviral activity of arbidol against influenza A, respiratory syncytial virus, rhinovirus, coxsackie virus and adenovirus in vitro and in vivo. *Arch. Virol.* Vol. 152(8): 1447-1455.

Schmidt, A.C. (2007). Progress in respiratory virus vaccine development. *Semin. Respir. Crit. Care Med.* Vol. 28(2): 243-252.

Schmidt, A.C., McAuliffe, J.M., Murphy, B.R. & Collins, P.L. (2001). Recombinant bovine/human parainfluenza virus type 3 (B/HPIV3) expressing the respiratory syncytial virus (RSV) G and F proteins can be used to achieve simultaneous mucosal immunization against RSV and HPIV3. *J. Virol.* Vol. 75(10): 4594-4603.

Schmidt, A.C., Wenzke, D.R., McAuliffe, J.M., St Claire, M., Elkins, W.R., Murphy, B.R. & Collins, P.L. (2002). Mucosal immunization of rhesus monkeys against respiratory syncytial virus subgroups A and B and human parainfluenza virus type 3 by using a live cDNA-derived vaccine based on a host range-attenuated bovine parainfluenza virus type 3 vector backbone. *J. Virol.* Vol. 76(3):1089-1099.

Sigurs, N., Gustafsson, P.M., Bjarnason, R., Lundberg, F., Schmidt, S., Sigurbergsson, F. & Kjellman, B. (2005). Severe respiratory syncytial virus bronchiolitis in infancy and asthma and allergy at age 13. *Am. J. Respir. Cri. Care Med.* Vol. 171(2), 137-141.

Simoes, E.A.F. (1999). Respiratory syncytial virus infection. *Lancet* Vol. 354(9181): 847-852.

Simoes, E.A., Carbonell-Estrany, X., Rieger, C.H., Mitchell, I., Fredrick, L. & Groothuis, J.R.; Palivizumab Long-Term Respiratory Outcomes Study Group. (2010). The effect of respiratory syncytial virus on subsequent recurrent wheezing in atopic and nonatopic children. *J. Allergy Clin. Immunol.* Vol. 126(2):256-262.

Simoes, E.A., Groothuis, J.R., Carbonell-Estrany, X., Rieger, C.H., Mitchell, I., Fredrick, L.M. & Kimpen, J.L.; Palivizumab Long-Term Respiratory Outcomes Study Group. (2007). Palivizumab prophylaxis, respiratory syncytial virus, and subsequent recurrent wheezing. *J. Pediatr.* Vol. 151(1): 34-42.

Simoes, E.A., Groothuis, J.R., Tristram, D.A., Allessi, K., Lehr, M.V., Siber, G.R. & Welliver, R.C. (1996). Respiratory syncytial virus-enriched globulin for the prevention of acute otitis media in high risk children. *J. Pediatr.* Vol. 129(2): 214-219.

Simoes, E.A., Sondheimer, H.M., Top, F.H., Jr., Meissner, H.C., Welliver, R.C., Kramer, A.A. & Groothuis, J.R. (1998). Respiratory syncytial virus immune globulin for prophylaxis against respiratory syncytial virus disease in infants and children with congenital heart disease. The Cardiac Study Group. *J. Pediatr.* Vol. 133(4): 492-499.

Singh, S.R., Dennis, V.A., Carter, C.L., Pillai, S.R., Jefferson, A., Sahi, S.V. & Moore, E.G. (2007a). Immunogenicity and efficacy of recombinant RSV-F vaccine in a mouse model. *Vaccine* Vol. 25(33): 6211-6223.

Singh, S.R., Dennis, V.A., Carter, C.L., Pillai, S.R. & Moore, E.G. (2007b). Respiratory syncytial virus recombinant F protein (residues 255-278) induces a helper T cell type 1 immune response in mice. *Viral Immunol.* Vol. 20(2): 261-275.

Smart, K.A., Paes, B.A. & Lanctôt, K.L. (2010). Changing costs and the impact on RSV prophylaxis. *J. Med. Econ.* Vol. 13(4): 705-708.

Spurling, G.K.P., Doust, J., Del Mar, C.B. & Eriksson, L. (2011). Antibiotics for bronchiolitis in children. *Cochrane Database Syst. Rev.* Vol. 6: CD005189.

Stein, R.T., Sherrill, D., Morgan, W.J., Holberg, C.J., Halonen, M., Taussig, L.M., Wright, A.L. & Martinez, F.D. (1999). Respiratory syncytial virus in early life and risk of wheeze and allergy by age 13 years. *Lancet* Vol. 354(9178): 541–545.

Stegmann, T., Kamphuis, T., Meijerhof, T., Goud, E., de Haan, A. & Wilschut, J. (2010). Lipopeptide-adjuvanted respiratory syncytial virus virosomes: A safe and immunogenic non-replicating vaccine formulation. *Vaccine* Vol. 28(34): 5543-5550.

Stewart, D.L., Romero, J.R., Buysman, E.K., Fernandes, A.W. & Mahadevia, P.J. (2009). Total healthcare costs in the US for preterm infants with respiratory syncytial virus lower respiratory infection in the first year of life requiring medical attention. *Curr. Med. Res. Opin.* Vol. 25(11): 2795-2804.

Sudo, K., Miyazaki, Y., Kojima, N., Kobayashi, M., Suzuki, H., Shintani, M. & Shimizu, Y. (2005). YM-53403, a unique anti-respiratory syncytial virus agent with a novel mechanism of action. *Antiviral Res.* Vol. 65(2): 125-131.

Szefler, S.J. & Simoes, E.A. (2003). Montelukast for respiratory syncytial virus bronchiolitis: significant effect or provocative findings? *Am. J. Respir. Crit. Care Med.* Vol. 167(3): 290-291.

Tang, R.S., MacPhail, M., Schikli, J.H., Kaur, J., Robinson, C.L., Lawlor, H.A., Guzzetta, J.M., Spaete, R.R. & Haller, A.A. (2004). Parainfluenza virus type 3 expressing the native or soluble fusion (F) Protein of Respiratory Syncytial Virus (RSV) confers protection from RSV infection in African green monkeys. *J. Virol.* Vol. 78(20): 11198-11207.

Tang, R.S., Schickli, J.H., MacPhail, M., Fernandes, F., Bicha, L., Spaete, J., Fouchier, R.A., Osterhaus, A.D., Spaete, R. & Haller, A.A. (2003). Effects of human metapneumovirus and respiratory syncytial virus antigen insertion in two 3' proximal genome positions of bovine/human parainfluenza virus type 3 on virus replication and immunogenicity. *J. Virol.* Vol. 77(20): 10819-10828.

Tayyari, F., Marchant, D., Moraes, T.J., Duan, W., Mastrangelo, P. & Hegele, R.G. (2011). Identification of nucleolin as a cellular receptor for human respiratory syncytial virus. *Nat. Med.* Epub ahead of print.

Techaarpornkul, S., Barretto, N. & Peeples, M.E. (2001). Functional analysis of recombinant respiratory syncytial virus deletion mutants lacking the small hydrophobic and/or attachment glycoprotein gene. *J. Virol.* Vol. 75(15): 6825-6834.

Thakur, C.S., Jha, B.K., Dong, B., Gupta, J.D., Silverman, K.M., Mao, H., Sawai, H., Nakamura, A.O., Banerjee, A.K., Gudkov, A. & Silverman, R.H. (2007). Small-molecule activators of RNase L with broad-spectrum antiviral activity. *Proc. Natl. Acad. Sci. USA* Vol. 104(23): 9585-9590.

Thompson, W.W., Shay, D.K., Weintraub, E., Brammer, L., Cox, N., Anderson, L.J. & Fukuda, K. (2003). Mortality associated with influenza and respiratory syncytial virus in the United States. *JAMA* Vol. 289(2): 179-186.

Tristram, D.A., Welliver, R.C., Mohar, C.K., Hogerman, D.A., Hildreth, S.W. & Paradiso, P. (1993). Immunogenicity and safety of respiratory syncytial virus subunit vacdcine in seopositive children 18-36 months old. *J. Infect. Dis.* Vol. 167(1): 191-195.

Trudel, M., Nadon, F., Séguin, C. & Binz, H. (1991a). Protection of BALB/c mice from respiratory syncytial virus infection by immunization with a synthetic peptide derived from the G glycoprotein. *Virology* Vol. 185(2): 749-757.

Trudel, M., Stott, E.J., Taylor, G., Oth, D., Mercier, G., Nadon, F., Séguin, C., Simard, C. & Lacroix, M. (1991b). Synthetic peptides corresponding to the F protein of RSV stimulate murine B and T cells but fail to confer protection. *Arch. Virol.* Vol. 117(1-2): 59-71.

Van Bleeck, G.M., Osterhaus, A.D. & de Swart, R.L. (2011). RSV 2010: Recent advances in research on respiratory syncytial virus and other pneumoviruses. *Vaccine* [Epub ahead of print].

Ventre, K. & Randolph, A.G. (2007). Ribavirin for respiratory syncytial virus infection of the lower respiratory tract in infants and young children. *Cochrane Database Syst Rev* Vol. 1: CD000181.

Vogel, A.M., Lennon, D.R., Harding, J.E., Pinnock, R.E., Graham, D.A., Grimwood, K. & Pattemore, P.K. (2003). Variations in bronchiolitis management between five New Zealand hospitals: can we do better? *J. Paediatr. Child Health.* Vol. 39(1): 40-45.

Wainwright, C. (2010). Acute viral bronchiolitis in children – a very common condition with few therapeutic options. *Paediatr Respir Rev.* Vol. 11(1): 39-45.

Waldman, W.J., Knight, D.A., Blinder, L., Shen, J., Lurain, N.S., Miller, D.M., Sedmak, D.D., Williams, J.W. & Chong, A.S. (1999). Inhibition of cytomegalovirus in vitro and in vivo by the experimental immunosuppressive agent leflunomide. *Intervirology*. Vol. 42(5-6): 412-418.

Wang, D., Bayliss, S. & Meads, C. (2011). Palivizumab for immunoprophylaxis of respiratory syncytial virus (RSV) bronchiolitis in high-risk infants and young children: a systematic review and additional economic modelling of subgroup analyses. *Health Technol. Assess.* Vol. 15(5):iii-iv, 1-124.

Weber, M.W., Mulholland, E.K. & Greenwood, B.M. (1998). Respiratory syncytial virus in tropical and developing countries. *Trop. Med. Int. Health* Vol. 3(4): 268-280.

Wedde-Beer K, Hu C, Rodriguez MM, Piedimonte G. (2002). Leukotrienes mediate neurogenic inflammation in lungs of young rats infected with respiratory syncytial virus. *Am. J. Physiol. Lung Cell Mol. Physiol.* Vol. 282(5): L1143-L1150.

Welliver, R.C. (2008). The immune response to respiratory syncytial virus infection: friend or foe? *Clinic. Rev. Allerg. Immunol.* Vol. 34(2): 163-173.

Welliver, T.P., Garofalo, R.P., Hosakote, Y., Hintz, K.H., Avendano, L., Sanchez, K., Velozo, L., Jafri, H., Chavez-Bueno, S., Ogra, P.L., McKinney, L., Reed, J.L. & Welliver, R.C.,Sr. (2007). Severe human lower respiratory tract illness caused by respiratory syncytial virus and influenza virus is characterized by the absence of pulmonary cytotoxic lymphocyte responses. *J. Infect. Dis.* Vol. 195(8): 1126-1136.

Weisman, L.E. (2003). Populations at risk for developing respiratory syncytial virus and risk factors for respiratory syncytial virus severity: infants with predisposing conditions. *Pediatr. Infect. Dis. J.* Vol. 22(2 Suppl): S33-37.

Weiss, W.J., Murphy, T., Lynch, M.E., Frye, J., Buklan, A., Gray, B., Lenoy, E., Mitelman, S., O'Connell, J., Quartuccio, S. & Huntley, C. (2003). Inhalation efficacy of RFI-641 in an African green monkey model of RSV infection. *J. Med. Primatol.* Vol. 32(2): 82-88.

Welliver, T.P., Garofalo, R.P., Hosakote, Y., Hintz, K.H., Avendano, L., Sanchez, K., Velozo, L., Jafri, H., Chavez-Bueno, S., Ogra, P.L., McKinney, L., Reed, J.L. & Welliver, R.C., Sr. (2007). Severe human lower respiratory tract illness caused by respiratory syncytial virus and influenza virus is characterized by the absence of pulmonary cytotoxic lymphocyte responses. *J. Infect. Dis.* Vol. 195(8): 1126-1136.

Whimbey, E., Couch, R.B., Englund, J.A., Andreeff, M., Goodrich, J.M., Raad, I.I., Lewis, V., Mirza, N., Luna, M.A., Baxter, B., Tarrand, J.J. & Bodey, G.P. (1995). Respiratory syncytial virus pneumonia in hospitalized adult patients with leukemia. *Clin. Infect. Dis.* Vol. 21(2): 376-379.

Williams, J.V., Harris, P.A., Tollefson, S.J., Halburnt-Rush, L.L., Pingsterhaus, J.M., Edwards, K.M., Wright, P.F. & Crowe, J.E., Jr. (2004). Human metapneumovirus and lower respiratory tract disease in otherwise healthy infants and children. *N. Engl. J. Med.* Vol. 350(5): 443-450.

Williams, J.W., Mital, D., Chong, A., Kottayil, A., Millis, M., Longstreth, J., Huang, W., Brady, L. & Jensik, S. (2002). Experiences with leflunomide in solid organ transplantation. *Transplantation*. Vol. 73(3): 358-366.

Wohl, M.E.B. & Chernick, V. (1978). Bronchiolitis. *Am. Rev. Respir. Dis.* Vol. 118(4): 759-781.

Wright, P.F., Karron, R.A., Belshe, R.B., Thompson, J., Crowe, J.E., Jr., Boyce, T.G., Halburnt, L.L., Reed, G.W., Whitehead, S.S., Anderson, E.L., Wittek, A.E., Casey, R., Eichelberger, M., Thumar, B., Randolph, V.B., Udem, S.A., Chanock, R.M. & Murphy, B.R. (2000). Evaluation of a live, cold-passaged, temperature-sensitive, respiratory syncytial virus vaccine candidate in infancy. *J. Infect. Dis.* Vol. 182(5): 1331-1342.

Wright, P.F., Karron, R.A., Madhi, S.A., Treanor, .J.J, King, J.C., O'Shea, A., Ikizler, M.R., Zhu, Y., Collins, P.L., Cutland, C., Randolph, V.B., Deatly, A.M., Hackell, J.G., Gruber, W.C. & Murphy, B.R. (2006). The interferon antagonist NS2 protein of respiratory syncytial virus is an important virulence determinant for humans. *J. Infect. Dis.* Vol. 193(4):573-581.

Wu, P., Dupont, W.D., Griffin, M.R., Carroll, K.N., Mitchel, E.F., Gebretsadik, T. & Hartert, T.V. (2008). Evidence of a causal role of winter virus infection during infancy inearly childhood asthma. *Am. J. Respir. Crit. Care Med.* Vol. 178(11): 1123-1129.

Wu, H., Pfarr, D.S., Johnson, S., Brewah, Y.A., Woods, R.M., Patel, N.K., White, W.I., Young, J.F. & Kiener, P.A. (2007). Development of motavizumab, an ultra-potent antibody for the prevention of respiratory syncytial virus infection in the upper and lower respiratory tract. *J. Mol. Biol.* Vol. 368(3): 652-665.

Wu, H., Pfarr, D.S., Losonsky, G.A. & Kiener, P.A. (2008). Immunoprophylaxis of RSV infection: advancing from RSV-IGIV to palivizumab and motavizumab. *Curr. Top. Microbiol. Immunol.* Vol. 317: 103-123.

Wyde, P.R., Chetty, S.N., Timmerman, P., Gilbert, B.E. & Andries, K. (2003). Short duration aerosols of JNJ 2408068 (R170591) administered prophylactically or therapeutically protect cotton rats from experimental respiratory syncytial virus infection. *Antiviral Res.* Vol. 60(3): 221-231.

Wyde, P.R., Laquerre, S., Chetty, S., Gilbert, B.E., Nitz, T. & Pevear, D.C. (2005). Antiviral efficacy of VP14637 against respiratory syncytial virus in vitro and in Cotton rats following delivery by small droplet aerosol. *Antiviral Res* . Vol. 68(1): 18-26.

Young D. (2010). FDA: MedImmune's Rezield has 3x allergic reactions as Synagis. *BioWorld Today* Vol. 21(104): 1-5.

Zamora, M.R., Budev, M., Rolfe, M., Gottlieb, J., Humar, A., Devincenzo, J., Vaishnaw, A., Cehelsky, J., Albert, G., Nochur, S., Gollob, J.A. & Glanville, A.R. (2011). RNA interference therapy in lung transplant patients infected with respiratory syncytial virus. *Am. J. Respir. Crit. Care Med.* Vol. 183(4): 531-538.

Zhang, L., Peeples, M.E., Boucher, R.C., Collins, P.L. & Pickles, R.J. (2002). Respiratory syncytial virus infection of human airway epithelial cells is polarized, specific to ciliated cells, and without obvious cytopathology. *J. Virol.* Vol. 76(11):5654-5666.